Nephrology Forum

Edited by

Jordan J. Cohen
University of Chicago School of Medicine
Michael Reese Hospital and Medical Center
Chicago, Illinois

John T. Harrington
Tufts University School of Medicine
New England Medical Center
Boston, Massachusetts

Jerome P. Kassirer
Tufts University School of Medicine
New England Medical Center
Boston, Massachusetts

Selected Installments from the Series
in *Kidney International*

Springer-Verlag New York Heidelberg Berlin

Jordan J. Cohen
Professor of Medicine
University of Chicago School of Medicine
Chairman of Medicine
Michael Reese Hospital and Medical Center
Chicago, Illinois 60616 U.S.A.

John T. Harrington
Professor of Medicine
Tufts University School of Medicine
Chief, General Internal Medicine Division
New England Medical Center
Boston, Massachusetts 02111 U.S.A.

Jerome P. Kassirer
Professor and Associate Chairman
Department of Medicine
Tufts University School of Medicine
Associate Physician-in-Chief
New England Medical Center
Boston, Massachusetts 02111 U.S.A.

Sponsoring Editor: Marie Low
Production: Anthony Buatti
With 53 Figures

Editorial Assistant: Cheryl J. Zusman, Managing Editor, "Nephrology Forum"

Library of Congress Cataloging in Publication Data
Nephrology Forum.
Nephrology Forum.
Transcriptions of discussions from Nephrology Forums originally published in Kidney international.
Includes index.
1. Kidneys—Diseases—Addresses, essays, lectures.
2. Nephrology—Addresses, essays, lectures.
I. Cohen, Jordan. J. II. Harrington, John T.
III. Kassirer, Jerome P. IV. Kidney international.
RC903.N46 1982 616.6′1 82-19327

Typeset by University Graphics, Inc.

9 8 7 6 5 4 3 2 1

ISBN-13: SOBA11072003531 e-ISBN-13: 978-1-4612-5465-2
DOI. 10.1007/978-1-4612-5465-2

Contents

Foreword

A few years ago, as the editor of *Kidney International*, I was approached by Drs. Cohen, Kassirer, and Harrington who suggested that a new feature should be included in each monthly issue of the journal. They suggested that it should employ a case discussion format such as that used frequently at specialty rounds in teaching hospitals, and that the discussion should place a special emphasis on the relationship between basic science and important problems in clinical nephrology. The summary of an actual patient history would first be presented to exemplify a particular clinical problem, a seasoned person of proven expertise would be invited to deliver a well-documented analysis of the relevant issues, and perhaps most ambitiously of all, a critical audience would be assembled to challenge the principal discussant in an open-ended, question-and-answer period. The entire affair would be recorded at the time of the live conference and transcribed subsequently in preparation for publication as a "Nephrology Forum."

I must confess that I was somewhat hesitant at first to endorse their proposal because, at the time, *Kidney International* had just begun to establish a solid reputation for the publication of high quality, peer-reviewed manuscripts dealing with the clinical and laboratory research interests of the international nephrological community. I worried that the Forum might be unable to sustain the high standards to which the journal aspired, that it might detract from the primary purpose to which the International Society of Nephrology had committed its official publication, or that logistical difficulties might preclude the inclusion of suitable international representation among the invited discussants. Recognizing, however, that the journal's circulation of almost 7000 included many clinical nephrologists and other specialists interested in the kidney, approval to launch the project on a trial basis was granted in June 1978.

It is now evident that even the most skeptical have been gratified by the success of the Forum over the ensuing years. Indeed, a recent poll of the journal's readership indicated that the Forum is now regarded as one of the most attractive and useful features of *Kidney International*. The roster of principal discussants contains some of the most eminent and respected authorities in the world; the wide range of clinical topics has been timely and challenging; the question-and-answer sessions that accompany each installment have been spirited and informative; and the references at the end of each Forum have provided a convenient and unusually current guide to further study. But perhaps most gratifying of all from an editor's point of view, the "Nephrology Forum" has also been fun to read. The informality of a live conference has been retained, thus giving the reader a feeling of actually "being there," while the structure and thoroughness of a published review have remained intact.

The success of "Nephrology Forum" as a regular feature of *Kidney International* has emboldened its trio of editors to venture forth with this volume. It is their view, and mine, that many of the Forums are deserving of a wider and more general audience. Not only do the clinical issues under consideration range far beyond the interests of nephrologists alone, the educational and practical value of this collection of Forums clearly warrant their inclusion in a book for generalists as well as specialists.

I take special pride in having played a small role in nuturing an educational venture that was conceived originally to enrich a rather small family of specialists but that now, in book form, promises to enlighten a broader medical community.

Roscoe R. Robinson, M.D.
Editor, *Kidney International*

Preface

This volume contains 15 "Nephrology Forum" installments selected from more than 50 that have been published in the monthly issues of *Kidney International*, the journal of the International Society of Nephrology. Designed to relate basic science principles to clinical nephrology, the Forum has attracted as discussants many outstanding clinical scholars who have produced exceptionally valuable reviews and critiques. Reception of the Forum by the nephrology community has been enthusiastic.

In preparing this initial compendium of "Nephrology Forums," we had two goals in mind. The first was to provide convenient access to selected installments of the Forum for those already familiar with the series. The second was to enable clinicians who do not make nephrology their "steady diet" to avail themselves of timely and authoritative expositions dealing with nephrologic topics of interest to the generalist.

We conceived "Nephrology Forum" in its original format several years ago. Having worked together at Tufts University School of Medicine and the New England Medical Center in Boston, the three of us were among a group of clinician-physiologists who gathered once a week at Renal Rounds to discuss interesting cases with other nephrologists, trainees, and house staff. The cases were selected for their teaching value, their relevance to important clinical issues, and the complexity of their pathophysiologic features. Discussions among the participants were always spirited, candid, and above all informative. An oft-heard lament, however, was that the interchanges were ephemeral, that the pedagogic value was simply too great not to be preserved in some way.

Our desire to capture and share some of the spirit and substance of our Renal Rounds gave birth to "Nephrology Forum" when *Kidney International* accepted our proposal to publish a monthly case discussion modeled on these informal conferences. While endeavoring to preserve the spontaneity characteristic of the original exercise, we chose to augment our local expertise with acknowledged leaders in nephrology. During the Forum's early phase the conferences were held in Boston, but subsequently many have been held abroad, giving the series a truly international scope.

Each installment is initiated by a description of a patient whose clinical course illustrates the pathophysiologic issues under consideration. The principal discussant uses the case as a point of departure for an in-depth analysis of clinical-physiologic correlations, diagnostic features, and therapeutic implications. After the discussion, a spontaneous question-and-answer period is recorded; during this segment of the Forum, many controversies and uncertainties surrounding the topic are exposed and examined.

If "Nephrology Forum" is as well received in book form as it has been as a journal feature in *Kidney International*, the credit must go to the principal discussants. It is through their efforts that this series has gained its currency and stature. As editors, our hope is that the readers of this volume will learn as much as we have from the Forums conducted by these exceptional teachers.

Jordan J. Cohen, M.D.
John T. Harrington, M.D.
Jerome P. Kassirer, M.D.

Principal Discussants

David S. Baldwin Professor of Medicine, New York University School of Medicine, New York, New York
Robert W. Berliner Dean, Yale University School of Medicine, New Haven, Connecticut
Neal S. Bricker Professor of Medicine, Director, Program in Kidney Diseases, UCLA School of Medicine, Los Angeles, California
George F. Cahill, Jr. Professor of Medicine, Harvard Medical School, Director of Research, Howard Hughes Medical Institutes, and Physician, Brigham and Women's Hospital, Boston, Massachusetts
J. Stewart Cameron Professor of Renal Medicine, Guy's Hospital Medical School, London, England
Jack W. Coburn Director, Nephrology Training Program, VA Wadsworth Medical Center, and Professor of Medicine, UCLA School of Medicine, Los Angeles, California
Ralph A. DeFronzo Associate Professor of Medicine, Yale University School of Medicine, New Haven, Connecticut
Alexander Leaf Professor of Medicine, Ridley Watts Professor of Preventive Medicine, Harvard Medical School, and Physician, Massachusetts General Hospital, Boston, Massachusetts
Norman G. Levinsky Chairman, Department of Medicine, Boston University Medical Center, Boston, Massachusetts
Francis P. Muldowney Research Professor of Medicine, University College, and Physician-in-Charge, Metabolism and Renal Unit, St. Vincent's Hospital, Dublin, Ireland
Eberhard Ritz Head, Division of Nephrology, University of Heidelberg, Heidelberg, Federal Republic of Germany
Roscoe R. Robinson Vice President for Medical Affairs, Vanderbilt University, Nashville, Tennessee
Robert W. Schrier Chairman, Department of Medicine, University of Colorado Medical Center, Denver, Colorado
Samuel O. Thier Chairman, Department of Medicine, Yale University School of Medicine, New Haven, Connecticut
Charles van Ypersele de Strihou Professor of Medicine, Head, Renal Service, University of Louvain Medical School, Cliniques Universitaires St-Luc, Louvain en Woluwe, Brussels

Part I
Intrinsic Renal Disease

Introduction

The five Forums in this section deal with intrinsic renal disease and span a wide spectrum of nephrologic problems. The section opens with a discussion by Dr. Roscoe R. Robinson of a case of well-documented, asymptomatic proteinuria of almost 2 decades duration. Dr. Robinson, for many years Director of the Nephrology Division at Duke University Medical Center, has had a longstanding interest in the problem of fixed and reproducible orthostatic proteinuria. His discussion reviews the excretion of protein by the normal kidney, the mechanisms of abnormal proteinuria, and the clinical significance of proteinuria in otherwise healthy individuals. He divides proteinuria in the latter setting into three qualitative patterns: constant proteinuria, fixed and reproducible orthostatic proteinuria, and transient orthostatic proteinuria. The histologic correlates of these patterns and their prognostic significance are thoroughly aired.

A case of idiopathic nephrotic syndrome associated with membranous glomerulopathy provides Dr. Stewart Cameron with an opportunity to review recent findings bearing on the pathogenesis and treatment of this important pathologic entity. Dr. Cameron, Professor of Renal Medicine at Guy's Hospital Medical School, London, England, has had extensive personal experience in the study and treatment of this disease. His discussion highlights the wide variety of circumstances associated with membranous nephropathy and reviews the several mechanisms thought to result in the formation of injurious immune complexes, including the most recent theories regarding in situ complex formation. A lively interchange follows, including comments by Dr. Cecil Coggins, Coordinator of the well-known U.S. Collaborative Study of Adult Nephrotic Syndrome.

Dr. David Baldwin, Professor of Medicine at New York University School of Medicine, examines two cases of glomerulonephritis, the first progressing to end-stage renal disease more than 5 decades after the onset of typical acute nephritis and the second recovering normal renal function despite 1 month of anuria. Dr. Baldwin uses these cases to exemplify his thesis that nonimmunologic mechanisms play at least as important a role in the progression of chronic glomerulonephritis as do various immunologic mechanisms. Among the potentially damaging nonimmunologic factors highlighted by Dr. Baldwin are glomerular hyperperfusion, secondary hypertension, and high protein and phosphorus diets. His discussion focuses attention on an increasingly attractive new hypothesis regarding the "nonspecific" pathogenesis of glomerulosclerosis and progressive renal failure.

Dr. Robert Schrier, Chairman of the Department of Medicine at the University of Colorado Medical Center, takes a case of acute tubular necrosis in a postoperative patient as a springboard for a scholarly review of the predisposing factors, the etiology, and the pathogenesis of acute renal failure. Dr. Schrier then uses this scientific base to construct a practical approach to the differential diagnosis of acute renal failure and to the modern treatment of this all-too-frequent, life-threatening condition. He emphasizes the potential importance of distinguishing between oliguric and nonoliguric forms of the disorder.

A puzzling case of acute interstitial nephritis leading to oliguric renal failure affords Dr. Charles van Ypersele an opportunity to review recent information gained both from experimental models and from clinical studies of this increasingly recognized condition. Dr. van Ypersele, Head of the Renal Service at the University of Louvain Medical School, Woluwe, Brussels, includes a detailed section on the differential diagnosis of interstitial nephritis in his discussion and stresses the importance of various drugs in the etiology of this disease. The question and answer period accompanying this Forum captures the spirited interchange among the physicians gathered in Brussels for this occasion. In a postscript to this Forum, Dr. van Ypersele answers the puzzle by providing retrospective but convincing evidence about the cause of the interstitial nephritis in the case presented.

Isolated Proteinuria in Asymptomatic Patients

Principal Discussant
Roscoe R. Robinson

Case Presentation

A 38-year-old man was evaluated at the Duke University Medical Center for routine follow-up of known proteinuria for 19 years. Qualitative proteinuria was first detected during routine urinalysis when he entered military service at age 19. Repetitive examination of randomly collected urine specimens over the next several days documented the presence of proteinuria, and the patient was then admitted to Wilford Hall USAF Medical Center for further evaluation.

On admission, the patient was asymptomatic. He had no history of signs or symptoms of any form of genitourinary disease. The patient denied any prior hospitalizations or health examinations. There was no family history of kidney disease. Physical examination revealed a healthy-appearing young man with a normal body build: height, 5′6″; weight, 147 lbs. Accentuated lumbar lordosis was not apparent. The supine blood pressure was 120/78 mmHg; the remainder of the physical examination was within normal limits. Laboratory examination showed a normal hemogram including a hematocrit of 44% and an erythrocyte sedimentation rate of 9 mm/h. Routine urinalysis was within normal limits except for 1+ proteinuria. Microscopic hematuria, pyuria, and casts were not present. Serum protein electrophoresis was normal. Blood chemistries were also normal, including a BUN of 16 mg/dl and a serum creatinine concentration of 0.9 mg/dl. Urine protein excretion was 0.64 g/day. Qualitative tests for protein on serial urine collections on 2 consecutive days revealed protein during maintenance of the quiet, upright ambulatory posture but none during recumbency. Inulin and PAH clearances in the recumbent posture were 135 and 655 ml/min/1.73 m^2 body surface area, respectively. Chest x-ray and excretory urography were normal. A percutaneous renal biopsy revealed normal renal tissue on light microscopy; electron microscopy was not performed. The patient was discharged to duty with a clinical diagnosis of "fixed and reproducible orthostatic proteinuria."

The patient remained asymptomatic without subsequent illness or hospitalization throughout the entire 19-year period. Routine follow-up evaluations were carried out subsequently at 4-, 9-, and 19-year inter-

vals. At 4 years he continued to exhibit qualitative proteinuria during assumption and maintenance of a quiet upright ambulatory posture. The urine sediment was normal. The 24-h excretion of protein was 0.42 g, and the endogenous creatinine clearance was 115 ml/min/1.73 m^2 body surface area. Maximum urine concentrating ability was normal. Physical examination at 9 years again was within normal limits. He continued to exhibit qualitative proteinuria only during the upright posture. The endogenous creatinine clearance was 98 ml/min/1.73 m^2 body surface area. At the 19-year follow-up, blood chemistries, chest x-ray, and electrocardiogram again were normal. Repeated qualitative tests of serial urine collections revealed proteinuria in the upright posture on one day, but not on another. The endogenous creatinine clearance was 145 ml/min/1.73 m^2 body surface area, and the 24-h excretion of total protein was less than 0.08 g.

Discussion

Dr. Roscoe R. Robinson (*Vice President for Medical Affairs, Vanderbilt University, Nashville, Tennessee*)*: This man has had qualitative proteinuria for at least 19 years. Prior to his most recent examination, he always had exhibited "fixed and reproducible" orthostatic proteinuria. On his last examination in 1979, however, qualitative evidence of upright proteinuria was detected on one day, but not on another; hence, the pattern of proteinuria became "transient" or "intermittent." The sporadic presence of upright proteinuria in this patient perhaps explains why only a small amount of protein was detected on quantitative examination of a 24-h urine sample. Qualitative proteinuria was the only clinically significant finding throughout this patient's 19-year observation period; at no time was its presence associated with urinary sediment abnormalities, evidence of a systemic disease known to affect the kidneys, or renal functional impairment. Proteinuria in this patient thus was always an "isolated" clinical phenomenon.

Diagnostic and prognostic uncertainty continue to surround the detection of qualitative proteinuria in asymptomatic individuals who seem to be in good health. The uncertainty is most pronounced when, as in this patient, the amount of proteinuria is modest, and when there is no evidence of systemic disease, impaired renal function, abnormal urine sediment, anatomic alteration as shown by excretory urography, and no history of renal or urologic disease. The unsuspected finding of qualitative proteinuria as an "isolated" event gives rise to two simple but important questions: (1) does proteinuria reflect the presence of

*At the time of the original forum, Dr. Robinson was Florence McAlister Professor of Medicine, and Director, Division of Nephrology, Duke University Medical Center, Durham, North Carolina.

underlying renal disease, and if so, (2) will the disease eventually cause morbidity or death? Unfortunately, neither of these questions can be answered with confidence in an individual patient because the causes and mechanisms of this type of proteinuric syndrome have not yet been clarified and are undoubtedly multiple.

Significant advances have been made in our understanding of the mechanisms of proteinuria in several experimental and clinical circumstances in the past decade. For this reason, before continuing our discussion of the clinical significance of "isolated" proteinuria, I would like to review briefly first, our present concepts regarding the manner in which a small amount of protein can enter the urine, and second, the mechanisms of pathologic proteinuria.

Excretion of Protein by the Healthy Kidney

The daily urinary excretion of protein in apparently healthy adults is 80 ± 24 mg according to Berggard [1]. Other estimates have differed slightly, but the total daily excretion of as much as 150 mg is probably within two standard deviations of the average, and this amount therefore can be accepted as a close approximation of the upper limit of normal. Nevertheless, the relatively inexact definition of the "normal" range of total protein excreted by the healthy kidney poses a practical problem as one attempts to distinguish between normal and abnormal excretion of protein, particularly in patients with only slight proteinuria. This definition is obscured further when complicating factors such as exercise and increased catecholamine activity are present. In a healthy individual, the small amount of protein in the urine is sufficient to permit detection with the usual qualitative tests if the urine is a concentrated specimen [2,3]. It is useful, therefore, if we have some estimate of urine concentration when considering the significance of a qualitative reaction for protein, because a concentrated urine can permit the detection of a normal amount of protein; conversely, a dilute urine can hinder the detection of an abnormal amount of protein.

Composition

Detailed analysis of the composition of normal urinary proteins requires physico- and immunochemical or radioisotopic techniques. Using these techniques, Poortman and Jeanloz have estimated that approximately 60% by weight of the total urine protein consists of normal plasma proteins in the healthy adult, whereas the remaining fraction derives directly from renal and other urogenital tissues [4]. The plasma proteins in healthy urine include albumin (about 40% of the total protein excretion), a large and heterogeneous array of small-sized immunoglobulins and their fragments, enzymes, peptide hormones, and other proteins. Normally, IgG or its fragments represents about 5 to 10% of the total urine protein, light chains comprise approximately 5%, and IgA accounts for approximately 3% (of which 90% is secretory IgA) [1,5]; IgM and IgD are not usually detectable [1]. Thus, the proteins in healthy urine include albumin (40%); tissue proteins and antigens or glycoproteins of uroepithelial origin, e.g., Tamm-Horsfall mucoproteins (40%); and immunoproteins and other plasma proteins (20%). This composition can be altered by both normal and abnormal events. For example, the increase in protein excretion after exercise is accounted for primarily by an increase in the excretion of proteins that are identical to those in plasma [4].

Anatomy of Ultrafiltration

The exact anatomic location of the glomerular ultrafiltration barrier for macromolecules is uncertain. On the one hand, histochemical localization of macromolecular enzymes suggests that the filtration slit membrane between the epithelial foot processes might be the primary filtration barrier [6]; electron microscopic localization of graded dextran particles suggests, on the other hand, that the subendothelial portion of the basement membrane might be the limiting barrier [7,8]. It seems most likely that all of the anatomic components of the capillary wall contribute to the limitation of transglomerular protein passage but that in a given experimental or clinical circumstance, molecular size, shape, or charge might be the determining factor [9]. For example, the presence of fixed glomerular anions within the endothelium and lamina rara interna might provide a major barrier to the filtration of larger circulating polyanions such as albumin, the substance of the basement membrane might restrict by size the passage of neutral macromolecules, and the slit diaphragm and lamina rara externa might prevent the passage of cationic macromolecules.

Filtration and Resorption

The amount and composition of normal urine protein are primarily the net consequence of filtration by the glomeruli and subsequent tubular reabsorption of proteins. Intraepithelial production and direct addition to tubule fluid account for some of the protein in healthy urine (e.g., Tamm-Horsfall protein and secretory IgA). Renal tubular secretion is another possible mechanism of proteinuria, but proof of its existence has not been established.

There is little question that most of the albumin and other plasma proteins in normal glomerular filtrate undergo subsequent renal tubular reabsorption along the nephron. Albumin concentrations of 0.1–3.0 mg/dl have been reported in fluid samples obtained by micropuncture from the proximal convoluted tubule and Bowman's space [10–13]. These concentrations indicate that the usual filtered load of protein far exceeds the amount in the urine; thus renal tubular reabsorption must take place along the nephron. Studies using micropuncture [11] and perfusion of isolated renal tubules [14] indicate that much of this protein is reabsorbed in the proximal tubule, although a small fraction might be reabsorbed in later nephron segments [11]. The mechanism of protein absorption, although unclear, probably involves selective endocytosis. Transport kinetics of the absorptive process are even less well understood, but some investigators have suggested that the absorptive maximum for albumin resides close to the plasma threshold, whereas the absorptive process for low-molecular-weight proteins exhibits considerable "splay" and its maximum might exceed the plasma threshold considerably [15]. In any case, when the proteins are absorbed, lysosomal combination and intracellular digestion occur and the resultant peptides or amino acids either disappear into the metabolic machinery of the cell or are returned to the contraluminal circulation. The number and nature of individual proteins that might be absorbed and returned intact to the peritubular circulation is in dispute. Similarly, controversy surrounds the magnitude of cellular uptake of protein from the peritubular circulation, although the existence of such a process seems well-established, at least for certain protein hormones such as insulin [15].

Physicochemical Factors

The transglomerular passage of plasma proteins has been examined in humans and experimental animals during the administration of several types of macromolecules. Dextran, a polymer of glucose with minimal tubular reabsorption, has been used most commonly. The use of dextrans of known molecular size to study the renal handling of macromolecules was pioneered by Wallenius [16] and recently was amplified by Chang et al. [17–19]. Wallenius demonstrated that the glomerular filtration of dextrans decreased sharply as their effective molecular radius increased above 20 Å and that transglomerular passage was minimal at molecular sizes greater than 34 Å. Small-sized plasma proteins such as ribonuclease and lysozyme also are known to traverse the glomerular capillary walls readily. In fact, some proteins have glomerular sieving coefficients as high as 0.9 [15]. Observations such as these have suggested that glomerular filtration involves molecular sieving through the functional equivalent of aqueous pores [20]. That is, molecular size and shape are the major determinants of the transglomerular passage of macromolecules. This physical phenomenon is summarized by the term *steric hindrance*, the value of which primarily depends on the ratio of the effective radius of the solute molecule to the radius of the pore. In addition to size and shape, however, electrical forces also are involved in macromolecular passage through the glomerular capillary wall. The electrical forces are summarized by the term *electrostatic hindrance*, the phenomenon whereby the mobility of macromolecules through the glomerular wall is hindered or facilitated by electrical interactions between cationic or anionic groups on the solute and areas of charge density on the channel wall. Chang et al. have demonstrated that the permeability of the normal rat glomerulus to polyanionic dextran sulfate is considerably lower than is the permeability to similarly sized molecules of neutral dextran [18]. Moreover, neutral dextrans having effective radii of 36 Å pass through the glomerular capillary wall more easily than does albumin, which has the same effective radius (36 Å), but which exists in plasma as a polyanion at physiologic pH. The addition of negatively charged sulfate radicals to the dextran molecule results in its passage across the glomerular barrier being impaired to the same degree as albumin. Conversely, the transglomerular passage of positively charged dextran molecules of the same size was facilitated [9,21–24]. Thus, among the physicochemical factors that influence the ability of a macromolecule to cross the glomerular ultrafiltration barrier, both electrostatic and steric hindrance must be considered. In relative terms, electrostatic factors probably play a lesser role in determining the transglomerular passage of the smallest macromolecules. Electrical charge probably assumes greater importance as the effective radius of the macromolecule approaches the diameter of the theoretical "pore." The magnitude of relative interplay between electrical charge versus molecular size and shape as determinants of transglomerular passage has not yet been established for any significant number of plasma proteins.

Hemodynamic Factors

In addition to physicochemical considerations, renal hemodynamic alterations provide other major influences on the transglomerular passage of macromolecules [20]. The mechanisms whereby hemodynamic changes affect urine protein excretion, however, are not well understood. One must remember that convective and diffusive forces are important theoretical determinants of macromolecular transport across the capillary wall, and that these forces are also influenced by glomerular hemodynamics. Administration of vasoactive compounds such as angiotensin [25,26] and norepinephrine [27], assumption of the upright posture [28,29], and exercise [4] all can lead to increased urine protein excretion. Proteinuria in these settings has been attributed to a function of the reduced renal blood flow and altered glomerular hemodynamics. Local increases in protein concentration along the glomerular capillaries (when glomerular plasma flow is reduced and filtration rate is relatively well maintained), increases in the permeability of the limiting glomerular membrane or its surface area available for transport, and increases in transglomerular pressure might be some of the mechanisms responsible.

Mechanisms of Abnormal Proteinuria

The major mechanisms whereby increased amounts of protein appear in the urine are: (1) elevated plasma concentrations of normal or abnormal proteins ("overflow" proteinuria such as lysozymuria in leukemia or Bence Jones proteinuria [30]; (2) direct addition of proteins to tubular fluid by the renal tubular epithelium (Tamm-Horsfall proteinuria) [31,32]; (3) altered renal tubular reabsorption of normal amounts of filtered proteins [33–36]; and (4) an altered capillary wall with a resultant increase in permeability secondary to a loss of glomerular polyanions or other causes of decreased permselectivity [9]. Whatever the cause of abnormal proteinuria, its magnitude can be increased by the same renal hemodynamic changes that are capable of increasing protein excretion by the healthy kidney. Little is known about the relative contribution of these mechanisms to the genesis of "isolated" proteinuria in asymptomatic patients. In view of the undoubted heterogeneity of the patient population with this syndrome, we logically can suspect that any of the possible mechanisms might be operative in a given patient at a given time.

Against this background, let us turn to a detailed consideration of the clinical significance and, when possible, the mechanisms of isolated proteinuria in asymptomatic and apparently healthy patients.

Clinical Significance of Proteinuria in Apparently Healthy Patients

Uncertainty still surrounds the clinical significance of "isolated" proteinuria. Several factors are responsible for this state of affairs. First, it has long been known that qualitative proteinuria occurs both in the presence and absence of underlying histologic alterations of renal structure [37–47]. Second, although progressive renal disease appears subsequently in some patients [37,48–49], one study has shown that the incidence of proteinuria in young adults is greater than the incidence of subsequent death from renal failure [50]. This finding strongly suggests that kidney disease might not exist in many such patients or that if it does, it does not cause death from renal failure. Third, we must recognize that conclusions derived from a study of one population are not necessarily applicable to another group. Finally, a profuse array of descriptive terms has been applied frequently to proteinuria observed in apparently healthy patients; juvenile, physiologic, orthostatic, constant, persistent, cyclic, intermittent, isolated, benign, minimal, and transient comprise only a partial list of the descriptive terms. In many instances, these terms have not been defined clearly; in others, the use of differing criteria has complicated the comparison of results between studies.

For these reasons, the exact definition of the clinical characteristics of the proteinuric population under consideration is of great importance. The remainder of the present discussion will focus exclusively on the clinical significance of proteinuria in a single, large, and arbitrarily defined adult population of patients in whom proteinuria is always first observed as an "isolated" clinical finding. It will apply only to patients who are asymptomatic and seemingly healthy at the time of initial examination, and who exhibit no evidence of systemic disease, impaired renal function, or *any* abnormality of the urine sediment. Excretory urography and nuclear or ultrasonic imaging are always within normal limits, and the patients have no history of kidney or genitourinary tract disease. In such patients, proteinuria is often first detected during a routine physical examination, perhaps in preparation for entrance into military service, participation in an athletic program, or application for life insurance or employment. Daily total protein excretion is usually, but not necessarily, less than 1.0 g. Most patients thus far described have been relatively young adults at the time of initial clinical presentation, but this fact might be related to the paucity of comparable survey observations in older populations. Neither the incidence nor prevalence of proteinuria as an isolated finding among various age or population groups is certain. Estimates of the incidence of qualitative proteinuria during casual or routine urinalysis in military inductees and other adult populations have varied widely, ranging from values of 0.6 to 8.8% [51–54].

Classification of Isolated Proteinuria

What methods should one use in assessing the clinical significance of isolated proteinuria in an individual patient? In general, proteinuria has been classified according to two clinical approaches, one without regard to body posture, and the other taking body posture into account. Using the first approach, the pattern of protein excretion on repeated qualitative testing is designated "transient" or "intermittent" if proteinuria comes and goes, and "persistent" if proteinuria is found on analysis of all specimens. In the second approach, "serial urine collection tests" identify proteinuria as "constant" if it is present both during recumbency and during quiet upright ambulation, "fixed and orthostatic" if it is present consistently only in the upright posture, and "transient" or "intermittent" and "orthostatic" when it is present inconsistently only in the upright posture [55,56]. Multiple urinalyses must be performed at the time of initial examination to identify the pattern correctly. The significance of many of these arbitrarily classified types is not certain: the various types probably should be viewed not as specific clinical entities, but as consequences of diverse causes and mechanisms. Further, even the relationship between persistent and constant proteinuria, as just defined, has not been delineated clearly. Although it seems likely that patients with these patterns are drawn from similar populations, studies using both approaches, i.e., with and without regard to posture, have not been performed in the same individuals. I would now like to discuss these two different approaches to the investigation and classification of isolated proteinuria.

Classification According to Repetitive Urinalysis without Control of Body Posture

As noted above, at least two distinct qualitative patterns of isolated proteinuria emerge when routine urinalyses are carried out repetitively over a short period: the persistent presence of qualitative proteinuria, or the intermittent or transient presence of qualitative proteinuria. Several years ago, Levitt performed a retrospective study to establish the clinical significance of these types of proteinuria [50]. The study group comprised graduates of the University of Minnesota who were given repetitive urinalyses on entrance to the university in 1925; each had qualitative proteinuria. By 1966, 41 years later, the mortality rate of this group was compared with that of presumably healthy 18-year-olds who had undergone examinations for life insurance in 1925, and whose urinalyses revealed no proteinuria qualitatively. The mortality rate was significantly higher in the patients who had had qualitative proteinuria in more than 80% of their initial urinalyses, i.e., those with persistent proteinuria. In contrast, no difference in mortality rate was noted in the patients who had had proteinuria in less than 50% of their initial specimens, i.e., those with intermittent or transient proteinuria. These findings imply that the long-term outlook is worse when repetitive examination reveals persistent proteinuria.

In France, Antoine et al. studied 16 patients in whom persistent proteinuria was an isolated finding [37]. Percutaneous renal biopsy revealed a heterogeneous spectrum of morphologic alterations in 12 of the 16 patients. Nevertheless, only two of these patients developed renal insufficiency after follow-up periods ranging from 8 to 28 years. The authors concluded that even in patients with documented renal pathology, the progression to renal failure is remarkably indolent. Included in Antoine's study were 10 other patients with the same clinical and histologic findings as the 16 patients described above, but these ten also had microscopic hematuria. This single additional indicator of disease activity was attended by more rapid progression of renal functional impairment.

Classification According to Repetitive Urinalysis with Control of Body Posture

For many years we have used a simple serial urine collection test to relate the qualitative appearance of proteinuria to changes of body posture [55,56]. When the test is conducted during moderate antidiuresis, results are reproducible in the same patient over short periods of time. On the morning after overnight fluid deprivation, two or more urine samples are collected consecutively during each of two sequentially assumed body postures: recumbency and quiet upright ambulation. Artificial upright lordosis is not induced. A qualitative test for protein (10% sulfosalicylic acid) and a measure of urine osmolality are performed on each urine sample.

As noted previously, one of three qualitative patterns emerges in an individual patient. Constant proteinuria occurs in approximately 5 to 10% of young men with proteinuria on routine urinalysis where posture is not controlled [56]. Fixed and reproducible orthostatic proteinuria occurs in approximately 15 to 20% of young men whose proteinuria is detected initially on routine urinalysis [56]. As I mentioned earlier, this type of proteinuria was initially exhibited by the patient under discussion today. Transient orthostatic proteinuria is claimed by King to be the most common of the three posturally defined patterns, perhaps occurring in 70 to 75% of young men with isolated proteinuria on routine urinalysis [56]. Unfortunately, transient orthostatic proteinuria has been studied far less thoroughly than have either fixed and reproducible orthostatic proteinuria or constant proteinuria. Approximate incidence figures for these types of proteinuria are available only for young men; similar figures are not available for women or other age groups.

Quantitative measurements of total protein excretion have been carried out in patients who have clear evidence of constant proteinuria and fixed and reproducible orthostatic proteinuria. Values for total protein excretion are often higher even during recumbency in patients with fixed and reproducible orthostatic proteinuria than in healthy patients whose qualitative tests are negative for protein in both the recumbent and upright postures [28,29]. But the amount of protein excreted is not sufficiently high to permit detection with the usual qualitative tests. The significance of this finding has not been established, nor is its occurrence known to be universal in patients with a qualitative pattern of orthostatic proteinuria other than that termed fixed and reproducible. Indeed, quantitative protein excretion during recumbency might well be within normal limits in patients with transient orthostatic proteinuria [57].

"Constant" Proteinuria For many years "constant" proteinuria, even as an isolated finding, has been regarded as *prima facie* evidence of kidney disease. Definite morphologic evidence of diverse forms of kidney disease is found by renal biopsy in most instances. Most of these patients probably have proteinuria that is persistent on repetitive routine urinalysis without postural control. In view of the marked diversity of the underlying renal pathology, it is illogical to expect that all such patients will follow an identical clinical course. Nevertheless, the clin-

ical course of constant proteinuria is remarkably indolent in the absence of other indicators of active disease such as microscopic hematuria. Although few long-term follow-up studies of patients with constant proteinuria have been performed, the results of one study demonstrated that approximately 80% of such patients still exhibited constant proteinuria after an average 6-year period. Of these, the majority had developed abnormal urine sediment, and almost 50% had developed mild hypertension, but very few had developed renal insufficiency [48,49].

Orthostatic Proteinuria The exact clinical significance of isolated orthostatic proteinuria remains controversial. In contrast to constant proteinuria, orthostatic proteinuria has been regarded as a benign and transient condition not associated with underlying kidney disease [58–60]. This concept of the disorder might be true in many patients, particularly in children. Other observations, however, have suggested that orthostatic proteinuria might be a reflection of incipient kidney disease, at least in some patients [49,61]. This controversy cannot be resolved until complex clinical and physiologic issues are clarified. To shed some light on the significance of orthostatic proteinuria, I would now like to examine the renal biopsy findings in these patients, the possible mechanisms involved in the proteinuria, and our long-term prospective studies.

Light-microscopic studies of kidney biopsy specimens from young adult males with fixed and reproducible orthostatic proteinuria revealed that 8% had unequivocal evidence of renal disease, 45% had subtle but definite alterations of glomerular structure (segmental or generalized capillary wall thickening without alteration of the basement membrane, or focal and segmental hypercellularity), and 47% exhibited a histologic pattern that appeared normal [45]. A limited number of electron-microscopic observations have confirmed a subtle form of segmental and focal glomerular alterations [46,62], and immunohistologic studies have shown that both immunoglobulin and complement are localized within such foci [63]. Recent histologic observations in patients with intermittent orthostatic proteinuria demonstrate minimal changes without immunoprotein on immunofluorescent microscopy, but only a small number of such patients have been studied [47].

The mechanism by which assumption of the quiet upright posture effects increased protein excretion is still uncertain. Regardless of the exact nature of the glomerular changes just described, their existence provides one possible explanation for the proteinuria, i.e., an underlying capillary wall defect, which facilitates an increased transglomerular passage of plasma proteins. By itself, however, the existence of an altered capillary wall does not explain abnormal protein excretion occurring only during quiet upright ambulation [57]. Earlier researchers postulated that any one of the several renal hemodynamic adjustments to standing might serve as the primary cause of orthostatic proteinuria; renal venous congestion or ischemia and a reduction of filtration rate all have been implicated [58,64]. This hypothesis became suspect when it was shown that the upright renal hemodynamic response was no different in patients with fixed orthostatic proteinuria than it was in normal subjects [20,65]. A quantitatively similar reduction of renal plasma flow and filtration rate, and an elevation of filtration fraction were observed in both groups. Of these three possible hemodynamic determinants of transglomerular protein transfer, the results of clearance studies [28] indicated to us that the normal reduction of plasma flow was of greatest importance. For example, experimentally induced renal vasodilation that obliterated the usual reduction of renal plasma flow was accompanied by a strikingly smaller rise of protein excretion than usual. We suggested that some function of the reduction of renal blood or plasma flow might secondarily permit an increased protein transfer across an altered capillary wall. According to this view, the combination of an altered capillary wall and the normal reduction of renal blood flow in the upright posture might be sufficient to effect an increased transglomerular passage of protein that readily exceeds the normal tubular reabsorptive capacity. One can speculate that the secondary hemodynamic contribution to fixed orthostatic proteinuria might be similar to that occurring during the administration of angiotensin in experimental animals [25,26]. This hypothesis is tentative and other possibilities exist. For example, an upright alteration of renal tubular reabsorption of protein has not yet been excluded. Alternatively, increased capillary permeability to plasma proteins during standing might be mediated via a direct effect of certain humoral agents on an altered capillary wall, agents whose release is also increased by postural changes. Such a role has been suggested for renin, angiotensin, and circulating vasoactive amines because of their capacity to produce proteinuria in animals [25–27,66,67].

Whatever the role of the alterations of glomerular structure in the pathogenesis of fixed and reproducible orthostatic proteinuria, only long-term prospective studies can determine their clinical significance. Our own 10-year follow-up study of young men with an initial diagnosis of fixed orthostatic proteinuria demonstrated that 49% still exhibited qualitative proteinuria [61]. No evidence of renal functional impairment or progressive renal disease had appeared in any of the patients, including the patient presented today. Furthermore, no relationship existed between the initial renal histology and the subsequent pattern of renal function of proteinuria. In short, the 10-year prognosis of young men with fixed and reproducible orthostatic proteinuria is excellent. A similarly benign intermediate-term course of 5–10 years has been described by other observers [67–69].

The significance of the subtle glomerular alterations that we found in 45% of our patients is uncertain, but the decreasing frequency of proteinuria and the preservation of normal renal function in this group suggests that the glomerular findings are not a manifestation of progressive renal disease. Until more time elapses, however, we cannot exclude the possibility that renal function will deteriorate in the patients who still had proteinuria when studied 10 years after the initial evaluation. As I mentioned previously, these results are not surprising in view of the heterogeneity of the histologic alterations.

Taken together, these findings suggest that fixed and reproducible orthostatic proteinuria does not necessarily represent a transient condition of adolescence—in some patients it might reflect the earliest expression of future renal disease. Continued observation is necessary to establish the validity of this hypothesis. In fact, our patient today is one whose return visit in 1979 was occasioned by his willingness to participate in the 20-year follow-up study of our original group of patients. Obviously, he has continued to do well. Because his proteinuria is now transient and his renal function has remained normal, I strongly suspect that his long-term prognosis is excellent. Our 20-year follow-up study, in cooperation with Drs. P. Springberg and L. Garrett at Wilford Hall USAF Medical Center and Dr. A. L. Thompson at the University of Nevada Medical Center, is just now underway so our observations are only preliminary. We have, however, reexamined 18 of the original 64 patients, and to date none has developed renal insufficiency. We hope the number of participants in the 20-year follow-up study will be large enough to permit meaningful comparisons with the earlier follow-up examinations [61].

Virtually no long-term data are available in patients with transient orthostatic proteinuria, but most clinicians believe that the prognosis of patients with this finding is excellent [50]. In many such patients, transient episodes of orthostatic proteinuria might reflect nothing more than fever, exercise, or exposure to environmental factors such as heat or cold. Indeed, as in angiotensin-induced proteinuria in the rat, this form of upright proteinuria might reflect nothing more than a transient and exaggerated renal hemodynamic response to these or other stimuli.

Summary of Renal Structural Alterations in Patients with "Isolated" Proteinuria

Renal biopsy specimens have been examined from patients in the five descriptive categories of isolated proteinuria I have used: persistent or intermittent proteinuria (defined on sequential routine urinalysis without control of body posture) [37,40,41]; constant proteinuria during both recumbent and upright postures [43]; and transient [47] or fixed and reproducible orthostatic proteinuria as defined during appropriate postural maneuvers [43,45]. In four of the five categories examined so far, a varying but important incidence of "definite" histologic alterations has been reported (about 10 to 70%), all of which have been sufficiently distinct to warrant a firm histologic diagnosis of renal disease ("definite" histologic alterations have not yet been reported in patients with transient orthostatic proteinuria). The lesions themselves have been extremely heterogeneous, and a consistent relationship has not been observed. The incidence of definite renal pathology has been found to be similarly high (about 40 to 70%) in patients with persistent, intermittent, or constant proteinuria [37,40,43,70], whereas a much lower figure (about 10%) has been found in patients with fixed orthostatic proteinuria [45]. In other patients from all five of the groups, the incidence of disparate but minimal alterations has been similarly variable (about 10 to 70%). In still others, perhaps most frequently in patients with transient or fixed orthostatic proteinuria, the renal architecture has appeared entirely normal on light microscopy [45,47], although subtle architectural "defects" of the glomerulus have been described on electron microscopy in a few patients [46,61]. It seems safe to conclude that, with the possible exception of transient orthostatic proteinuria, (1) each of these five types of proteinuria is associated with a broad spectrum of histologic findings ranging from normal renal architecture to definite evidence of disease; (2) a similarly heterogeneous display of underlying renal pathology or architectural alteration occurs in each type but the frequency of definite disease is lowest by far in patients with transient or fixed orthostatic proteinuria; and (3) no absolute relationship exists between the type of proteinuria and the presence or absence of renal pathology. Renal biopsy remains the only means of distinguishing between the patient with structural renal disease and the one without.

Unfortunately, the description of definite pathologic alterations per se does not provide any necessary insight into their actual clinical significance as a cause of subsequent morbidity or mortality. One still must determine whether a particular lesion is static, resolving, or progressing. Prospective studies are clearly required. We also must continue our search for functional indexes of disease activity as an aid to determining the activity of the pathologic lesions.

In our approach to the management of patients with isolated proteinuria, we emphasize yearly follow-up evaluation. The initial evaluation includes a thorough physical examination, a determination of the persistence of a given qualitative pattern, urinalysis, and measurements of quantitative protein excretion and endogenous creatinine clearance. Ultrasonography is sometimes performed as well. Renal biopsy usually is not undertaken unless there is a distinct change in the clinical course, such as an abrupt and definite increase in daily protein excretion, the appearance of distinct and persistent abnormalities of the urine sediment, or impairment of renal function.

It is interesting to speculate that a persisting pattern of qualitative proteinuria over several years—whether it be persistent, intermittent, fixed, or transient orthostatic or constant in type—might be attended by an important incidence of underlying renal pathology [41–46,50,51]. In fact, it would not be surprising to observe in the same patient at different times over a relatively long period different types of proteinuria, because its detection depends on the simultaneous interaction of many variables (e.g., posture, urine concentration, and the natural history of an underlying disease process) [71]. Figure 1 depicts a hypothetical patient whose disease progression is accompanied by a variable but steady increase of total protein excretion during both recumbency and upright ambulation. Depending on the relationship between the lower limits of qualitative urine protein detection and the changing influences on urine protein excretion, an everchanging pattern of qualitative proteinuria will emerge. At various times, a patient might exhibit intermittent or transient orthostatic proteinuria, or perhaps it might seem to become fixed for a variable period [71]. Eventually, quantitative protein excretion might rise sufficiently to permit its qualitative detection in both recumbent ard upright specimens, i.e., the proteinuria becomes constant. Some patients move through this sequence so explosively that constant proteinuria seems to exist from the very onset of disease. In others, the disease progresses so slowly that a variable but generally

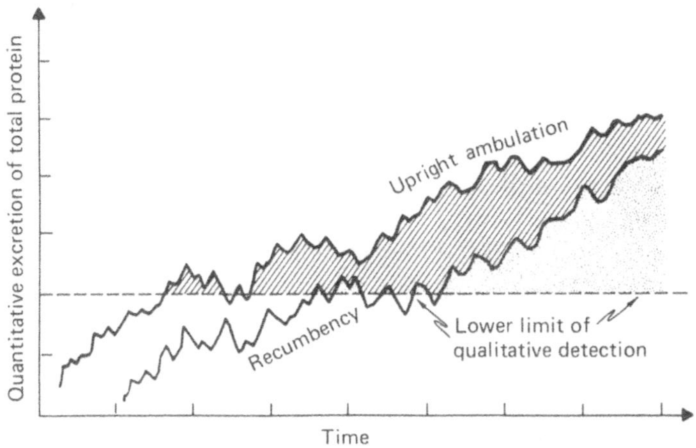

Fig. 1. Sequential relationship between quantitative protein excretion and qualitative tests for urine protein in a hypothetical patient with progressive renal disease. (Reprinted with permission from S. Karger [71].)

orthostatic pattern is observed for years. Eventually, if the underlying disease progresses sufficiently, protein excretion can rise during recumbency and yield the pattern of constant proteinuria; alternatively, the disease process can heal, and proteinuria disappears completely. Considerations such as these should underscore the difficulties that beset any attempt to relate a given clinical observation to any particular pattern of qualitative proteinuria. Nevertheless, although the long-term prognosis still must be regarded with reservation, if persistent proteinuria is the *sole* alteration, the 10-year outlook is excellent in most patients, as in the patient presented today.

Questions and Answers

Dr. Jerome P. Kassirer: Our approach to the diagnosis of orthostatic proteinuria has been to measure protein excretion using a quantitative sulfosalicylic acid method during 8 h of recumbency and again during 16 h of routine activites in the upright posture. Using this method we have diagnosed orthostatic proteinuria when protein excretion is abnormal only in the upright posture. Do you think there is any advantage to this quantitative approach over the qualitative method you used?

Dr. Robinson: I don't know. Unfortunately, too few descriptions have been published about the relationship between recumbent and upright quantitative values for total urinary protein excretion and the qualitative patterns I have described. At least in patients with fixed orthostatic proteinuria, however, quantitative excretion seems usually to be increased during recumbency, but the protein excretion does not rise sufficiently to permit qualitative detection. I cannot say whether that is the case in transient or intermittent proteinuria. Resolution of the question also depends on the sensitivity of our methods for quantifying small amounts of proteinuria and the adequacy of our definition of the "normal" range of protein excretion in the recumbent posture.

Dr. Kassirer: We occasionally observe patients who, in the course of recovering from the nephrotic syndrome or poststreptococcal nephritis, show an orthostatic pattern of protein excretion. These patients seem to have a benign long-term prognosis. Is there any solid evidence to support this contention?

Dr. Robinson: I don't know the answer to that question either. I know of no solid data that relate prognosis in those disorders to the presence or absence of orthostatic proteinuria at some time during the clinical course.

Dr. Cecil H. Coggins *(Clinical Director, Renal Unit, Massachusetts General Hospital, Boston)*: In reviewing the literature on patients with mild to moderate proteinuria, I cannot find very much good data correlating the clinical information with sophisticated histologic analysis. In a few surveys, patients were biopsied but not followed, and even in these studies the biopsies usually were not examined by electron microscopy or immunofluorescence. I believe that you and your colleagues have carried out the few studies that do correlate reliable clinical information with solid pathologic analysis.

Dr. Robinson: Thank you, Dr. Coggins. I agree that there are too few prospective follow-up studies. Parenthetically, insofar as our own studies are concerned, most of the paraffin blocks containing the original biopsy specimens are still available. In the near future, I hope that we can reexamine new sections from these blocks for comparison with those cut originally. It will be interesting to note the similarity or lack thereof between our original morphologic interpretations and those made independently 20 years later.

Dr. Jordan J. Cohen: Let us assume that your reexamination of the original biopsy material confirms your initial impression that asymptomatic patients with mild proteinuria often have detectable histologic changes. To interpret such a finding, one would have to know the spectrum of histologic findings in truly normal persons without proteinuria. Are sufficient histologic data available to define what the normal spectrum is?

Dr. Robinson: I think we have a far better understanding today than we did in 1958 to 1960. For instance, kidney biopsies performed 1 h after renal transplantation in well-matched siblings offer one basis for comparison. Nevertheless, determining a precise definition of normal can be a very difficult task.

Dr. Kenneth Shapiro *(Renal Fellow, NEMC)*: You alluded to the possible role of angiotensin in the pathogenesis of postural proteinuria. Are you aware of any studies using angiotensin blockers or indomethacin to treat this condition?

Dr. Robinson: No, there are none to my knowledge.

Dr. John T. Harrington: Dr. Robinson, your studies on postural proteinuria have given us a great deal of insight into the significance of proteinuria of less than 1 g/day. Dr. Coggins recently published the first full results of the Adult Idiopathic Nephrotic Syndrome Collaborative Study analyzing patients with proteinuria greater than 3.5 g/day [72]. I am interested in your thoughts regarding the group in the middle, i.e., those who excrete 1–3 g of protein per day.

Dr. Robinson: In general, it is my bias that the greater the degree of proteinuria, the higher the likelihood of underlying kidney disease. Depending on the results of the urine sediment examination, I might wish to further test a patient who excretes 1–3 g of urinary protein per day. Some clinicians would say that renal biopsy should be performed if the excretion rate is greater than 2.0 g/day. If proteinuria of such magnitude is an isolated finding, I believe that one can postpone biopsy until the first appearance of a change in clinical status. Overall, I suspect that the subsequent appearance of such changes will be much more frequent and earlier than it is in patients with lesser degrees of proteinuria. A good study of these patients, which correlates long-term clinical information with modern renal pathology, is needed.

References

1. Berggard I: Plasma proteins in normal human urine. In Manuel Y, Revillard JP, Betuel H (eds.): Proteins in Normal and Pathological Urine. Basel, Karger, 1970
2. Free AH, Rupe CO, Metzler I: Studies with a new colorimetric test for proteinuria. Clin Chem 3:716–727, 1957
3. Hinberg IH, Katz L, Waddell L: Sensitivity of in vitro diagnostic dipstick tests to urinary protein. Clin Biochem 11:62–64, 1978
4. Poortman J, Jeanloz RW: Quantitative immunological determination of plasma proteins excreted in human urine collected before and after exercise. J Clin Invest 47:386–393, 1968
5. Castenfors J, Piscator M: Renal haemodynamics, urine flow and urine protein excretion during exercise in supine position at different loads. Acta Med Scand (Suppl) 472:231–244, 1967
6. Ryan GB, Karnovsky MJ: An ultrastructural study of the mechanisms of proteinuria in aminonucleoside nephrosis. Kidney Int 8:219–232, 1975
7. Caulfield JF, Farquhar MG: The permeability of glomerular capillaries to graded dextrans: Identification of the basement membrane as the primary filtration barrier. J Cell Biol 63:883–903, 1974
8. Farquhar MG: The primary glomerular filtration barrier—Basement membrane or epithelial slits? Kidney Int 8:197–211, 1975
9. Brenner BM, Bohrer MP, Baylis C, Deen WM: Determinants of glomerular permselectivity: Insights derived from observations in vivo. Kidney Int 12:229–237, 1977
10. Dirks JH, Clapp JR, Berliner RW: The protein concentration in the proximal tubule of the dog. J Clin Invest 43:916–921, 1964
11. Leber PD, Marsh DJ: Micropuncture study of concentration and fate of albumin in rat nephron. Am J Physiol 219:358–363, 1970
12. Oken DE, Flamenbaum W: Micropuncture studies of proximal tubule albumin concentrations in normal and nephrotic rats. J Clin Invest 50:1498–1505, 1971
13. Van Liew JB, Buentig W, Stolte H, Boylan JW: Protein excretion: Micropuncture study of rat capsular and proximal tubule fluid. Am J Physiol 219:299–305, 1970
14. Bourdeau JE, Carone FA, Ganote CE: Serum albumin uptake in isolated

perfused renal tubules: Quantitative and electron microscope radioautographic studies in three anatomical segments of the rabbit nephron. J Cell Biol 54:382–398, 1972
15. Maack T, Johnson V, Kau ST, Figueirdo J, Sigulem D: Renal filtration, transport, and metabolism of low-molecular-weight proteins: A review. Kidney Int 16:251–270, 1979
16. Wallenius G: Renal clearance of dextran as a measurement of glomerular permeability. Acta Soc Med Upsal 59(Suppl 4):1–19, 1954
17. Chang RLS, Ueki IF, Troy JL, Deen WM, Robertson CR, Brenner BM: Permselectivity of the glomerular capillary wall to macromolecules. II. Experimental studies in rats using neutral dextran. Biophys J 15:887–906, 1975
18. Chang RLS, Deen WM, Robertson CR, Brenner BM: Permselectivity of the glomerular capillary wall. III. Restricted transport of polyanions. Kidney Int 8:212–218, 1975
19. Chang RLS, Deen WM, Robertson CR, Bennett CM, Glassock RJ, Brenner BM: Permselectivity of the glomerular capillary wall: Studies of experimental glomerulonephritis in the rat using neutral dextran. J Clin Invest 57:1272–1286, 1976
20. Deen WM, Bohrer MP, Brenner BM: Macromolecule transport across glomerular capillaries: Application of pore theory. Kidney Int 16:353–365, 1979
21. Rennke HG, Cotran RS, Venkatachalam MA: Role of molecular charge in glomerular permeability: Tracer studies with cationized ferritins. J Cell Biol 67:638–646, 1975
22. Rennke HG, Venkatachalam MA: Glomerular permeability: In vivo tracer studies with polyanionic and polycationic ferritins. Kidney Int 11:44–53, 1977
23. Rennke HG, Patel Y, Venkatachalam MA: Glomerular filtration of proteins: Clearance of anionic, neutral, and cationic horseradish peroxidase in the rat. Kidney Int 13:278–288, 1978
24. Bohrer MP, Baylis C, Humes HD, Glassock RJ, Robertson CR, Brenner BM: Permselectivity of the glomerular capillary wall: Facilitated diffusion of circulating polycations. J Clin Invest 61:72–78, 1978
25. Eisenbach GM, Van Liew JB, Boylan JW: Effect of angiotensin on the filtration of protein in the rat kidney: A micropuncture study. Kidney Int 8:80–87, 1975
26. Bohrer MP, Deen WM, Robertson CR, Brenner BM: Mechanism of angiotensin II-induced proteinuria in the rat. Am J Physiol 2:F13–F21, 1977
27. Lathem W: Renal circulatory dynamics and urinary protein excretion during infusions of 1-norepinephrine and 1-epinephrine in patients with renal disease. J Clin Invest 36:1277–1285, 1957
28. Robinson RR, Lecocq FR, Phillippi PJ, Glen WG: Fixed and reproducible orthostatic proteinuria. III. Effect of induced renal hemodynamic alterations upon urinary protein excretion. J Clin Invest 42:100–110, 1963
29. Robinson RR, Glenn WG: Fixed and reproducible orthostatic proteinuria. IV. Urinary albumin excretion in healthy human subjects in the recumbent and upright positions. J Lab Clin Med 64:717–721, 1964

30. Boylan J: Introduction to the symposium on proteinuria and renal protein catabolism. Kidney Int 16:247–250, 1979
31. Tamm I, Horsfall FL: A mucoprotein derived from human urine which reacts with influenza, mumps, and Newcastle disease viruses. J Exp Med 95:71–97, 1952
32. Hoyer JR, Seiler MW: Pathophysiology of Tamm-Horsfall protein. Kidney Int 16:279–289, 1979
33. Butler EA, Flynn FV: The proteinuria of renal tubular disorders. Lancet 1:978–980, 1958
34. Butler EA, Flynn FV: The occurrence of post-gamma protein in urine: A new protein abnormality. J Clin Pathol 15:172–178, 1961
35. Peterson PA, Ervin PE, Berggard I: Differentiation of glomerular, tubular, and normal proteinuria: Determinations of urinary excretion of β_2-microglobulin, albumin, and total protein. J Clin Invest 48:1189–1198, 1969
36. Piscator M: Proteinuria in chronic cadmium poisoning. III. Electrophoretic and immunoelectrophoretic studies on urinary proteins from cadmium workers, with special reference to the excretion of low molecular weight proteins. Arch Environ Health 12:335–344, 1966
37. Antoine B, Symvoulidis A, Dardenne M: La stabilité évolutive des états de proteinurie permanente isolée. Nephron 6:526–536, 1969
38. Antoine B, Symvoulidis A, Dardenne M, De Montera H, Bach JF: L'état de proteinurie permanente isolée. I. Diversité histologique. Presse Med 77:9–14, 1969
39. Manuel Y, Revillard JP, Francois R, Traeger J, Gaillard L, Salle B, Freycon MT, Borenstein I: Trace proteinuria. In Manuel Y, Revillard JP, Betuel H (eds.): Proteins in Normal and Pathological Urine. Basel, Karger, 1970, pp. 198–208
40. Morel-Maroger L, Leroux-Robert C, Richet G: Renal histology in 30 cases of isolated proteinuria: Frequency of hyaline and fibrinoid deposits in renal arterioles. Isr J Med Sci 3:98–105, 1967
41. Muth RG: Asymptomatic mild intermittent proteinuria: A percutaneous renal biopsy study. Arch Intern Med 115:569–574, 1965
42. Pollak VW, Pirani CL, Muehrcke RC, Kark RM: Asymptomatic persistent proteinuria: Studies by renal biopsies. Guy's Hosp Rep 107:353–372, 1958
43. Phillippi PJ, Reynolds J, Yamauchi H, Beering SC: Persistent proteinuria in asymptomatic individuals: Renal biopsy studies on 50 patients. Milit Med 131:1311–1317, 1966
44. Revillard JP, Fries D, Salle B, Blanc N, Traeger J: Proteinuria in glomerular disease. In Manuel Y, Revillard JP, Betuel H (eds.): Proteins in Normal and Pathological Urine. Basel, Karger, 1970, pp. 188–197
45. Robinson RR, Glover SN, Phillippi PJ, Lecocq FR, Langelier PR: Fixed and reproducible orthostatic proteinuria. I. Light microscopic studies of the kidney. Am J Pathol 39:291–306, 1961
46. Robinson RR, Ashworth CT, Glover SN,, Phillippi PJ, Lecocq FR, Langelier PR: Fixed and reproducible and orthostatic proteinuria. II. Electron and microscopic study of renal biopsy specimens from five cases. Am J Pathol 39:405–417, 1961

47. Sinniah R, Law CH, Pivee HS: Glomerular lesions in patients with asymptomatic persistent and orthostatic proteinuria discovered on routine medical examination. Clin Nephrol 7:1–14, 1977
48. King SE: Albuminuria in renal diseases. II. Preliminary observations on the clinical course of patients with orthostatic proteinuria. NY State J Med 59:825–835, 1959
49. King SE: Diastolic hypertension and chronic proteinuria. Am J Cardiol 9:669–674, 1962
50. Levitt JI: The prognostic significance of proteinuria in young college students. Ann Intern Med 66:685–696, 1967
51. Diehl HS, McKinlay CA: Albuminuria in college men. Arch Intern Med 49:45–55, 1932
52. Wolman IJ: The incidence, causes and intermittency of proteinuria in young men. Am J Med Sci 210:86–100, 1945
53. Lyall A: The classification of cases of albuminuria. Br Med J 2:113–117, 1941
54. Burden HJ: Persistent functional albuminuria. Am J Med Sci 188:242–247, 1934
55. Derow HA: The diagnostic value of serial measurements of albuminuria in ambulatory patients. N Engl J Med 227:827–830, 1942
56. King SE: Patterns of protein excretion by the kidney. Ann Intern Med 42:296–308, 1955
57. Mery JP, Berger J, Milhaud A, Crosnier J: La proteinurie orthostatique: A propos de 300 observations. Rev Prat (Paris) 11:3115–3118, 1961
58. Bull GM: Postural proteinuria. Clin Sci 7:77–108, 1948
59. Fishberg AM: Orthostatic proteinuria. In: Hypertension and Nephritis, 5th ed. Philadelphia, Lea & Febiger, 1954, pp. 396–407
60. Prince CL: Orthostatic albuminuria. J Urol 50:608–615, 1954
61. Thompson AL, Durrett RR, Robinson RR: Fixed and reproducible orthostatic proteinuria. VI. Results of a 10-year follow-up evaluation. Ann Intern Med 73:235–244, 1970
62. Ruckley VA, MacDonald MK, MacLean PR, Robson JS: Glomerular ultrastructure and function in postural proteinuria. Nephron 3:153–166, 1966
63. Lang K, Treser G, Sagel I, Ty A, Wasserman E: Routine immunohistology in renal diseases. Ann Intern Med 64:25–36, 1966
64. Greiner T, Henry JP: Mechanism of postural proteinuria. JAMA 157:1373–1378, 1955
65. King SE, Baldwin DS: Renal hemodynamics during erect lordosis in normal man and subjects with orthostatic proteinuria. Proc Soc Exp Biol Med 86:634–638, 1954
66. Tobian L, Nason P: The augmentation of proteinuria by an acute sodium depletion that stimulates the secretion of renin. J Clin Invest 43:1301–1309, 1964
67. Montoliu J, Botey A, Torras A, Darnell A, Revert L: Renin-induced massive proteinuria in man. Clin Nephrol 11:267–271, 1979
68. Chaptal J, Jean R, Bonnet H, Pages A: Etude histologique du rein dans 33 cas de proteinurie isolée de l'enfant. Arch Fr Pediatr 23:385–390, 1966

69. Lagrue G, Bariety J, Druet PH, Mieliez P: Les divers types de proteinuries. In: Les Proteinuries. Paris, Sandoz, 1969
70. McLaine PN, Drummond KN: Benign persistent asymptomatic proteinuria. Pediatrics 46:548–552, 1970
71. Robinson RR: Proteinuria in asymptomatic patients. In: Proc 5th Int Cong Nephrol, Vol. 3. Basel, Karger, 1974, pp. 27–33
72. Collaborative Study of the Adult Idiopathic Nephrotic Syndrome: A controlled study of short-term prednisone treatment in adults with membranous nephropathy. N Engl J Med 301:1301–1306, 1979

Pathogenesis and Treatment of Membranous Nephropathy

Principal Discussant
J. Stewart Cameron

Case Presentation

A 19-year-old woman was admitted to New England Medical Center Hospital (NEMCH) for evaluation of the nephrotic syndrome. The patient was in excellent health until proteinuria was first detected 10 months earlier during the third month of her first pregnancy. Twenty-four-hour urine protein excretion remained in the 5–10-g range, and progressive pedal, hand, and periorbital edema developed. During the final weeks of the pregnancy, hypertension was present (systolic blood pressure, 140–150 mmHg; diastolic blood pressure, 90–96 mmHg). A healthy infant girl was delivered approximately 3 months prior to admission. Following delivery, the edema persisted. The patient's serum albumin concentration varied between 3.1 and 2.0 g/100 ml, serum creatinine concentration remained normal, and 24-h urine protein excretion varied between 4 and 15 g.

There was no history of dysuria, gross hematuria, urinary frequency, flank pain, or fever. There was no history of previous streptococcal infections or prior renal disease. She had no known allergies and was using no medications.

On admission to NEMCH, the patient was in no distress. The physical examination revealed the following: blood pressure, 132/80 mmHg; pulse, 60/min without postural change; respirations, 12/min; and temperature, 37 °C; the head, eyes (including optic fundi), ears, nose, and throat were unremarkable; the chest was clear to auscultation and percussion. The cardiac examination and peripheral pulses were normal. The abdominal, pelvic, and rectal examinations were unremarkable. Presacral edema and pitting edema (2+) from the knees to the ankles were present. The neurologic examination was within normal limits. There were no skin rashes, petechiae, or eruptions present. Laboratory findings disclosed the following data: hemoglobin, 14.5 g/100 ml; white blood cell count, 10,400/mm^3 with a normal differential; platelet count, 265,000/mm^3; serum creatinine, 0.9 mg; blood urea nitrogen, 11 mg/100 ml; serum sodium, 141 mEq; serum potassium, 4.3 mEq; serum chloride, 107 mEq; serum bicarbonate, 26 mEq/liter; total serum protein, 5.5 g; serum albumin, 3 g; serum cholesterol, 315 mg; serum calcium, 9.1 mg;

serum phosphorus, 4.4 mg; and serum uric acid, 5.3 mg/100 ml. Liver enzymes were normal. Fasting and 2-h postprandial blood sugar concentrations were normal. Results of chest x-ray and electrocardiogram were unremarkable. Results of urinalysis revealed the following: specific gravity, 1.023; pH, 6; protein, 4+; no glucose; white blood cells, 10–15/high power field (HPF); red blood cells, 4–5/HPF; no casts were present. Two urine cultures revealed less than 30,000 colonies of staph species and diptheroids. The 24-h urine protein excretion was 4.4 g. An i.v. urogram revealed kidneys of normal size with prompt bilateral function and no evidence of obstruction. An antinuclear antibody test was negative, and serologic tests for rheumatoid factor, syphilis, and streptozyme level were negative. The total hemolytic complement activity was 195 U (normal, 150–250 U) and the complement 3 (C3) concentration was 0.73 mg/ml (normal, 0.87–2.2 mg/ml).

Results of an open renal biopsy revealed membranous nephropathy (Fig. 1).

The patient was entered into the interhospital Study of Adult Idiopathic Nephrotic Syndrome (120 mg/day of prednisone versus placebo). The patient began her assigned "medication" (which later was disclosed to be placebo) 2 months after admission and continued for 8 weeks. She developed mild-to-moderate acne and gained weight. At the end of the treatment period, the serum creatinine concentration was unchanged at 0.8 mg/100 ml, and the serum albumin concentration remained at 2.8 g/100 ml; the 24-h urine protein excretion was 15 g. Since there was no evidence of any response to therapy, the medication was discontinued in accordance with the experimental protocol.

Presently, approximately 3.5 years after biopsy, the patient is in the second trimester of her second pregnancy and doing well clinically although she continues to have heavy proteinuria and significant hypoalbuminemia. Her renal function, however, as measured by her serum creatinine concentration of 0.6 mg/100 ml, remains normal and she is normotensive.

Discussion

Dr. J. Stewart Cameron *(Professor of Renal Medicine, Guy's Hospital Medical School, London, England)*: This woman presented at age 19 approximately 4 years ago. She had proteinuria in the nephrotic range then and since, but edema only during her pregnancy. One of the questions that arises immediately is, How far can one work up such a patient in the middle of pregnancy? Clearly, there was no great problem for this patient because she went through to a full-term normal delivery. One can, of course, do a needle renal biopsy during pregnancy in the sitting position if necessary. The problem of localizing the kidneys is increased, however, because of the radiation dose to the fetus. Like the

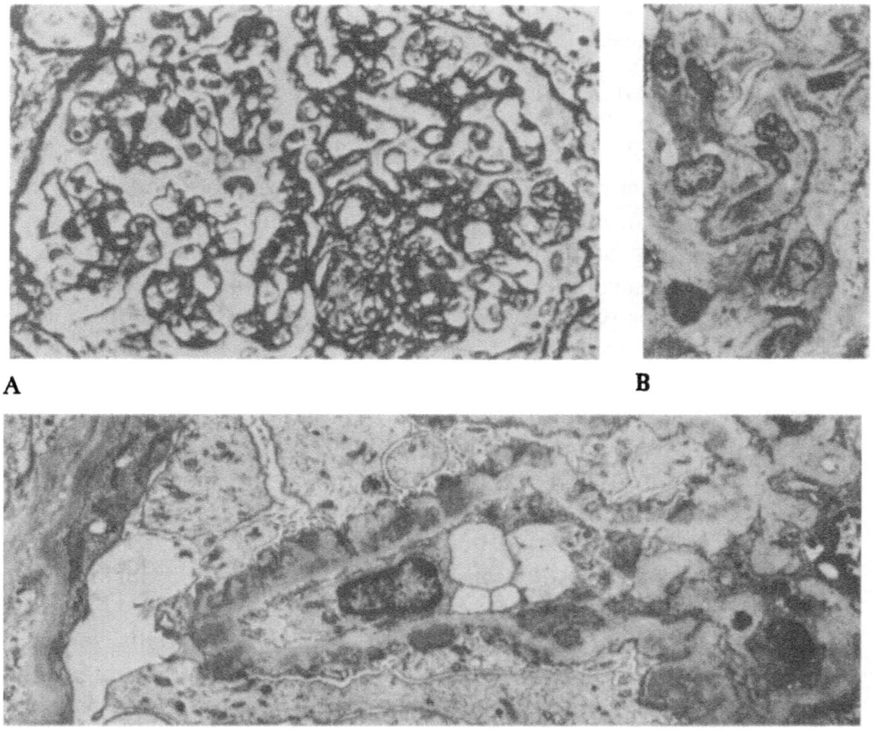

Fig. 1. Renal biopsy. **A**: In this silver methenamine preparation, segmental glomerular sclerosis, mild mesangial hypercellularity, and a focal basement membrane spike pattern can be observed (×570). **B**: The subepithelial deposits are distinct in the stained 1-μm epon section (×1068). **C**: Subepithelial electron-dense deposits, basement membrane projections, and extensive foot fusion are noted in this electron micrograph (×3204).

physicians treating this patient, we tend not to biopsy during pregnancy, but to wait for delivery and then do the full investigation. One of the other questions that arises at this point is: How long had she had proteinuria? As with so many patients with glomerular disease, the answer is that we don't know. All we can say is that the condition was found at this point, and we can suspect rather strongly that it preceded her pregnancy and was not precipitated by it. First pregnancy is one of the occasions, like induction into the Armed Forces or insurance examinations, when we discover proteinuria. When we talk about follow-up and we show long-term survival statistics, we have to remember that these data are all related to the *apparent clinical onset* of the disease. The biologic onset of the disease is something we never know.

A renal biopsy was done early in the patient's workup and showed according to the report typical optical and immunofluorescent findings of membranous nephropathy. I thought perhaps we might pause and review this biopsy first.

Dr. Seymour Rosen *(Associate Professor of Pathology, Harvard Medical School; Associate Pathologist and Head, Surgical Pathology at Beth Israel Hospital, Boston Massachusetts)*: The renal biopsy, obtained through an open surgical procedure, was an excellent specimen containing much renal cortex (Fig. 1). The glomerular tufts had apparent diffuse thickening of peripheral capillary walls and mild mesangial hypercellularity accompanied by matrical increase. In scattered glomeruli the process was more severe, and segmental capillary lumenal obliteration, adhesions, and fibrocellular crescents were observed. A typical spike pattern of the glomerular capillary wall was noted in silver methenamine preparations. Focal interstitial fibrosis, tubular atrophy, and chronic inflammation were seen; the vessels were unremarkable. Immunofluorescent findings were that of a glomerular 3+ IgG coarse peripheral granular pattern with a slightly less intense B_1C and a trace to 1+ IgM deposition in a similar distribution. The 1-μm epon sections stained with methylene blue-azure II-basic fuchsin clearly delineated glomerular capillary subepithelial deposits. Electron microscopic studies disclosed diffuse subepithelial electron-dense deposits and extensive foot process fusion; no subendothelial or mesangial deposits were recognized. Mesangial hypercellularity and matrical increase, as seen by light microscopy, were also noted. In conclusion, this pattern is that of membranous nephropathy with mild proliferation and focal sclerosis.

Dr. Cameron: This biopsy showed mesangial hypercellularity and segmental sclerosing lesions. I think most people now would accept both these features [1] as complications or associated features of membranous nephropathy, the latter especially in advanced cases. On the other hand, the combination of these observations makes one wonder, based on the findings of optical microscopy alone, about systemic lupus erythematosus (SLE). I think perhaps we might usefully discuss at this point what is for or against SLE in this particular biopsy and how to tell the difference between an SLE membranous biopsy and an idiopathic one.

Does this patient have SLE? The obvious answer is to do the appropriate tests: look for antibodies to double-stranded native DNA by either the Farr test or the more recently introduced *Crithidia luciliae* kinetoplast test, which is cheap, quick, and easy as opposed to the Farr test. Finally, our decision as to whether or not a patient with no obvious clinical stigmata of SLE can be called SLE depends on this information. I assume that the tests in this patient were and remain negative, and that she does *not* have SLE. Usually, even in a patient with SLE membranous nephropathy, there are some subendothelial or mesangial deposits. Pure membranous nephropathy, however, *can* occur in SLE without any mesangial or subendothelial deposits. Can immunofluorescence help us to distinguish SLE membranous from idiopathic membranous nephropathy? The answer is yes, but only to a limited extent. Most of us expect to find a "full house" of immunoglobulins—IgG, IgM, and IgA—together with early components of complement, such as Clq and C4 [2], which were not looked for in this particular biopsy. Their absence makes one suspicious that the patient does not have SLE. This isn't an invariable rule, and certainly we have some patients who seem to have idiopathic membranous nephropathy with a "full house" of immunoglobulins—about 20–30% of our patients. Of 42 of our patients with idiopathic membranous nephropathy, all biopsies showed IgG, and 75% showed C3, as everyone reports. About 30% of patients had IgA, or IgM, or both; about 30% had fibrin deposition; and 20% had early complement components. Thus, if the kidney biopsy in a patient who appears to have idiopathic membranous nephropathy shows all complement components and immunoglobulins, it raises the question of whether the patient has SLE. IgA was absent in the patient presented today.

I assume that this patient was screened for Australian antigenemia [3], and that she is not C2 deficient [4], which are two clinical associations one can detect. I am just mentioning these because later on we will be talking about the circumstances associated with membranous nephropathy. Our own series of membranous nephropathy patients is now just around 100 patients: two-thirds male and one-third female. A woman 19 years old is a prime subject for SLE. We should not forget that idiopathic membranous nephropathy with no tests positive for SLE may evolve into florid clinical and immunologic SLE [5,6]. We had two such cases, and I think this possibility justifies doing tests for SLE and complement concentrations not just once, but from time to time.

We should also ask whether this biopsy falls into the group described by Burkholder et al. [7] as mixed membranous and proliferative glomerulonephritis, type III. The study described a small group of patients with mesangial proliferation, sometimes some segmental accentuation of the proliferation, and not only epimembranous deposits but also subendothelial and mesangial deposits. Since we have seen the electron microscopy, we can say that the present patient doesn't fit into this category. Had we not had that available to us, I think we might have just wondered whether she was one of this group of patients. Because they have been little discussed, I thought I would briefly mention our experience with ten such patients. All their tests for SLE were negative, all their complement concentrations were normal, and they did not have the complement abnormalities we associate with mesangiocapillary glomerulonephritis (MCGN). Rather than consider this disorder an extra variety of MCGN or membranoproliferative glomerulonephritis

(MPGN), we regard it as a separate variety: "glomerulonephritis with deposits at multiple sites." Both of the well-known forms of MCGN, of course, may show some subepithelial deposits, but these are rather infrequent. Nobody talks about these patients, and they are excluded from published papers. Some regard them as an atypical form of membranous nephropathy.

Could we have diagnosed membranous nephropathy on clinical grounds? I don't think there are any specific characteristics in the differential diagnosis of nephrotic patients that will allow you to pick out membranous patients from the others. Patients with membranous nephropathy are more often male, usually have microscopic hematuria as this patient did, and even in mild cases differential protein clearances are usually nonselective. Renal function and blood pressure may both be normal or abnormal. Recently, two attempts to predict histologic data on clinical grounds have been published. One was in adults using a sequential bayesian analysis [8], and the other was in children using discriminant function analysis [9]. Both suggested that you could progress a long way clinically toward discriminating among different patients using these analyses on all the data available. I think that while this may be possible in children, our current attitude is that all adult nephrotics should have renal biopsy as part of their evaluation, if only so that we can give the patient or relatives a more accurate prognosis apart from the question of treatment. I would be interested in learning your views about renal biopsy in nephrotic patients.

The patient under discussion was entered in the collaborative Study of Adult Idiopathic Nephrotic Syndrome [10,65], and we will hear more about this later. I gather that despite developing acne and gaining weight, she was receiving a placebo! Four years since she was first documented as having proteinuria, her renal function remains within normal limits, and profuse proteinuria without edema persists. Now she is pregnant again with delivery expected in a few months, and I think we might pause to consider the management of the nephrotic patient who becomes pregnant. During the second trimester, the patient was still normotensive without edema, but had urinary protein excretion of 3.2 g/24 h. Her serum creatinine concentration was only 0.6 mg/100 ml, which I take as an indication that she had achieved the supranormal glomerular filtration rate (GFR) and creatinine clearance that one would expect as part of the normal second trimester of pregnancy. Her urine is being cultured every month as a routine appropriately. There are few data on this. In one study, however, of 31 pregnancies in 19 patients with the nephrotic syndrome [11], 11 were complicated by bacteriuria, or overt clinical infections, or both, which is of course a much higher figure than the 7% or so that you expect in normal pregnant women. I am frankly not very worried about a patient like this in pregnancy [11,12], so long as the patient has normal renal function and above all normal blood pressure. I think previous reports in the literature on pregnancy and renal disease have not clearly distinguished the different effects of different renal diseases and the effects of hypertension and diminished renal function on pregnancy. In fact, renal function isn't necessary to become pregnant and carry to term. We (and others) have had a patient on dialysis who delivered a normal child [13]. The dangerous thing is *hypertension*, especially if it is present before the pregnancy begins and above all if it is accompanied, as it was fortunately not in the case of this patient, by reduced renal function. Patients with GFR of around 40 ml/min and fairly vicious hypertension are, to my mind, about the limit at which one can expect to get a pregnancy through to an early conclusion with a live baby. In patients with membranous nephropathy, our own experience and that in the literature [11,13] is very good. Very few patients have aborted or developed severe hypertension and lost the baby, and I would hope that this patient's second pregnancy will be as successful as the first one was. There is an association between hypoalbuminemia and small babies [11], and since her serum albumin concentration is low (3 g/100 ml), we can expect her baby to be a little smaller than normal. I don't think this indicates dysmaturity or that all of these women are having their babies early; I suspect that it simply reflects the fact that the infants are slightly protein-malnourished, although there is no good evidence for this.

I think this patient will go to term and have a normal baby because she has been "road-tested" once already and both her renal function and blood pressure are normal. We will discuss her long-term outlook when we discuss membranous nephropathy in general.

Are there any questions so far?

Dr. John T. Harrington: Of interest is your comment about the long time-lag between the onset of apparently idiopathic membranous nephropathy and the subsequent development of SLE in some patients. Could you be more specific?

Dr. Cameron: Well, one of our patients took between 2 and 3 years, and Libit et al. [5] document cases of 1, 3, and 5 years. Simenhoff and Merrill's [6] patients took 5 months and 7 years. One of these was a C2 deficient patient, whose course they had earlier published as an association between C2 deficiency and membranous nephropathy. Of course, if the possibility of SLE had not been investigated adequately, some of these patients could have had SLE all the time. I have only mentioned patients in whom it was carefully assessed at the beginning of their illness.

Dr. Jordan J. Cohen: Dr. Coggins, does your recent Study of Adult Idiopathic Nephrotic Syndrome [10] indicate whether or not patients with membranous nephropathy can continue longer than 5 years and then develop SLE?

Dr. Cecil H. Coggins *(Clinical Director, Renal Unit, Massachusetts General Hospital, Boston)*: There were three patients in the study in whom pathologic reports indicated SLE from the outset, but the serologic tests were negative. Within a fairly short period of time in each case the serologic tests became positive. The patients did not, however, have membranous nephropathy; they had "mixed deposit disease."

Dr. Cameron: We looked very hard at the pathologic reports of a patient with atypical membranous nephropathy who subsequently developed SLE. She had only subepithelial deposits on the plastic-embedded material. We looked carefully at the mesangium and the subendothelial space, and no deposits were seen initially. Our pathologist commented on the great irregularity in size and number of the deposits around the different capillary loops in our patients, compared with the monotonous regularity of the typical idiopathic membranous biopsy. He suspected SLE, and he was later proven to be right.

Does anyone feel that the patient under discussion should have been biopsied in pregnancy?

Dr. Harrington: We were not caring for this patient at the time of her first pregnancy, but we have never biopsied a patient during pregnancy. In answer to your earlier question about biopsying adults with nephrotic syndrome, I believe most nephrologists in the United States prefer to biopsy virtually all adult patients with nephrotic syndrome, except those with diabetes.

Dr. Cameron: Perhaps I might add what we do in patients with diabetes. We require some clinical clue, such as the absence of retinopathy or the presence of persistent microscopic hematuria, that suggests something else besides the presence of diabetic nephropathy. Undoubtedly, if you do biopsy these suspicious patients with diabetes, then you find a good portion of them do not have diabetic nephropathy. Wass et al. [14] think that most units are biopsying too few patients with diabetic nephropathy. There is no real answer to this. Certainly a lot of *clinically* unnecessary biopsies would be performed if every diabetic with proteinuria were biopsied.

Churg has found a very high incidence of diabetes in his series of patients with membranous nephropathy [15]. In contrast, we only have one patient with clinical diabetes in 100 patients with membranous nephropathy. Clearly, the New York population differs in this respect from the London population, or the selection of patients differs markedly.

Dr. Coggins: That incidence would, of course, depend heavily on whether you decide to biopsy patients with diabetes. An abnormal glucose tolerance test eliminates a patient from our study. I might add that in trying to decide whether to biopsy patients with diabetes we also use the absence of retinopathy as a clinical clue. Recently, a patient in our hospital, who had no retinopathy detectable by fluorescein study, had a nephrectomy (before transplantation) and had clear histologic findings of diabetic nephropathy.

Dr. Cameron: Rather than discussing in detail the histopathology of membranous nephropathy, which is interesting but very well-documented [16], I want to talk more about what we do and do not know about the immunopathogenesis of this disease. Membranous nephropathy can be found in a variety of circumstances, some of which suggest that like other forms of glomerulonephritis it may be a consequence of glomerular deposition of circulating soluble complexes. Until recently this seemed to be the likely explanation for the pathogenesis of this condition. There are two salient features in membranous nephropathy, however, that require an explanation. *First,* most investigations fail to find, by the various techniques for detecting circulating immune complexes, material in many patients with membranous nephropathy [17–19]. The highest percentage I have been able to find is in Border's [20] series from the Collaborative Study of Adult Idiopathic Nephrotic Syndrome in which, by one method at least out of the three they employed, almost half the patients with membranous nephropathy were shown to have complex-like material. Most people score less than 20%, and some zero [17]. Second, despite the glomerular deposition of immunoglobulins and complement components, as in other forms of nephritis, there is a striking absence of obvious glomerular proliferation in the majority of patients.

The relationship of membranous nephropathy to possible immune complex deposition is a fascinating one. First, we must consider Dixon and Germuth's work. It was demonstrated that a pattern remarkably like that of membranous nephropathy could be induced in rabbits given chronic serum sickness by repeated daily injections of a foreign protein using a constant low-dosage schedule (2.5 mg/day) [21,22]. Germuth showed further that the deposition of complexes in the peripheral capillaries giving a membranous-like pattern was associated with the presence in the circulation of smaller immune complexes. In contrast, rabbits given foreign protein according to different schedules showed deposition of larger complexes principally in the mesangium. You will note that I have avoided saying that these complexes were necessarily being deposited in the glomeruli; but they were in the circulation, and Germuth presumed like many other investigators that this was indeed the case. Further study suggests that the membranous pattern was associated with small quantities of complexes in the circulation [22]. Kuriyama [23], working with ovalbumin-induced nephritis in rabbits, and Koyama et al. [24], who injected preformed complexes of bovine serum albumin into mice, suggested that the animals, which produced principally low avidity antibody, showed peripheral membranous-like deposition of complexes rather than mesangial deposition.

One can postulate, then, that human glomerulonephritis might arise from the presence in the circulation of small amounts of complexes formed from low avidity antibody, and that this explains the relative difficulty of detecting immune complexes in this disorder. This contrasts with mesangiocapillary or postinfectious glomerulonephritis and SLE, in which complexes are easily found in large amounts in the majority of patients.

Could it be that membranous nephropathy is not the result of the deposition of circulating complexes at all, and that this explains why we cannot find them? I would now like to review some work done during the past few years which supports the idea that complexes may form by combination of antibody and antigen in situ within the glomerulus, and that this may be one mechanism—perhaps the principal mechanism—by which membranous nephropathy arises.

For a time after the work of Dixon and Germuth, we became used to thinking that there were fundamentally two contrasting varieties of nephritis (Fig. 2). One variety was that in which deposition of antibody

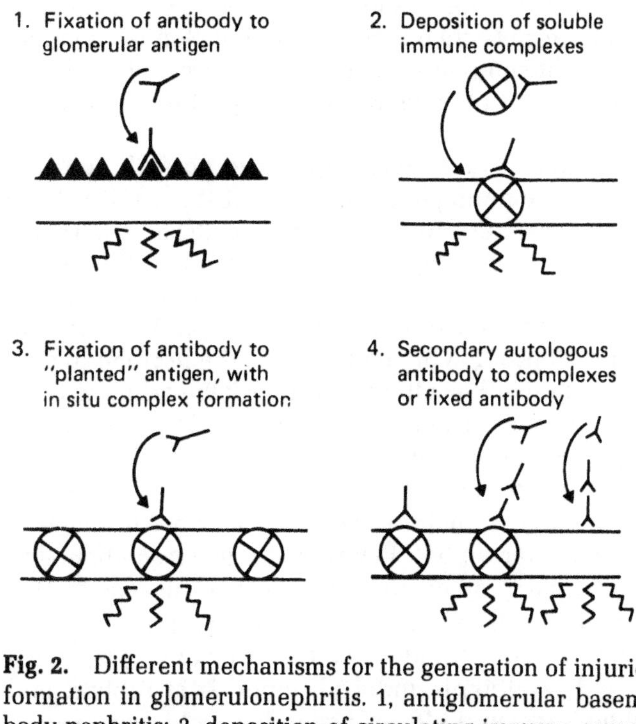

Fig. 2. Different mechanisms for the generation of injurious immune complex formation in glomerulonephritis. 1, antiglomerular basement membrane antibody nephritis; 2, deposition of circulating immune complexes; 3, in situ complex formation; 4, secondary autologous antibody deposition. (See text for explanation.)

against glomerular antigens induced the inflammation; the other variety was that due to the deposition in the glomerular capillary walls of immune complexes formed in the circulation, and again inflammation was induced. What we are talking about now is the possibility that a new antigen "planted" either in the glomerular capillary wall or the mesangium might combine with circulating antibody to induce inflammation. In retrospect, of course, the autologous phase of antiglomerular basement membrane antibody nephritis is an example of this: The heterologous antibody fixes to the glomerular basement membrane, and after several days autologous antibody to this foreign protein (in this case heterologous IgG) forms, and it is during the fixation of this autologous antibody that the inflammation and renal damage takes place.

Some of the earlier observations in this field were those of Mauer et al. [25]. They localized aggregated immunoglobulin in the mesangium in experimental animals and then injected an antibody directed against this immunoglobulin. The result was a brisk nephritis. More recently, another experiment was reported by Golbus and Wilson [26] in which Concanavalin A was attached to the glomeruli, an antibody against it injected, fixed, and again a nephritis was produced.

It has become clear that in another of the hallowed models of presumed soluble complex disease—acute serum sickness in rabbits—one of the earliest events that can be detected in the glomerulus is the deposition of the foreign protein *without* any antibody or complement. After a couple of days as the antibody against the foreign protein appears in the circulation, it then appears in the glomeruli. Finally after another 2 or 3 days, immune elimination of the circulating foreign antigen by the antibody occurs with extensive deposition of complexes. It is quite possible, therefore, in even an old-fashioned disease such as acute serum sickness (which has been with us since Von Pirquet in 1908), that the renal injury is partly mediated through in situ immune complex formation.

The first suggestion (so far as I am aware) that human membranous nephropathy might result from in situ formation of complexes in the capillary wall came from Evans in 1974 [27]. He suggested that differential filtration of various antigens and antibodies through the capillary wall, to produce an antibody-antigen ratio in the subepithelial space suitable for complex formation, might account for the formation of deposits at this site. He further pointed out that once deposited such complexes might be in equilibrium with the antigen and antibody in the circulation. Although more recent work on other determinants of molecular penetration into the glomerular capillary wall besides molecular size, in particular charge [28], has rendered his detailed arguments obsolete, the idea remains a fruitful one.

This brings us to a discussion of the model usually thought to resemble human membranous glomerulonephropathy most closely—Heymann nephritis. In brief, the original descriptions of this model by Glassock et al. [29] showed that when rats were given injections of isologous kidney, a nephritogenic antigen could be found in the renal tubular brush border, called renal tubular epithelial (RTE) antigen. When this was prepared crudely and injected, antibody was induced in the host rat, and a chronic membranous nephropathy appeared with the glomerular deposits containing RTE antigen. The antigen was detected in a particular fraction of the tubule preparation called FX 1A, and hence it is referred to as FX 1A in many publications. This fraction contains several antigens, and most work has been done with relatively crude preparations.

Initially it was assumed that this disease resulted from the formation of FX 1A–antiFX 1A immune complexes in the circulation and their subsequent deposition within the kidney. Barabas et al. [30], however, showed that a single injection of antiFX 1A antibody could also lead to prolonged proteinuria. They postulated that the FX 1A released from tubules following the injection led to the formation of complexes with the injected antibody; the complexes thus formed then deposited in the glomeruli. This form of the disease is usually referred to as "passive" Heymann nephritis [31]. Van Es et al. [32] showed later that the chronic proteinuria that followed the single injection of rabbit antiFX 1A depended upon secondary autologous antibody directed against the heterologous rabbit antiFX 1A antibody present in the glomeruli, the immune complex thus acting as a "planted" antigen.

Even more fascinating, it has been shown that the glomerular basement membrane contains antigens that cross-react with antiFX 1A, and that formation of complexes within the glomerular wall follows within seconds of injection of the antiFX 1A antibody [33,34]. The crucial experiments involved in vivo perfusion of the isolated kidney with antiFX 1A antibodies both from the circulation and eluted from the kidneys of rabbits with nephritis, both of which fixed, and FX 1A–antiFX 1A complexes, which did not. This work has been confirmed recently by Steinmuller et al. [35] using an in vitro isolated perfused kidney system.

All of this may be relevant to human membranous nephropathy, although the extent to which in situ complex formation contributes is unknown. It is quite possible that both mechanisms—deposition of complexes formed in the circulation and in situ complex formation—aré important. In other forms of glomerulonephritis, deposition of soluble complexes may predominate, but membranous nephropathy *may* be a disease in which the majority of the immune material is formed within the subepithelial space. This could explain why one cannot find complexes in the circulation in the majority of patients, and might explain the failure of membranous nephropathy to transmit to grafted kidneys, unlike other forms of glomerulonephritis such as MCGN or mesangial IgA disease [36]. In passing, it is also interesting to remember that SLE, rather surprisingly, does not transmit to grafted kidneys. A priori, this is one of the forms of glomerulonephritis that one would think might transmit with regularity. A suggestion from Izui et al. [37], however, is relevant here. These workers proposed that DNA might bind to basement membrane collagen and then react in situ with circulating antiDNA antibody; this might then allow other complexes in the circulation access to the capillary wall from which they were otherwise excluded. Whether there are antiDNA-DNA complexes in the circulation at all is the subject of present debate [38,39].

One can begin to play with these new ideas to speculate on what determines the initiation and progression of nephritis. Certainly, events that might modify the glomerular capillary wall permeability [29] become crucial if antigen and antibody are to gain access to the subepithelial space. Low-affinity antibody could certainly exist in the circulation alongside free antigen and form complexes in the capillary wall while there were few or none in the circulation, as suggested by Evans [27]. It may be that only some special sorts of antigen can do this, but the variety of circumstances in which membranous nephropathy may be found suggests that many antigens must be capable of this. This speculation may lead us not to chase complexes in the circulation, but to go to the kidney to study the actual site where the damage is taking place.

Turning back to human membranous glomerulopathy, Table 1 shows some antigens that are implicated in the human disease. The most interesting, in view of the discussion today, is the possibility that some patients may have membranous nephropathy arising from immune complexes with RTE as the antigen. Naruse et al. [40,41] first discussed this possibility, but we [42] were unable to confirm this either in idiopathic or in drug-induced membranous nephropathy using antisera to a slightly different nephrogenic antigen extracted from human urine. I believe other studies have also failed to confirm this interesting finding although Ozawa et al. [43] suggested that, as one might expect, RTE was

Table 1. Antigens and circumstances reported to be associated with membranous nephropathy.

Intrinsic Antigens	Extrinsic Antigens	Debatable Associations
DNA	Hepatitis B	Renal venous thrombosis
Renal tubular epithelial	Tuberculosis pallidum	Diabetes
Carcinoembryonic	Filarial	Rheumatoid arthritis
Other tumor	Mercury and mercurials	Sjögren's syndrome
Thyroglobulin	Gold	Sarcoidosis
	Penicillamine	Tuberculosis
	Tridione	

involved in the membranous nephropathy secondary to renal venous thrombosis. Costanza et al. [44] described a patient in whom carcinoembryonic antigen (CEA) appeared to be the antigen involved. We [45] and others have been unable to confirm this association, which is surprising since it is now 5 years since that paper was published, and a number of patients have been studied using several different antigenic determinants of the CEA to prepare the antisera. Also with reference to Table 1, it should be pointed out that membranous nephropathy may be associated with Hodgkin's disease, as well as the more usual "minimal change" pattern.

The extrinsic antigens are also listed in Table 1. There are a number of infectious agents and drugs that are particularly associated with membranous nephropathy. The patients with this variety of membranous nephropathy are particularly important because they teach us two things: First, the continued deposition of *something* in the glomerulus is necessary for the continuing disease, because if you take away the drug these patients almost invariably get better although it can take 1 or 2 years. Second, there is some mechanism by which the glomerulus can remove the subepithelial or intramembranous deposits; the nature of this is obscure.

Finally, some more general and debatable associations of membranous nephropathy are shown in Table 1. We have already discussed the possible association with diabetes mellitus. I will end the discussion of the possible associations of membranous nephropathy by simply stating that my own prejudice is that renal venous thrombosis is in all probability secondary to the glomerular disease in every case.

As I mentioned earlier, I do not wish to discuss the histopathologic changes in detail. They have been well described by Ehrenreich and Churg [15] and by Bariéty et al. [46]. I will only make three points: First, oil immersion on immunofluorescent material may be necessary to demonstrate the finest granular deposits in stage 1 membranous nephropathy, and one may be tempted to diagnose linear immunofluorescent studies erroneously unless immersion is used. Second, the classical "spikes" of stage 2 membranous nephropathy may not be present in early stage 1 cases. To differentiate these from "minimal change" lesions, the capillary walls cut obliquely are more helpful, because if silver preparations under the oil immersion are used one can see a "bubbly" appearance of deposits cut through horizontally. Third, after clinical resolution of membranous nephropathy and a normal biopsy appearance on optical microscopy, electron microscopy may still reveal lucent areas within the apparently normal basement membrane, which we believe represent the sites of leached-out deposits. Gärtner et al. [47], who described this appearance, have called this stage 5 membranous nephropathy. It is already clear from the lack of correlation between renal function and renal biopsy grading [16] that stages 1 through 4 do not represent progressively worse manifestations of the disease, although 1 through 3 may represent a histologic evolution. In general, GFR does not correlate well with glomerular changes in glomerular diseases, but correlates much better with interstitial and tubular changes.

Perhaps we can finish by considering the long-term outlook for patients with membranous nephropathy. Figure 3 shows the actuarial survival for all the published series of membranous nephropathy up to 1976, including our own data [48]. You can see that by and large this is a slowly progressive disease with renal failure and other causes of death coming in 3 to 5 years from onset. Figure 4 summarizes data from all the patients with membranous nephropathy whom we biopsied more than 10 years ago. All these 33 patients had at least 10 years of potential follow-up. These data are percentages of those analyzed at that particular point, not actuarially calculated figures. The proportion of patients in remission apparently decreases as we lose a few patients from follow-up around the decade mark. I suspect that the proportion in remission would be around 40% at 10 to 15 years. We lost mainly

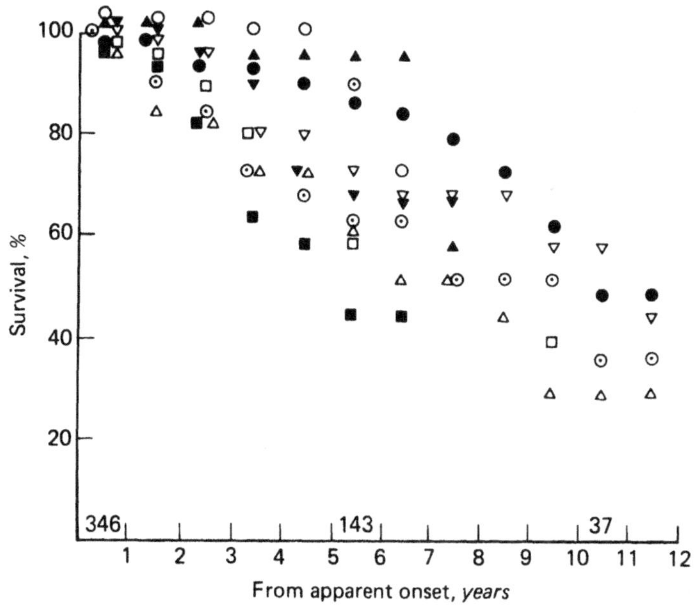

Fig. 3. Actuarial survival of patients with membranous nephropathy, calculated from series published up to 1976. Deaths and the requirement for dialysis or transplantation have been included as "deaths." Deaths from "nonrenal" causes (e.g., myocardial infarction) have been included. All series predominantly or entirely of adult patients, except data taken from Ref. 51, represented by *solid triangle* (▲). Data taken from Ref. 48 represented by *solid circle* (●).

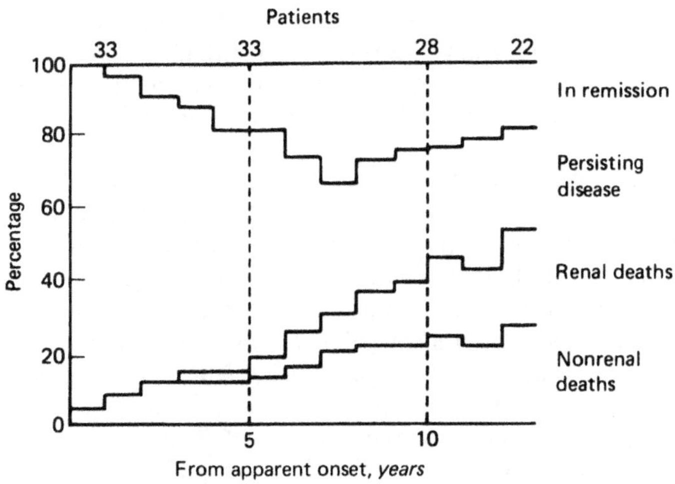

Fig. 4. The status at last follow-up of 33 patients with membranous nephropathy biopsied before 1968. The percentage of patients in each follow-up category is indicated at *left*, and the number of patients available for analysis (including all those then or previously listed as dead or on dialysis) is indicated at *top*.

patients who were fit and well, which is what always happens. Another point I particularly want to make is that there are *no* renal deaths in our series until after 3 years, and that any study with an end-point based on terminal renal failure is going to have to run at least 5 or 10 years. Finally, there are quite large numbers of nonrenal deaths, particularly from cardiovascular disease.

Figure 5 is my summary of what probably happens to patients with membranous nephropathy from the literature and from our own series. By 15 years, there are probably very few patients with active disease and none with a continuing nephrotic syndrome. From our own data, most of the patients who go into renal failure appear to suffer a persisting nephrotic syndrome and transfer from this category to that of renal death.

Recently, Hopper et al. [49] have suggested that male patients do much worse than female patients with membranous nephropathy when renal failure is considered. This has not been the case in our own series of 94 patients. Of 59 men, eight have died (or required substitution therapy), and only three of these deaths (5%) have been from renal failure as against eight deaths among 35 women, four of them (12%) from renal failure. The mean follow-up in our series is similar to Hopper's, and the mean ages almost identical. In his series, one-third of male patients had gone into terminal renal failure before 7 years had passed. Even excluding the few children in our series, the difference persists.

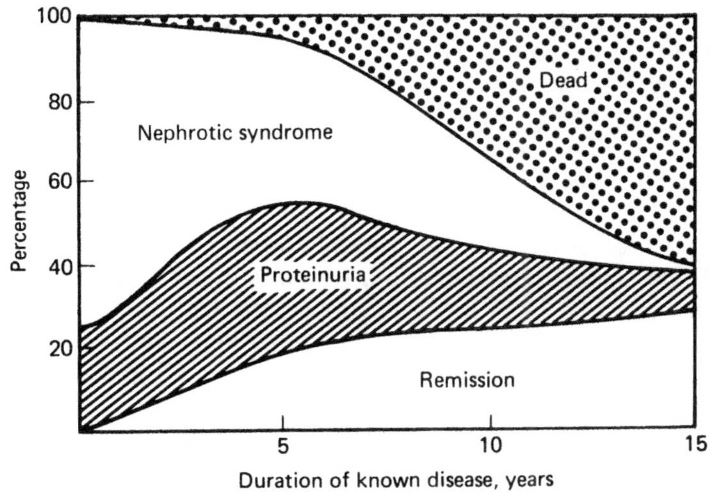

Fig. 5. A synthesis of the probable long-term outcome of adult patients with membranous nephropathy. An increase in the proportion of patients with minor proteinuria at apparent onset (i.e., clinical discovery), for example by a change in biopsy policy in isolated proteinuria, would improve the prognosis of the group. A diagram for children would probably be similar, but the proportion with persisting nephrotic syndrome and renal death would be smaller. (Derived from data in Figs. 3 and 4.)

An interesting observation is that younger patients do better than older patients. Table 2 shows an analysis of data on adults and children from the literature [48]. This is true even though the proportion of nephrotic patients is about the same in either group. The percentage in renal failure at about 5 years is only 4% in the children, but 20% in the adults. Also the remission rate (i.e., the complete absence of proteinuria or clinical signs of renal disease) is almost 50% in the children, but much lower in the adults. The proportion of remissions might be depen-

Table 2. Comparison of outcome in adult and childhood onset patients with membranous nephropathy.

	NS	F/U >5 years	Deaths in CRF	Remissions (Treatment)	Remissions (No Treatment)
Adults (N = 435)[a]	85%	207	82 (19%)	34	35
Children (N = 82)[b]	79%	29	4 (4%)	15	25

[a]Adult, >15 years old at apparent onset.
[b]Children, <15 years old at apparent onset.
Note: N, number of patients studied; NS, nephrotic syndrome; F/U, follow-up; CFR, chronic renal failure.
Source: data from Ref. 48.

dent on how many patients were treated if treatment works, but in crude figures 35% of the children and 8% of the adults went into remission without any treatment whatsoever except diuretics. In our own series (Table 3), about 25% of the patients went into remission without any treatment. You can compare these data with the more extensive data from Ehrenreich et al. [50], which caused such a stir because they suggested an effect of corticosteroids on membranous nephropathy (Table 3). As you can see in our data, out of 26 patients who received nothing at all eight went into remission, which is approximately 25% (Table 3). We, certainly, have not been impressed with the idea that steroids make any difference at all to these patients and we have stopped treating our patients with membranous nephropathy with corticosteroids.

Using current measurement of GFR or creatinine clearance as the end-point for a trial of therapy, many years will be necessary to demonstrate an effect if one is present. Any tool we have is going to be a blunt instrument in under 5 years. This must be remembered when we examine the essentially negative results that have emerged from the trials carried out so far (Table 4). Most of these trials lasted for only a year or two, and in several the numbers were small; in the Medical Research Council trial, neither the dosage nor the duration of treatment was standardized.

At this point, we must raise the data of the Collaborative Study of Adult Idiopathic Nephrotic Syndrome [10]. With Dr. Coggins present, I will only say that at first I viewed these data with great skepticism, but the randomization and analysis seem to have been impeccably performed and appear to show an effect of corticosteroids in delaying renal failure and diminishing proteinuria in adult patients with membranous nephropathy. I am reminded of the epigraph of Toulmin: "A man demonstrates his rationality . . . by the manner in which, and the occasions on which he *changes* [his] ideas, procedures and concepts" (italics added) [54]. I hope that I will be able to demonstrate my rationality by changing my belief on the absence of specific treatment for membranous nephropathy, but we need more data and must take steps to generate them.

Questions and Answers

Dr. John T. Harrington: Dr. Coggins, will you lead off by briefly summarizing and commenting on the results of the Study of Adult Idiopathic Nephrotic Syndrome?

Dr. Cecil H. Coggins: For the past several years we have been conducting a prospective cooperative study on the effect of prednisone compared to placebo in adults with the idiopathic nephrotic syndrome

Table 3. The effect of treatment with corticosteroids on long-term follow-up in patients with membranous nephropathy.

	Group I[a] (N = 48)		Group II[b] (N = 103)		Group III[c] (N = 67)		Group IV[d] (N = 26)	
	Rx	No Rx	Rx	No Rx	Rx	No Rx	Rx	No Rx
Dead	5	7	6	22	6	1	5	12
Persistent NS	5	2	12	11	15	5	0	0
Persistent proteinuria	8	9	24	11	0	0	0	0
Remission	4	8	17	0	25	15	5	4
	22	26	59	44	46	21	10	16
Follow-up	5.4 years, mean		5.8 years, mean		1 to 15 years		0 to 23 years	
Duration of Rx	2 to 38 months (mean 7 months)		6 weeks to 39 months		NA		NA	

[a]Seven patients also received immunosuppressants, and analysis confined to NS since only nephrotic patients treated. Data taken from Ref. 48.

[b]Sixteen patients also received immunosuppressants. Data taken from Ref. 50.

[c]Twenty-four patients also received immunosuppressants, and seven of these did not receive corticosteroids. Data taken from Ref. 51.

[d]All NS, data taken from Ref. 52.

Note: N, number of patients studied; Rx, administration of corticosteroids; NS, nephrotic syndrome; NA, data not available.

Table 4. Results of controlled studies of immunosuppressant drugs in patients with membranous nephropathy.

Agent	Duration	Result
Corticosteroids	2 to 4 years	None
Azathioprine plus Corticosteroids	2 years	None
Azathioprine	1 year	None
Cyclophosphamide	2 years	None
Chlorambucil	1 year	P and C_{cr}, same[a]

[a]P, proteinuria; C_{cr}, creatinine clearance.
Source: data from Ref. 53.

[10,65]. Patients were randomly allocated either to a treatment or control group.

The patients in the group receiving prednisone underwent therapy for 2 months during which they received prednisone every second day. This was followed by tapering of medication for approximately 1 month at the discretion of the individual physician. All patients who remitted and then relapsed again received additional treatment. Of the group of 34 patients, however, only five patients received more than one course. The treated group had significantly more remissions, less proteinuria, and, of the greatest import, better maintenance of creatinine clearance during the follow-up period. We were surprised to find an observable difference and tried to find some way in which the groups were not comparable, or whether the therapeutic group initially contained patients with a better prognosis. We compared a large number of clinical, laboratory, and histologic characteristics of the patients in both groups and found no correlation between the prognosis and these characteristics. Further, we found no selection bias between the treatment and control groups. There seems to be no other explanation for the differences other than the prednisone therapy. The duration of observation of both groups was the same on the average, and each had an equal opportunity to develop problems. It may be a bit surprising that some of the control patients developed renal failure so quickly.

Dr. Cameron: Yes, I was going to ask you about that. The data (Fig. 3) reveal that it is very unusual for patients to develop renal failure in less than 4 years from apparent onset. The "stop point" in your trial is a doubling of serum creatinine concentration, but I think you have 11 patients who are in renal failure in the control group and only one in the treatment group. Is that right?

Dr. Coggins: Yes, the renal failure for nine of the 11 patients was rather severe. For two patients, however, it shouldn't be called renal failure; their serum creatinine concentrations simply doubled.

Dr. Cameron: Certainly from our own experience and the published literature, it is unusual for one-third of the 35 control patients with nephrotic syndrome to develop renal failure so soon.

Dr. Coggins: Within about 2.5 years, one-third of the group doubled their serum creatinine concentrations. During the same time, two-thirds of the patients did not raise their serum creatinine concentrations significantly. It sounds less dramatic when stated that way and doesn't seem surprising. Many patients in both groups are doing well as the years go by with no sign at all of progression of their renal disease. There is another point, which you mentioned earlier, that we can confirm. Any patient who has *any* kind of remission, even a partial remission defined as a reduction in proteinuria to below 2 g/day, has an excellent chance of maintaining GFR in the future, confirming the findings of Idelson et al. [55].

Dr. Cameron: Yes. When the prognosis for patients with proteinuria only is examined and compared with that of patients with a full nephrotic syndrome, a consistent pattern appears with the single exception of patients with SLE, where there is no difference. Patients with mesangiocapillary, membranous, and focal segmental sclerosing lesions and a nephrotic syndrome show almost identical survival curves with about 30 to 40% having 10-year survival. Those that were never nephrotic showed about 90% survival at the same point. In other words, simple clinical observation at the beginning of the disease, the presence of swelling in the ankles or more than 3 g of proteinuria, gives a useful prognostic index although it is a gloomy one.

Dr. Harrington: Of those patients who developed renal failure within 5 years, how many of those patients unequivocally had normal renal function at 3 years as this patient does? It is my feeling that if a patient survives 3 years and still has unequivocal normal function, the long-term prognosis is very good [55]. Do you have any information on this point?

Dr. Cameron: We do have data on this [48]. We have seen patients like the patient under discussion who maintain perfectly normal renal function for several years, but then very slowly develop renal failure. I suspect, however, that you are right; if a patient maintains normal renal function for 3 to 5 years, the prognosis could be considered generally good but not invariably so.

Dr. Coggins: One of the questions that we asked of patients in our study was, When did edema or proteinuria first develop? It is very "soft" data because often the patients don't know but will give an answer. In looking at those answers, we found no difference between the patients with persistence of normal renal function and those in whom renal function deteriorated rather rapidly.

Dr. Cameron: We have one patient who has had proteinuria for 22 years generally short of the nephrotic range [48]. There are several patients in the literature with similar courses [56]. Certainly, a few patients can persist for long periods with membranous nephropathy without decline in renal function but with persisting urine abnormalities short of a nephrotic syndrome [57]. As we agreed earlier, the presence of a nephrotic syndrome does not necessarily indicate that the patient will do poorly even if it persists for 4 or 5 years, but by and large it marks the individual as a higher-risk patient. Looking at the survival curves in Fig. 3, it is an indolent disease. The survival curves are in general flat for the first few years, then bend over, which is rather different from other forms of glomerulonephritis in which a mortality is seen in the first few years.

Dr. Jordan J. Cohen: The hypothesis that glomerular disease develops because of the in situ formation of immune complexes is a very intriguing one. If true, would such a pathogenesis suggest to you a different therapeutic strategy from that presently used?

Dr. Cameron: It might at the theoretical level, but I don't think at the practical level as yet. If we believe that the generation of immune complexes in the circulation is the crucial event with both the antibody and the antigen in solution, then one can examine a number of things, including the quantity of antibody or the avidity with which the antibody combines with the antigen, and try to modify these with therapeutic agents. If combination takes place on a surface, however, in this case the outside of the glomerular basement membrane, then the nature of the combination may be very different. We already know, for example, that we can do things in a tube with immune reactants in solution which, probably for reasons of steric hindrance, can't be done if some of the reactants are fixed to the wall of the tube.

Instead of asking how complexes get into the sites they do, in or on the capillary wall, we must now ask how we might influence the access of free antigen and free antibody to the site of reaction. Recently, the influence of charge on the access of immune materials and events that affect the charged molecules within the glomerular capillary wall have been explored. For example, aminonucleoside nephrosis induced in the kidney *denies* access of circulating immune complexes to the capillary wall [58], whereas several other manipulations permit access of the complexes.

I think the real implication for therapy is that anyone who thinks about the therapy of established glomerulonephritis in simplistic terms is in difficulty. Certainly, the old idea of using immunosuppressants because glomerulonephritis was supposed to be a disease of hyperimmunity seems laughable now. The new idea that we might simply "activate the T cells" with something like levamisole and thus improve things is equally naive. Not only at the level of cellular control, but even at the level of local assembly of complexes, it is probably very complicated. The in situ formation of complexes also implies that the material in the circulation may not tell us a thing about what is going on in the kidney; it might even mislead us.

Dr. John Donohoe *(Renal Services, University Hospital, Boston)*: Could I ask you about the comment that you made concerning the pathogenesis of membranous nephropathy? I think you said that it is unusual for membranous nephropathy to recur in a transplant patient.

Dr. Cameron: Yes. There are several de novo cases in patients who undoubtedly had problems other than nephritis as a cause of renal failure [59,60], but there are only two patients so far whose courses are reasonably well documented in whom membranous nephropathy recurred following renal transplantation [61,62].

Dr. Donohoe: Don't those cases strengthen the argument in favor of circulating immune complexes rather than in situ formation?

Dr. Cameron: I suspect that *both* mechanisms—deposition of circulating immune complexes and in situ complex formation—operate in several types of glomerulonephritis, but possibly the balance is in favor of in situ immune complex formation in membranous nephropathy. Unpublished work by Border and Glassock unequivocally demonstrates circulating immune complexes in Heymann nephritis of rats, the same disease in which some others have shown in situ immune complex formation, and I am sure that both are right. There is in this model for the first time good evidence for the operation of both mechanisms. It is almost certainly true, although the evidence is less clear, that both mechanisms operate in acute serum sickness nephritis in rabbits. I suspect that it is a question of predominance of one mechanism or the other in some conditions. One would therefore expect that the minority of patients with membranous nephropathy and large amounts of soluble immune complexes in their circulation might have an aggressive recurrence of the disorder in the graft.

Dr. Cohen: It has recently been suggested that complement receptors for C3b on the glomerular capillary wall play a role in some forms of immune complex deposition. What do you think about this suggestion?

Dr. Cameron: It *may* be important in human renal disease, but of course we know that rats and many other animals who do not have glomerular C3b receptors can develop membranous nephropathy and other forms of glomerulonephritis that closely resemble the human disease. So, while the possession in humans and a few closely related primates of the C3b receptors (in the interstitium incidentally as well as in the glomerulus) may have an influence on the initiation and progression of disease, I can't believe it is a dominant mechanism. In fact, human beings are a little resistant to the induction of nephritis compared with the incidence of nephritis found in dogs, rats, and mice; we are a relatively nephritis-resistant rather than nephritis-prone species. The presence of C3b receptors *could* relate to this, but it should work exactly the other way around. C3b receptors should allow the more avid fixation of complement-fixing immune complexes in the kidney.

With membranous nephropathy, it is interesting that the C3b receptors are believed to be on the epithelial cells of the glomeruli, and of course in membranous nephropathy the immune deposits are subepithelial. We do know also that these C3b receptors may become undetectable and then return in diseases that are exclusively subendothelial, such as mesangiocapillary glomerulonephritis during complement fixation. I am inclined to think that at the moment C3b receptors are a very nice phenomenon in search of a relation to something clinically important!

Dr. David Bernard *(Renal Service, University Hospital, Boston)*: Dr. Cameron, you mentioned that in your experience the drug-induced varieties of membranous nephropathy will invariably fade away, perhaps over a period of years. Recently, we had a patient who was treated with gold therapy and subsequently developed severe nephrotic syndrome. After some 9 months, the disease persists despite some steroid therapy. Would you give this patient a good prognosis?

Dr. Cameron: I think I would. Clearly, there is the possibility of a secondary mechanism, such as autologous antibody to immune complexes formed in situ or deposited in the glomerulus. This may happen in malarial nephropathy, for example. There is also evidence in the literature suggesting that not all cases of penicillamine-induced nephropathy remit [63]. The problem is that the patients may not have been followed long enough. I think the best report is by Gärtner et al. [64]. They followed 31 patients with penicillamine-induced nephropathy for more than 2 years and found that all patients got better after 2 years although many of them had been fully nephrotic even after 1 year (Neild, personal communication). What might still be causing the nephrotic syndrome at 1 year is fascinating. When you imply that this patient hasn't improved, you have not yet waited for 24 months when many patients finally remit.

References

1. Gärtner HV, Fischbach H, Wehner H, Bohle A, Edel HH, Kluthe R, Scheler F, Schmulling RM: Comparison of clinical and morphological features of peri-(epi-, extra-) membranous glomerulonephritis. Nephron 13:288–301, 1974

2. Sinniah R, Feng PH: Lupus nephritis: Correlation between light, electron microscopic and immunofluorescent findings and renal function. Clin Nephrol 6:340–351, 1976
3. Combes B, Stastny P, Shorey J, Elgenbrodt EH, Barrera A, Hull AR, Carter NW: Glomerulonephritis with deposition of Australia antigen-antibody complexes in glomerular basement membrane. Lancet 2:234–237, 1971
4. Pickering RJ, Michael AF, Herdman RC, Good RA, Gewurz H: The complement system in chronic glomerulonephritis—three newly associated aberrations. J Pediatr 78:30–43, 1971
5. Libit SA, Burke B, Michael AF, Vernier RL: Extramembranous glomerulonephritis in childhood: Relationship to systemic lupus erythematosus. J Pediatr 88:394–402, 1976
6. Simenhoff ML, Merrill JP: The spectrum of lupus nephritis. Nephron 1:348–375, 1964
7. Burkholder PM, Hyman LR, Krueger RP: Characterization of mixed membranous and proliferative glomerulonephritis. Recognition of three varieties. In Kincaid-Smith P, Mathew TH, Becker EL (eds.): Glomerulonephritis I. New York, Wiley, 1973, pp. 557–559
8. World MJ: Variables discriminating between cryptogenic glomerular lesions in adults with the nephrotic syndrome. Q J Med 45:451–468, 1976
9. International Study of Kidney Disease in Children. Nephrotic syndrome in childhood: Prediction of histopathology from clinical and laboratory charactersitics at time of diagnosis. Kidney Int 13:159–165, 1978
10. Coggins CH: Study of adult idiopathic nephrotic syndrome. Abstr Int Congr Nephrol, Montreal, 1978, p. D36
11. Studd JWW, Blainey JD: Pregnancy and the nephrotic syndrome. Br Med J 1:276–280, 1960
12. Strauch BS, Hayslett JP: Kidney disease and pregnancy. Br Med J 4:578–582, 1974
13. Editorial: Pregnancy after treatment for renal failure. Lancet 1:861, 1978
14. Wass JAH, Watkins PJ, Dische FE, Parsons V: Atypical glomerular disease in diabetes mellitus. Proc EDTA 13:546–552, 1976
15. Churg J, Ehrenreich T: Membranous nephropathy. In Kincaid-Smith P, Mathew TH, Becker EL (eds.): Glomerulonephritis I. New York, Wiley, 1973, pp. 443–448
16. Ehrenreich T, Churg J: Pathology of membranous nephropathy. Path Ann 3:145–168, 1968
17. Ooi YM, Ooi BS, Pollak VE: Relationship of levels of circulating immune complexes to histologic patterns of nephritis: A comparative study of membranous glomerulopathy and diffuse proliferative glomerulonephritis. J Lab Clin Med 90:891–898, 1977
18. Stuhlinger WD, Verroust PJ, Morel-Maroger L: Detection of circulating immune complexes in patients with various renal diseases. Immunology 30:43–47, 1976
19. Woodroffe AJ, Border WA, Theofilopoulos AN, Gore O, Glassock RJ, Dixon FJ, Wilson CB: Detection of circulating immune complexes in patients with glomerulonephritis. Kidney Int 12:268–278, 1977
20. Border W, Abrass C, Hall C, Brown C, Glassock R, Coggins C: Detection of circulating immune complexes (iCK) in adult idiopathic nephrotic syndrome (AINS). Kidney Int 13:58A, 1978

21. Germuth FG, Rodriguez E: The immunopathology of the renal glomerulus. Boston, Little, Brown, 1973
22. Germuth FG, Taylor TJ, Siddiqui SY, Rodriguez E: Immune complex disease. VI: Some determinants of the varieties of glomerular lesions in the chronic bovine serum albumin-rabbit system. Lab Invest 37:162–169, 1977
23. Kuriyama T: Chronic glomerulonephritis induced by prolonged immunization in the rabbit. Lab Invest 28:224–235, 1973
24. Koyama A, Niwa Y, Shigematsu H, Taniguchi M, Tada T: Studies on passive serum sickness. II. Factors determining the localization of antigen-antibody complexes in the murine renal glomerulus. Lab Invest 38:253–262, 1978
25. Mauer SM, Sutherland DER, Howard RJ, Fish AJ, Najarian JS, Michael AF: The glomerular mesangium. III. Acute immune mesangial injury. A new model of glomerulonephritis. J Exp Med 137:553–570, 1973
26. Golbus S, Wilson CB: Glomerulonephritis (GN) produced by the in situ formation of immune complexes on the glomerular basement membrane. Kidney Int 13:61A, 1978
27. Evans DJ: Pathogenesis of membranous nephropathy. Lancet 1:1143–1144, 1974
28. Brenner BM, Bohrer MP, Baylis L, Deen WM: Determinants of glomerular permselectivity: Insights derived from observations in vivo. Kidney Int 12:229–237, 1978
29. Glassock RJ, Edgington TS, Watson JI, Dixon FE: Autologous immune complex nephritis induced with renal tubular antigen. II. The pathogenic mechanism. J Exp Med 127:573–587, 1968
30. Barabas AZ, Nagi AH, Lannigan R: Induction of autologous immune complex nephritis in rats by heterologous antikidney mitichondrial serum. Int Urol Nephrol 2:303–308, 1970
31. Feenstra K, Van Der Lee R, Greben HA, Arenos A, Hoedemaeker PJ: Experimental glomerulonephritis in the rat induced by antibodies directed against tubular antigens. I. The natural history of a histologic and immunohistologic study of light microscopic and ultrastructural level. Lab Invest 32:235–242, 1975
32. Van Es CA, Blok APR, Schoenfeld L, Glassock RJ: Chronic nephritis induced by antibodies reacting with glomerular bound immune complexes. Kidney Int 11:106–115, 1977
33. Fleuren GJ, Lee RVD, Greben HA, Van Damme BJC, Hoedemaeker PHJ: Experimental glomerulonephritis in the rat induced by antibodies directed against tubular antigens. IV. Investigations into the pathogenesis of the model. Lab Invest 38:496–501, 1978
34. Van Damme BJC, Fleuren GJ, Bakker WW, Vernier RL, Hoedemaeker PHJ: Experimental glomerulonephritis in the rat induced by antibodies directed against tubular antigens. Lab Invest 38:502–509, 1978
35. Steinmuller DR, Belok S, Salant DJ, Stilmant MM, Lowenstein LM, Couser WG: Subepithelial (SE) immune complex (IC) deposits in experimental membranous nephropathy (MN) are formed in situ. Abstr Int Congr Nephrol, Montreal, 1978, p. G10
36. Cameron JS, Turner DR: Recurrent glomerulonephritis in allografted kidneys. Clin Nephrol 7:47–54, 1977

37. Izui S, Lambert P-H, Miescher PA: In vitro demonstration of a particular affinity of glomerular basement membrane and collagen for DNA. A possible basis for local formation of DNA-anti-DNA complexes in systemic lupus erythematosus. J Exp Med 144:428–443, 1976
38. Izui S, Lambert P-H, Miescher PA: Failure to detect circulating DNA-anti-DNA complexes by four radioimmunological methods in patients with systemic lupus erythematosus. Clin Exp Immunol 30:384–392, 1978
39. Davis JS, Godfrey SM, Winfield JB: Direct evidence for circulating DNA/anti-DNA complexes in systemic lupus erythematosus. Arthr Rheum 21:17–22, 1978
40. Naruse T, Kitamura K, Miyakawa Y, Shibata S: Deposition of renal tubular epithelial antigen along the glomerular capillary walls of patients with membranous glomerulonephritis. J Immunol 110:1163–1166, 1973
41. Naruse T, Miyakawa Y, Kitamura K: Membranous glomerulonephritis mediated by renal tubular epithelial antigen-antibody complex. J Allerg Clin Immunol 54:313–318, 1974
42. Whitworth JA, Leibowitz S, Kennedy MC, Cameron JS, Evans DJ, Glassock RJ, Schoenfeld LS: Absence of glomerular renal tubular epithelial antigen in membranous glomerulonephritis. Clin Nephrol 5:159–162, 1976
43. Ozawa T, Boedecker EA, Schorr W, Guggenheim S, McIntosh RM: Immune-complex disease with unilateral renal vein thrombosis. Arch Pathol Lab Med 100:279–282, 1976
44. Costanza ME, Pinn V, Schwartz RS, Nathanson L: Carcinoembryonic antigen-antibody complexes in a patient with colonic carcinoma and nephrotic syndrome. N Engl J Med 289:520–522, 1973
45. Whitworth JA, Unger A, Cameron JS: Carcinoembryonic antigen in tumour-associated membranous nephropathy. Lancet 2:611, 1975
46. Bariéty J, Druet PH, LaGrue G, Samarq P: Milliez P: Les glomerulopathies "extramembraneuses" (GEM). Etude morphologique en microscopie optique electronique et en immunofluorescence. Path Biol (Paris) 18:5–32, 1970
47. Gärtner HV, Watanabe T, Ott V, Adam A, Bohle A, Edel HH, Kluthe R, Renner E, Scheler F, Schmulling RM, Sieberth HG: Correlations between morphologic and clinical features in idiopathic perimembranous glomerulonephritis. A study on 403 renal biopsies of 367 patients. Curr T Pathol 65:1–29, 1977
48. Row PG, Cameron JS, Turner DR, Evans DJ, White RHR, Ogg CS, Chantler C, Brown CB: Membranous nephropathy. Long-term follow-up and association with neoplasia. Q J Med 44:207–239, 1975
49. Hopper J, Trew PA, Biava CG: Membranous nephropathy (MN) relative benignity in woman. Abst Int Congr Nephrol, Montreal, 1978, p. D2
50. Ehrenreich T, Porush JG, Churg J, Garfinkel L, Glabman S, Goldstein MH, Grishman E, Yunis SL: Treatment of idiopathic membranous nephropathy. N Engl J Med 295:741–746, 1976
51. Kleinknecht C, Broyer M, Habib R: Steroids for idiopathic membranous nephritis. N Engl J Med 296:49, 1977
52. Pierides AM, Malasit P, Morley AR, Wilkinson R, Uldall PR, Seere DNS: Idiopathic membranous nephropathy. Q J Med 46:163–177, 1977
53. Cameron JS: The treatment of immunological renal disease. In Zabriskie J, Villareal H, Becker EL (eds.): Immunological Renal Disease.

54. Toulmin S: Human Understanding. Oxford, Clarendon Press, 1972, p. vi
55. Idelson BA, Smithline N, Smith GW, Harrington JT: Prognosis in steroid-treated idiopathic nephrotic syndrome in adults. Arch Intern Med 137:891–896, 1977
56. Pollak VE, Pirani CL, Muehrcke RC, Kark RM: Asymptomatic persistent proteinuria: Studies by renal biopsies. Guy's Hosp Rep 107:353, 1958
57. Franklin WA, Jennings RB, Earle DP: Membranous glomerulonephritis: Long-term serial observations on clinical course and morphology. Kidney Int 4:36–56, 1973
58. Couser WG, Jermanovich NB, Belok S, Stilmant MM, Hoyer JR: Effect of aminonucleoside nephrosis on immune complex localization in autologous immune complex nephropathy in rats. J Clin Invest 61:561–572, 1978
59. Olsen S, Bohman SO, Petersen VP: Ultrastructure of the glomerular basement membrane in long-term renal allografts with transplant glomerular disease. Lab Invest 30:176–189, 1977
60. Steinmuller DR, Stilmant MM, Idelson BA, Monaco AP, Sahyoun AI, Lewis EJ, Davis RC, Couser WG: De novo development of membranous nephropathy in cadaver renal allografts. Clin Nephrol 9:210–218, 1978
61. Crosson JT, Wathen L, Raij L, Andersen C, Anderson R: Recurrence of idiopathic membranous nephropathy in a renal allograft. Arch Intern Med 135:1101–1106, 1978
62. Rubin RJ, Pinn VW, Barnes BA, Harrington JT: Recurrent idiopathic membranous glomerulonephritis. Transplantation 24:4–9, 1977
63. Bacon PA, Tribe CR, Mackenzie JC, Verrier Jones J, Cumming RH, Amer B: Penicillamine nephropathy in rheumatoid arthritis. A clinical, pathological and immunological study. Q J Med 45:661–684, 1976
64. Gärtner HV, Neild GH, Bohle A, Hallauer W, Hoppe-Seyler G, Lüttgen FM, Schollmeyer P: Peripmembranöse glomerulonephritis nach penicillamin-therapie. Bericht uber 31 fälle. Klin Wochenschr 53:835–837, 1975
65. Collaborative Study of the Adult Idiopathic Nephrotic Syndrome: A controlled study of short-term prednisone treatment in adults with membranous nephropathy. N Engl J Med 301:1306, 1979

Chronic Glomerulonephritis

Nonimmunologic Mechanisms of Progressive Glomerular Damage

Principal Discussant
David S. Baldwin

Case Presentations

Patient 1. A 66-year-old man was first evaluated in the Renal Clinic of the New England Medical Center (NEMC) at age 53. At age 9, he developed periorbital and peripheral edema, gross hematuria, cylindruria, and proteinuria. He was told he had acute glomerulonephritis and was confined to bed for 1 month; the edema and hematuria resolved. He remained asymptomatic for the next 4 decades although urinalyses performed during Army and insurance examinations consistently revealed trace to 1+ protein.

At the age of 53, he noted intermittent pedal edema over a 3-month period. Physical examination revealed a blood pressure of 130/90 mmHg. The ocular fundi were normal. Cardiovascular examination was unremarkable. No abdominal organomegaly was present. There was 1+ pitting edema of the feet. Urinalysis revealed a specific gravity of 1.012, a pH of 5, no sugar, 1+ protein, 3 to 5 red blood cells per high-power field, no white blood cells, and rare granular casts. Twenty-four-hour urine protein excretion measured on three occasions ranged between 400 and 900 mg; no significant postural component to the protein excretion was evident. Urine culture was sterile. The serum albumin was 4.5 mg/dl. The serum creatinine was 1.1 mg/dl and the BUN was 17 mg/dl. The patient was believed to have "latent glomerulonephritis" for which no specific therapy was recommended. His edema resolved spontaneously during the next several weeks.

During the ensuing 13 years, serial measurements of serum creatinine revealed a slowly progressive decline in renal function (Table 1). During this period, urinalyses continued to reveal 1+ to 3+ protein and occasional red blood cells. The patient developed mild hypertension, treated initially with alpha-methyldopa, and later with propranolol. The latter drug was discontinued 2 years ago because of mild hyperkalemia (serum potassium, 5.8 mEq/liter); however, the serum potassium concentration

Table 1. Clinical course of patient 1.

Age	Blood Pressure (mmHg)	Serum Creatinine (mg/dl)	24-h Urine Protein (g)
53	120/85	1.4	3.0
54	140/90	1.5	
55	115/80	1.5	1.4
56	138/90	1.7	0.75
57	130/95	1.9	
59	172/92	2.0	6.1
60	150/96	2.3	0.4
61	160/102	2.4	1.77
62	140/85	2.7	2.29
63	160/90	3.4	
64	170/100	3.8	
64.5	150/90	4.3	0.44
65	160/100	6.0	
66	160/100	7.2	0.49

remained in the range of 5.0 to 5.4 mEq/liter subsequently. Because of recent increasing fatigue, intermittent nausea, and pruritus, plans are being made to initiate chronic hemodialysis.

Patient 2. A 44-year-old woman was first admitted to NEMC 12 years ago because of acute renal failure. Three weeks earlier she had complained of a mild sore throat lasting only a few days. One week before admission she noted fever, palpitation, and painful erythematous lesions and swelling over the anterior lower legs. Physical examination at another hospital disclosed mild pharyngitis, erythema nodosum, and tachycardia. Blood pressure was 134/82 mmHg. Neither a heart murmur nor edema was noted. An electrocardiogram revealed nonspecific T-wave abnormalities, and β-hemolytic streptococcus was recovered from a throat culture. The BUN was 12 mg/dl, and a urinalysis revealed no protein and 2 to 3 red blood cells per high-power field. Acute rheumatic fever was diagnosed, and treatment with erythromycin and aspirin was begun. Fever, tachycardia, and cardiac abnormalities improved, but edema developed. After 5 days, the urine output suddenly ceased. The BUN rose swiftly to 117 mg/dl and the serum creatinine increased to 4.7 mg/dl. The patient was transferred to NEMC for further evaluation and treatment.

Her first pregnancy had been complicated by hypertension and postpartum hemorrhage 10 years earlier. She denied a history of renal disease, hypertension, diabetes, urinary tract infection, renal calculi, or hematuria. She was allergic to penicillin.

Physical examination revealed a blood pressure of 120/70 mmHg; mild periorbital, sacral, and ankle edema; and erythema nodosum. Urinalysis demonstrated 3+ protein, many red blood cells, and 3 to 4 red blood cell casts. Serum complement (C3) was subnormal; ANA and LE preps were negative. Nephrotomography demonstrated 15.5-cm kidneys. She was treated with peritoneal dialysis, oral Kayexalate, and a Giovanetti diet. An open renal biopsy 2 days later revealed diffuse, exudative, and proliferative glomerulonephritis typical of acute poststreptococcal glomerulonephritis. During the next 3 weeks, the patient remained anuric and required 2 peritoneal dialyses. Despite normal blood pressure (110–140/70–90 mmHg), papilledema occurred. The neurologic examination was otherwise normal.

One month after her illness began, urinary volume progressively increased and she noted less fatigue. Renal function improved and peritoneal dialysis was discontinued. Blood pressure rose to 150/115 mmHg and therapy with alpha-methyldopa was begun. After another month, the BUN had fallen to 11 mg/dl and the serum creatinine to 1.1 mg/dl. During the next 2 months she continued to feel well, and her renal function remained normal. Hypertension persisted; the urinary sediment contained 50 to 75 red blood cells per high-power field and occasional red blood cell and granular casts. Urinary protein excretion declined from 4.7 to 2.3 g daily. A second renal biopsy revealed one-third of the glomeruli to be hyalinized, with more than one-half normal or only slightly sclerotic. No cellular proliferation or exudation remained. Hyaline droplet degeneration of proximal tubular cells and protein casts within tubules were evident. The biopsy was interpreted as revealing chronic, inactive proliferative glomerulonephritis.

During the next 6 months, the serum creatinine remained unchanged and hematuria disappeared. Retinopathy and hypertension resolved, and antihypertensive therapy was withdrawn. Urinary protein excretion fell to 1 g daily.

Nine years ago, hypertension reappeared (the blood pressure was 150/115 mmHg), and treatment with alpha-methyldopa was reinstituted. A symptomatic proteus urinary tract infection 7 years ago was treated with sulfonamides. An intravenous pyelogram was normal (kidneys were 14.2 cm), the serum creatinine was 0.8 mg/dl, and proteinuria was unchanged. Since then, urinary protein excretion has gradually declined to 200 mg daily. Alpha-methyldopa was discontinued because of fatigue. She takes 50 mg of hydrochlorothiazide daily and 40 mg of propranolol 4 times daily, and her blood pressure remains relatively well controlled. Six months ago, physical examination was normal. The BUN was 12 mg/dl and the serum creatinine was 0.9 mg/dl. Urinalysis revealed 1+ proteinuria; no cells or casts were found in the urinary sediment.

Discussion

Dr. David S. Baldwin *(Professor of Medicine, New York University School of Medicine, New York, New York)*: The first patient's story began when, at 9 years of age, he had an illness labeled "acute glomerulonephritis." The early features of the disease resolved in 1 month, but proteinuria persisted. He developed hypertension 44 years later at age 53, and by the time he was 66 years old—57 years after the apparent onset of his renal disease—advanced renal failure necessitated the use of hemodialysis. Is this clinical progression consistent with the long-term course of acute glomerulonephritis, or should we scrutinize the clinical features of this patient's disease to determine whether another diagnosis would fit better?

The term acute glomerulonephritis implies the presence of a disease characterized morphologically by diffuse endocapillary proliferation in glomeruli, often with exudative features, and occasionally with extracapillary proliferation as well. These are the histologic features of immune complex-mediated, postinfectious glomerulonephritis, of which poststreptococcal glomerulonephritis (PSGN) is the prototype. Let us examine the course of this patient's disease as compared with 185 patients with sporadic (i.e., nonepidemic) PSGN observed at Bellevue Hospital, in whom a poststreptococcal cause was established in all, and in whom the diagnosis was confirmed by renal biopsy in two-thirds [1]. Most of the patients in this series were adults; all were hospitalized at onset.

We are given no information relative to the possible cause of this patient's disease, so one cannot use failure to document an antecedent group-A, β-hemolytic streptococcus infection to dismiss the diagnosis of PSGN. The early features that were used to establish the clinical diagnosis of "acute nephritis" included edema, gross hematuria, and proteinuria. Having no further details, I will not dispute the likelihood that the clinical features at least were compatible with acute glomerulonephritis. What about the patient's subsequent clinical course? Persistent proteinuria was observed in about one-half of our patients with PSGN, but it has been described less often by other observers, especially in series of children, and only rarely in reports of epidemic PSGN. The recurrence of hypertension many years after the onset of PSGN also is compatible with our experience. The development of uremia was quite unusual in our patients, although it did occur in a few. Persistent proteinuria, moderate hypertension, and minimal impairment of renal function were common. In our study, which began in 1960 and includes new patients added throughout the subsequent 20 years, ten of 185 patients now have advanced renal failure [2].

The only feature of this patient's clinical course that does not appear compatible with postinfectious diffuse proliferative glomerulonephritis is the recurrence of edema many years after the onset of the disease. In PSGN, edema typically occurs at onset, may at times be associated with the nephrotic syndrome, and subsides within days to weeks in association with remission of the other initial manifestations in well over 90% of patients studied. Edema may persist in the unusual patient in whom severe, active renal disease continues and in whom progression to irreversible renal failure occurs shortly after the onset of PSGN or within 1 year or so. However, when the initial features remit, as they typically do, neither edema nor the nephrotic syndrome recurs except in those rare instances in which the patient experiences a second episode of acute nephritis. Of course, edema also can reappear in the terminal stage of renal failure as a manifestation of the patient's marked functional impairment and limited ability to handle salt and water.

What other possibilities should we consider in the patient whose early clinical features were compatible with acute nephritis? Do any other glomerular diseases better explain this patient's subsequent course than does postinfectious, diffuse, proliferative glomerulonephritis? When this patient first became ill, Berger's IgA nephropathy had not yet been described. Yet one can easily understand how patients with gross hematuria, whom we now know might possibly have IgA nephropathy or non-IgA focal glomerulonephritis, might have been thought to have "acute glomerulonephritis." The occurrence of edema at onset, however, is rare (although not unheard of) in IgA nephropathy. As our increasing experience with Berger's nephropathy has taught us, the patient's slowly progressive clinical course would be compatible with this diagnosis, but the fact that the later development of edema and heavy proteinuria was not associated with progression of renal failure over a relatively short period of time virtually eliminates Berger's nephropathy from the differential diagnosis. Another morphologic entity that is occasionally marked by symptoms of "acute nephritis" at onset is mesangiocapillary glomerulonephritis (MCGN). We do not know the serum complement level, which might be helpful in this differential diagnosis if persistent or intermittent depression of C3 beyond the acute stage had occurred. In the course of MCGN, however, the nephrotic syndrome is common, especially when the patient is becoming uremic. I believe this patient's protracted clinical course and particularly the absence of the nephrotic syndrome definitely rule out the diagnosis of MCGN. Finally, extracapillary proliferative (or crescentic) glomerulonephritis can have an "acute nephritic" onset, but the diagnosis is highly unlikely in this patient; he was much too young, and his disease was too indolent. Actually, the spectrum of crescentic glomerulonephritis does include patients whose course is "not so rapidly progressive," but a mild and brief acute episode followed by slow progression over decades is not compatible with this diagnosis.

Diffuse endocapillary proliferative glomerulonephritis, therefore, is probably the correct morphologic diagnosis. Slow progression to glomerular sclerosis and end-stage renal failure occurred even though the initial episode was mild, and minimal proteinuria was the only manifestation for more than 40 years. We know from similar observations in patients with documented PSGN that, during the years following the acute stage, proliferation is no longer present in glomeruli, and immunopathologic evidence of immune-complex disease is no longer demonstrable. Yet the disease progresses. In a moment we will consider possible nonimmunologic mechanisms by which glomerulonephritis might progress in such patients.

The second patient described today provides a fascinating contrast with the first. In this woman, PSGN was documented by bacteriologic, clinical, and morphologic criteria at age 44 years. Although her disease was severe enough to necessitate dialysis during the initial 3 weeks, her course has been relatively benign over the subsequent 12 years of follow-up. On the other hand, our first patient, who seemed to have mild acute nephritis, ultimately developed uremia. For more than 4 decades, however, he showed only minimal evidence of glomerular disease, and his clinical course was very similar to the experience of our second patient during the 12 years since her initial episode. In relating the severity of disease at onset in PSGN to the eventual outcome, we have observed a correlation between the severity of initial clinical and morphologic manifestations and the presence of hypertension, proteinuria, renal functional impairment, and glomerular sclerosis 2 or more years from onset [1]. Patients who had mild disease initially were not protected from developing chronic disease, however. It is even more interesting that most of the patients who eventually became uremic experienced periods of several years with only minor manifestations of disease: little or no proteinuria, normal blood pressure or mild hypertension, and creatinine clearance in the normal range [2].

The classic episode of acute PSGN in the second patient occurred in concert with acute rheumatic fever and erythema nodosum following a documented group-A, β-hemolytic streptococcus pharyngitis. Not only was the infectious cause established, but in addition a renal biopsy showed the typical findings of diffuse endocapillary proliferative glomerulonephritis, and serum complement was decreased. The patient, who became anuric at the onset and remained so for 3 weeks, required peritoneal dialysis. With PSGN of this severity, one would expect the presence of extracapillary as well as endocapillary proliferation, but this finding was not described.

Although most patients with acute PSGN who have oliguria or anuria for more than a few days usually have extensive extracapillary proliferation and often do not regain renal function, a diuresis occurred after 3 weeks and renal function returned to normal during the next month. Because hypertension and heavy proteinuria persisted, another renal biopsy was performed 4 months from onset; this time the biopsy revealed remitted acute PSGN, now with sclerosis of one-third of glomeruli but without proliferation. During the next 6 months, hypertension and retinopathy subsided and the urinary protein excretion diminished; renal function remained normal. Hypertension reappeared 3 years after onset, and for the subsequent 9 years of follow-up the patient's hypertension has been controlled with medication, she has had minimal but persistent proteinuria, and she has maintained normal renal function.

Despite the severity of the disease at onset, this patient's course has been relatively benign thus far. The development of glomerular sclerosis and the reappearance and persistence of hypertension and proteinuria indicate, however, that irreversible damage accompanied the acute episode. The features of the long-term course in this patient are typical of those we have observed in the majority of our adult patients who have been followed for 10 years or more [3]. In many, the evidence of progressive disease is lacking, but hypertension and proteinuria, both sequelae of the acute attack, persist. In others, manifestations that remitted early have reappeared, and slow progression has occurred. A few have advanced to end-stage renal failure. In today's first patient, 44 years elapsed between the onset of the disease and terminal uremia. The second patient, whose disease began when she was in her 40s and who has evidence of chronic disease 12 years later, can be expected to have a slowly progressive course, but she probably never will have clinically significant renal insufficiency.

The importance of these two case histories is not that they merely teach us that PSGN can insidiously lead to uremia over many years after the early features of the disease subside. After all, PSGN is now an uncommon disease, as is acute rheumatic fever, the other sequel of β-hemolytic streptococcal infection. But these observations on the continued progression of PSGN after the initial immune process has subsided have provided the stimulus for us to speculate on what factors, other than immune mechanisms, might be capable of producing glomerular damage. It seems highly likely to me that if nonimmunologic mechanisms of glomerular injury are responsible for progression in PSGN, these mechanisms probably play a role in other glomerular diseases as well. I'd now like to turn to a discussion of these mechanism's.

An immunopathogenetic mechanism—immune complex or anti-glomerular basement membrane antibody—is held responsible for most forms of primary glomerular disease in humans. Although immunologic mechanisms and the mediators of glomerular damage that they induce might form the basis for initiating most glomerular diseases, certain clinical observations and experimental data suggest that the progression of these diseases is influenced by several nomimmunologic factors.

Intrarenal Vascular Disease

Sclerosis of arterioles and prearterioles, a common finding in advanced glomerular disease, has long been recognized at postmortem examination and conventionally has been interpreted as an effect of hypertension. Researchers thus have assumed that ischemic glomerular sclerosis resulting from intrarenal vascular disease contributes to the progression of renal failure during the hypertensive stage of glomerular disease and, consequently, the importance of control of blood pressure has been stressed [4–8].

Malignant hypertension can occur with glomerulonephritis, and the associated necrotizing arteriolitis of the renal vessels might justifiably be attributed to the marked elevation of diastolic blood pressure. The frequent occurrence of intrarenal vascular sclerosis early in the course of glomerulonephritis prior to the advent of hypertension, or with only mild elevation of blood pressure, however, suggests a particular susceptibility of the renal arterioles to the effects of hypertension in glomerulonephritis, or perhaps indicates that vascular disease even might be a primary feature of the disease rather than a secondary manifestation of hypertension.

We have studied biopsies in patients in intermediate stages of poststreptococcal glomerulonephritis [9] and in Berger's IgA nephropathy [10], when renal function is normal or minimally impaired and hypertension is mild or absent. The results demonstrate a high incidence of arteriolar and prearteriolar sclerosis. Similar observations have been made in a variety of other glomerular diseases in which vascular sclerosis exceeded the damage that one would anticipate for the age of the patient and the duration and severity of hypertension. Kincaid-Smith reported that the incidence of renal arterial and arteriolar lesions ranged from 54 to 82% in normotensive patients under age 40 years who had various forms of glomerulonephritis [11] (Table 2).

In our studies, vascular changes closely correlated with glomerular sclerosis and suggested to us a cause-and-effect relationship in which ischemia was responsible for glomerular damage. As shown in Figure 1, 21 renal biopsy specimens from patients with poststreptococcal glo-

Table 2. Arterial and arteriolar lesions in normotensive patients with glomerulonephritis (age under 40 years).

Glomerular Histology	Vascular Lesions	
Minor glomerular lesions	44/68	64.7%
Membranous nephropathy	20/37	54.1%
Diffuse proliferative glomerulonephritis	91/123	74.0%
Focal and segmental glomerulonephritis	96/116	82.6%

Source: data from Ref. 11.

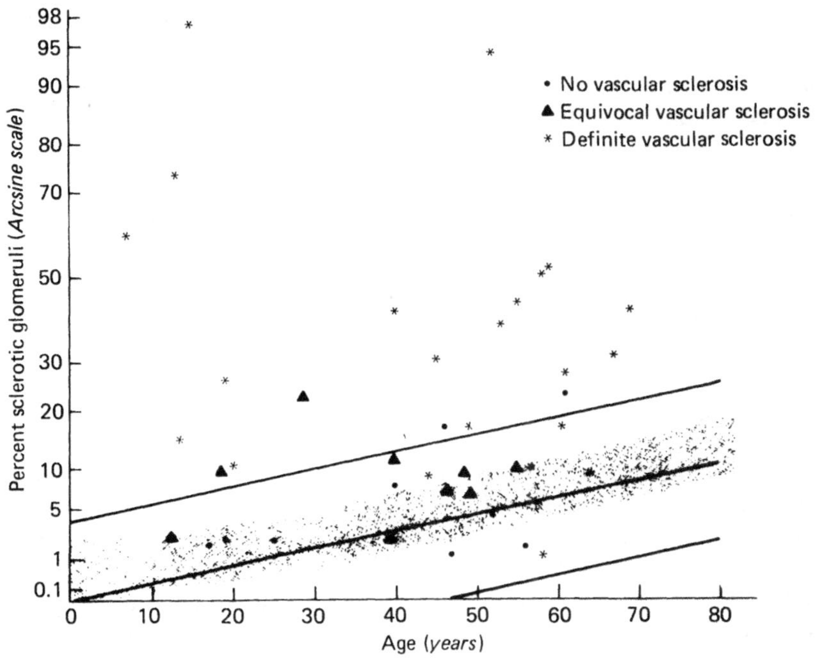

Fig. 1. Correlation between glomerular sclerosis and vascular sclerosis in poststreptococcal glomerulonephritis. Percentage of sclerotic glomeruli on renal biopsy is plotted against age of the patient. The mean *(shaded band)* and the 95% population confidence limits are shown for the regression of glomerular sclerosis against age in normals [61]. Appropriate symbols indicate for each datum whether vascular sclerosis was absent, equivocal, or definitely present. The correlation between glomerular sclerosis and vascular sclerosis is highly significant ($P < 0.002$). Data from Ref. 9.

merulonephritis were judged to have a significantly greater frequency of glomerular sclerosis than did specimens from age-matched controls; 17 of the 21 also showed arteriolar sclerosis. In 19 specimens unaffected by glomerular sclerosis, only five showed arteriolar sclerosis. A similar correlation was demonstrated for Berger's IgA nephropathy. Sixteen of 20 specimens with significantly more glomerular sclerosis than expected showed arteriolar sclerosis as well; of 26 specimens without glomerular sclerosis, only four had arteriolar sclerosis.

The frequent presence of ischemic or "collapse-type" sclerosis of the glomeruli rather than disorganization of glomerular structure seemed to lend further support to a causative role for vascular sclerosis in the progression of these glomerular diseases [9,10]. Such an hypothesis is especially attractive for our understanding of PSGN in which immune damage almost certainly abates within 1 year or so from onset, as evidenced by the usual absence of immunoglobulins in glomeruli beyond this time [12]. Under these circumstances, progressive glomerular sclerosis requires the operation of nonimmunologic mechanisms, and the clinical and pathologic evidence just cited supports the theory that vascular disease and resultant ischemia cause progressive renal damage. Recent hemodynamic and morphologic observations in the remnant kidney and in experimental nephritis suggest, however, that adaptive increases in perfusion following nephron loss or injury can be responsible for further glomerular damage. The emphasis thus has shifted away from ischemic glomerular sclerosis to hyperperfusion as a possible mechanism for both vascular and glomerular injury in chronic glomerulonephritis.

Adaptive Changes in Glomerular Hemodynamics

Studies in experimental animals show that removal of about five-sixths of renal mass results in proteinuria, hypertension, progressive renal failure, and advanced glomerular sclerosis [13–15]. This finding suggests that adaptive alterations in renal hemodynamics, or other factors related to reduced renal mass and its biochemical consequences, can cause further renal damage. Such mechanisms could contribute to ongoing parenchymal destruction in patients with renal disease regardless of the initial cause of reduced renal parenchymal mass.

Brenner and co-workers, in studies of glomerular hemodynamics in the remnant kidney, have demonstrated adaptive increments in glomerular blood flow and single-nephron GFR [16–18] (Table 3). Despite only a minimal increase in systemic arterial pressure, transcapillary hydraulic pressure significantly increased as a result of elevated glomerular capillary hydraulic pressure. Adaptive reductions in afferent arteriolar resistance must account for the increased transmission of systemic pressure to the glomerular capillaries and for the increments in glomerular perfusion. The authors suggest that these adaptive changes might have an adverse effect on renal function by accelerating glomerular sclerosis in the remaining glomeruli. The alterations in glomerular

Table 3. Increased glomerular pressure and flow in remnant kidneys.

	$\overline{AP}^a$ (mmHg)	BUN (mg/dl)	GFR (ml/min)	SNGFR[b] (nl/min)	Q_A^c (nl/min)	$\overline{\Delta P}^d$ (mmHg)
Remnant kidney	128 ± 4	94 ± 9	0.21 ± .03	62 ± 6	187 ± 20	44.2 ± 2.2
Control kidney	111 ± 3	20 ± 3	0.70 ± .07	27 ± 4	75 ± 12	36.6 ± 1.7

[a] $\overline{AP}$ refers to systemic pressure.
[b] SNGFR refers to single nephron GFR.
[c] Q_A refers to glomerular plasma flow.
[d] $\overline{\Delta P}$ refers to transcapillary hydraulic pressure.
Source: data from Ref. 18.

hemodynamics that occur in the remnant kidney resemble those that Azar et al. have described in one-kidney, "post-salt" hypertension, in which glomerular sclerosis was associated with reduced arteriolar resistance and increases in transcapillary pressure, glomerular blood flow, and single-nephron GFR [19].

Maddox et al. have shown that Munich-Wistar rats with recently induced, mild to moderate nephrotoxic serum nephritis (NSN) maintain normal glomerular plasma flow rates and single-nephron GFR despite morphologic evidence of widespread glomerular injury [20]. Transcapillary hydraulic pressure was considerably elevated due to increased glomerular capillary pressure, and single-nephron GFR failed to increase only because of a reduction in the ultrafiltration coefficient; the authors attribute these results to the loss of patent capillaries in NSN. Allison et al. found that these same pressures remain elevated in rats with chronic glomerulonephritis [21]. Thus, adaptive decreases in afferent arteriolar resistance must occur in the course of glomerulonephritis as they do in reduced renal mass, thereby exposing the glomeruli to increased intracapillary pressures.

Further evidence of secondary glomerular damage in the remnant kidney has been provided by Olson et al., who found that endothelial and epithelial cell abnormalities occur along with altered charge and size-selective properties of the glomerular wall [22]. These authors showed a reduction in the charge-selective barrier to filtration in the remnant kidney by demonstrating that the fractional clearance of anionic horseradish peroxidase was increased, whereas that of the cationic form was decreased. Fractional clearance of low-molecular-weight neutral dextrans was not affected, but the clearance of higher-molecular-weight neutral dextrans was practically doubled; these changes suggested impairment of glomerular size selectivity as well.

Utilizing cationic probe molecules, Shea et al. showed that proteinuria in the subtotally nephrectomized rat was not accompanied by changes in the ultrastructural distribution of anionic sites in the glomerular basement membrane [23]. These investigators have suggested, rather, that proteinuria in the remnant kidney results from sustained rises in glomerular capillary pressure that, in turn, cause an increase in pore size.

Direct Effect of Hypertension on Glomerular Structure and Function

The occlusive effect of hypertension on the renal arterioles and prearterioles is generally accepted as the mechanism by which hypertension aggravates the course of glomerulonephritis. Vascular narrowing is thought to accelerate glomerular sclerosis through ischemia. The "vicious cycle in Bright's disease" as proposed by Wilson and Byrom alludes to this mechanism [24]. However, a number of recent studies in experimental hypertension and in hypertension superimposed on a variety of glomerular diseases provide evidence that glomerular damage might be produced directly by hypertension rather than secondarily through ischemia resulting from occlusive small vessel alterations.

Knowlton et al., in 1946, administered DOCA to rats with nephrotoxic serum nephritis and produced severe hypertension and a worsening of the glomerular disease; the authors reported no change in proteinuria [25]. In a series of studies in which NSN was induced in animals with preexisting hypertension, Masuyama and associates observed increased severity of hypertension and more persistent proliferative and sclerotic changes in glomeruli; vascular alterations were not described [26–28]. Motoki et al. produced hypertension with DOCA and salt-loading in the unilaterally nephrectomized rat with NSN and noted increased glomerular proliferation and sclerosis [29]. Teodoru, et al. showed that more rabbits with NSN develop severe glomerulonephritis and die of uremia if they have been unilaterally nephrectomized or salt loaded beforehand [30]. Blood pressure measurements were not performed in this study, but one can presume that the salt-loaded rabbits were hypertensive. Increased proteinuria and proliferative-sclerotic glomerular changes were reported by Tikkanen and associates, who superimposed DOCA-salt hypertension on autologous immune glomerulonephritis (Heymann nephritis) in the rat; vascular sclerosis and necrosis occurred infrequently in this model [31]. Using DOCA-salt hypertension in heterologous immune glomerulonephritis (passive Heymann nephritis), Iversen and Ofstad noted more marked glomerular basement membrane thickening, greater proteinuria, and a shortened life span of the experimental animals [32].

In a study of steroid-induced hypertension in the uninephrectomized rat, Hill and Heptinstall first suggested in 1968 that failure of adequate arteriolar constriction rather than excessive narrowing was responsible for the hypertensive lesions that developed in insufficiently hypertrophied vessels and their "unprotected" glomeruli [33]. The following year, Still and Dennison demonstrated, in a study of DOCA-salt hypertension in the uninephrectomized rat, that glomeruli could undergo cell swelling and sclerosis that resembled changes in arterioles; they suggested that hypertension might directly damage the glomerular capillary [34]. The vascular and glomerular damage described by these authors probably was attributable to malignant hypertension, but they introduced a new and important concept—that glomerular vessels are affected directly by hypertension and do not suffer merely as a secondary result of arteriolar narrowing and ischemia.

Azar et al., in studies of one-kidney, "post-salt" hypertension in the rat, recently showed proliferation and sclerosis of glomeruli in association with reduced arteriolar resistance and increases in transcapillary pressure, glomerular blood flow, and single-nephron GFR [19]. These investigators suggested that adaptive decreases in afferent resistance following uninephrectomy overrode the ability of arterioles to increase their resistance in the presence of superimposed hypertension, thus exposing the glomerular capillaries to damaging increases in hydraulic pressure. In a subsequent study, these authors demonstrated that salt-sensitive rats who develop hypertension with both kidneys intact show similar increases in single-nephron GFR that result from elevated glomerular blood flow and glomerular transcapillary hydraulic pressure [35]. The authors propose that the glomerular lesions in these rats are attributable to high glomerular capillary pressures that occur when hypertension and nephrosclerosis are superimposed on the genetically reduced number of adapted nephrons known to exist in this strain.

In related studies, Mauer and associates examined the effect of hypertension produced by renal artery clipping on streptozotocin-induced diabetes mellitus in the rat. They observed increased mesangial matrix material and heavier deposits of IgG, IgM, and C3 in the unclipped "diabetic" kidney [36]. Additional evidence for the possible role of glomerular hemodynamic factors in diabetic glomerulosclerosis was adduced by Azar, who demonstrated that glomerular capillary pressure is increased prior to any morphologic changes in rats with short-term diabetes induced by pancreatectomy [37]. Finally, Hosteter et al. recently reported glomerular hyperfiltration in moderately hyperglycemic Munich-Wistar rats made diabetic with streptozotocin [38]. This hyperfiltration resulted from elevations in glomerular plasma flow and increases in transcapillary hydraulic pressure difference.

We have examined the effect of superimposed renal artery clip hypertension (CH) on the clinical and morphologic features of NSN in the Sprague-Dawley rat [39]. Our objective was to determine (1) whether the effects on the renal arterioles of a given elevation in blood pressure were increased in the nephritic animal; and (2) whether the glomerular abnormalities of NSN would be aggravated by concomitant hypertension. To avoid the catastrophic effects of necrotizing vasculitis that would be anticipated with marked elevations in blood pressure and which could obscure differences between hypertension alone and hypertension superimposed on NSN, we selected animals for comparison that had mean systolic blood pressures ranging between 120 and 160 mmHg. Further, we attempted to induce a mild form of NSN to facilitate the recognition of any magnified effects of superimposed hypertension on the severity of glomerular lesions.

Table 4 includes data for all animals sacrificed at 3, 4, and 5 months after application of the renal artery clip, which followed injections of nephrotoxic serum by 1 month. Data for control animals and those with NSN alone and CH alone are given for comparison. The mean systolic blood pressures in the two hypertensive groups were almost identical;

Table 4. Effect of clip hypertension on nephrotoxic serum nephritis.

	No.	Blood Pressure (mmHg)	Cardiac Index[a] (%)	Proteinuria (mg/24 h)
Control	17	102 ± 2	0.27 ± .01	2 ± 2
NSN	12	105 ± 2	0.25 ± .01	24 ± 12
CH	16	145 ± 3	0.36 ± .01	27 ± 11
NSN + CH	15	142 ± 6	0.36 ± .03	144 ± 28

[a]Cardiac index refers to the heart weight to body weight ratio (%).
Note: NSN, nephrotoxic serum nephritis; CH, clip hypertension.

the similarity in heart weight to body weight ratios lends support to the close correspondence in measured blood pressures in the CH and NSN + CH groups. As Table 4 shows, the superimposition of hypertension on NSN markedly increased the level of protein excretion at the time of each monthly sacrifice. The incidence and severity of glomerular and vascular lesions similarly were aggravated by the superimposition of hypertension on NSN (Figs. 2–5). Whereas the occurrence of glomerular proliferation and tuft necrosis never exceeded approximately 20% in rats with CH or NSN alone, when CH was combined with NSN, the incidence of these glomerular abnormalities exceeded 80% in the latter stages of the experiment. The incidence and severity of glomerular sclerosis similarly increased in rats with CH superimposed on NSN. Arteriolar medial hypertrophy was not noted in rats with NSN and occurred mildly and only occasionally in rats with CH; the incidence of severe arteriolar sclerosis reached almost 100% when hypertension was combined with NSN.

Our studies demonstrate that the superimposition of hypertension in the rat with NSN markedly aggravates the glomerular abnormalities and induces changes in the renal arterioles that do not occur in NSN alone or in CH alone at comparable levels of systolic blood pressure. The results suggest that the intrarenal vessels in experimental nephritis might be abnormal in a way that renders them more susceptible to the effects of increased intraluminal pressure, even though these vessels appear morphologically unaffected by the disease. The diseased glomerular capillaries might be showing a similar increased susceptibility to damage. On the other hand, one could hypothesize that the glomerulus in experimental nephritis actually is exposed to greater hydraulic pressure and flow than might normally occur at a given systemic pressure. Such increases could be due to adaptive alterations in renal resistance that accompany glomerular disease. The failure of arteriolar con-

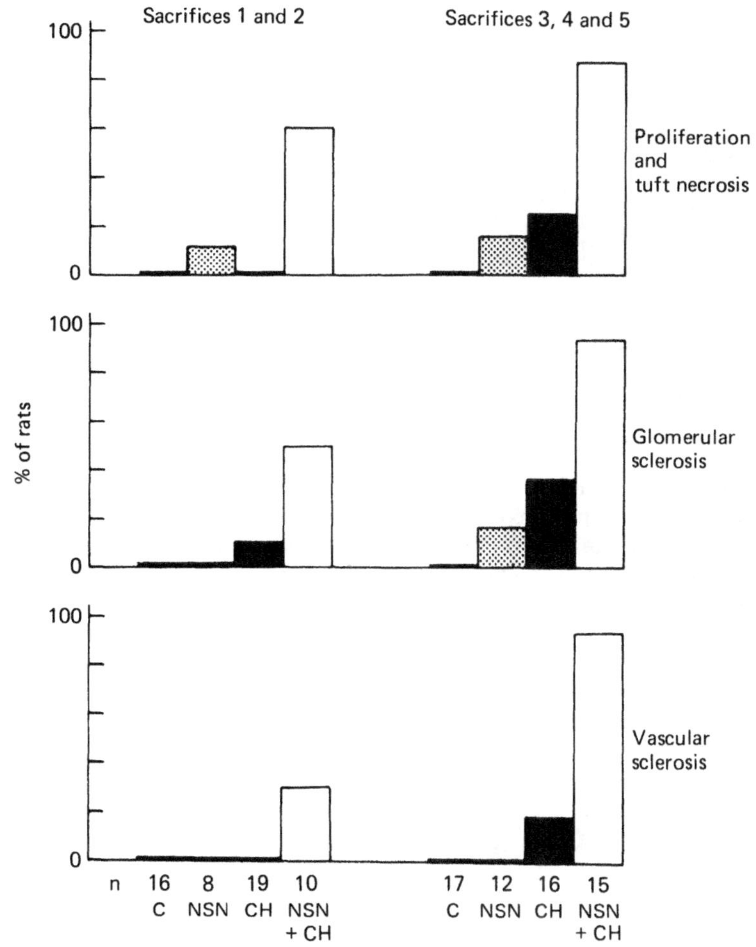

Fig. 2. Incidence of glomerular and vascular morphologic lesions in nephrotoxic serum nephritis, in clip hypertension, and in the combination of nephrotoxic serum nephritis with clip hypertension. The superimposition of clip hypertension (CH) in nephrotoxic serum nephritis (NSN) increased the incidence of glomerular proliferation, tuft necrosis, and sclerosis, and resulted in the appearance of vascular sclerosis (arteriolar medial hypertrophy) in almost every instance.

striction to occur in the presence of systemic hypertension could lead to hyperfiltration and resultant acceleration of glomerular proliferation and sclerosis. This afferent arteriolar "failure" also might be responsible for the markedly increased frequency and severity of small vessel damage that occurs at a given level of systemic pressure when hypertension is combined with glomerulonephritis.

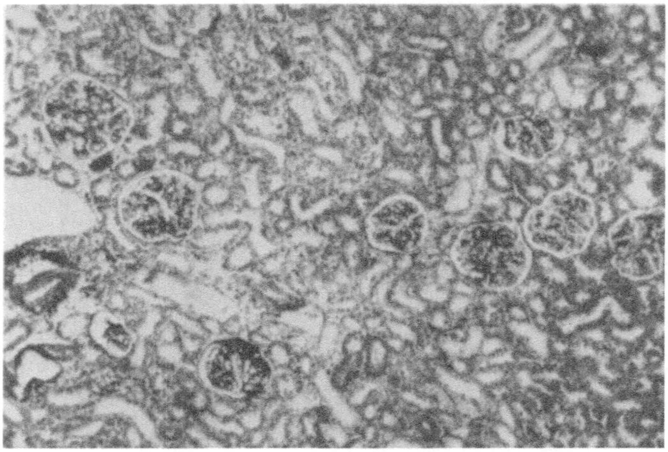

Fig. 3. Nephrotoxic serum nephritis. Photomicrograph of rat kidney 3 months after administration of nephrotoxic serum. Blood pressure was 98 mmHg. Glomeruli show increased mesangial matrix; a single glomerulus is sclerotic. Several small arteries present in the field are normal. Periodic acid-silver methenamine counterstained with hematoxylin and eosin (×180).

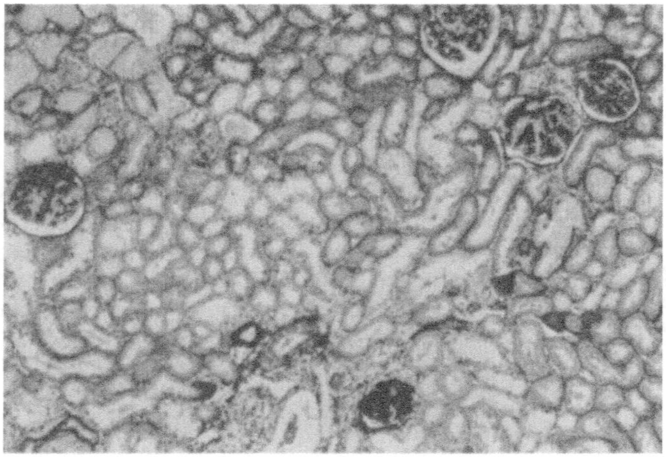

Fig. 4. Clip hypertension. Photomicrograph of unclipped right kidney 4 months afrer application of clip to left renal artery. Blood pressure was 149 mmHg. Glomeruli show increased mesangial matrix; a single glomerulus is sclerotic. A normal small artery is shown. Periodic acid-silver methenamine counterstained with hematoxylin and eosin (×180).

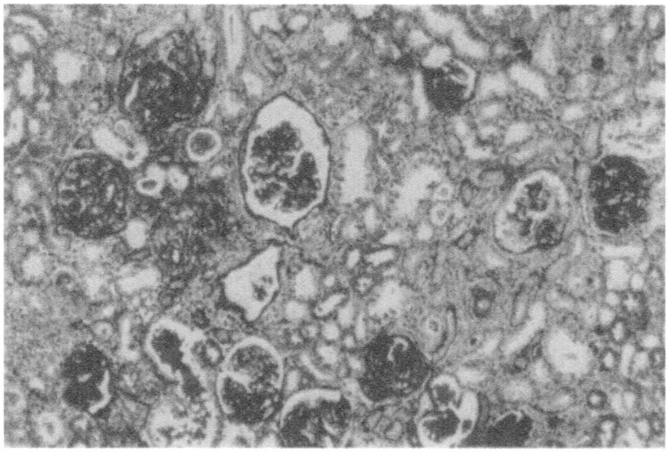

Fig. 5. Nephrotoxic serum nephritis with superimposed clip hypertension. Photomicrograph of unclipped right kidney 3 months after administration of nephrotoxic serum and 2 months after application of clip to left renal artery. Blood pressure was 140 mmHg. Glomeruli show widespread sclerosis and severe intra- and extracapillary proliferation. Medial hypertrophy and intimal hyaline are present in prearterioles; there are no necrotizing vascular lesions. Periodic acid-silver methenamine counterstained with hematoxylin and eosin (×180).

Adverse Role of Dietary Protein in Experimental Nephritis and in a Model of Renal Ablation

Numerous investigators have explored a possible deleterious effect of dietary protein on the course of experimental nephritis and on the progressive renal failure that occurs with subtotal renal ablation. On balance, the available evidence indicates that high protein intake accelerates renal failure in both models. In 1939, Farr and Smadel showed that in rats with NSN given a 5% protein intake, clinical renal disease subsided rapidly and glomerular and tubular injury resolved [40,41]. By contrast, rats fed a diet containing 40% protein uniformly developed renal failure and died within 1 year. Postmortem examination revealed progressive scarring and destruction of tubules and glomeruli. Rats fed a basal or mixed-stock diet followed a course that was intermediate between results from the extremes of protein intake.

Earlier, Medlar and Blatherwick [42,43] and Kennedy in 1957 [44] had suggested that sclerosis occurring with aging, uninephrectomy, or both could be accelerated by high-protein feeding. Lalich and Allen studied unilaterally nephrectomized rats fed diets containing 30% protein and found excessive proteinuria followed by ultrastructural changes leading to eventual sclerosis of glomeruli [45]. In a recent study, Kleinknecht and associates examined the effects of various protein diets on growth, renal function, and survival in Wistar rats who were subjected to ablation of seven-eighths of their renal mass [46]. A diet containing 37% protein led to anorexia, growth failure, and rapid deterioration of renal function in these rats. Although the content of sodium, phosphate, and calcium also was higher in the high-protein diets, none of the dietary regimens was low in these minerals, so an important, albeit not exclusive, deleterious role for protein was established in these studies.

The mechanism by which high protein intake accelerates glomerular sclerosis in animals with experimental nephritis, subtotal renal ablation, or aging has not been elucidated. However, studies by Shannon et al. [47], Van Slyke et al. [48], and Pitts [49] in the 1930s might be relevant to this issue. These authors showed that urea clearance, filtration rate, and renal blood flow could be increased two- to threefold in the dog by high-protein feeding. Once again, a possible role for increased glomerular perfusion and hyperfiltration in the causation of sclerosis is suggested. There are as yet no adequate clinical studies in humans that examine the relationship between protein intake and the course of parenchymal renal disease.

Phosphorus Restriction and Preservation of Renal Function

Preservation of renal function by phosphorus restriction has been demonstrated in the renal ablation model by Ibels and associates [50] and in nephrotoxic serum nephritis in the rat by Karlinsky et al. [51]. Ibels and colleagues reported prevention of proteinuria, renal calcification, histologic changes, functional deterioration, and death from uremia (Table 5). Similar salutary effects were noted in the phosphorus-restricted rat with experimental nephritis. The mechanism by which phosphorus restriction prevents functional deterioration in the remnant or the diseased kidney is not known [52]. One obvious possibility is that dystrophic and metastatic renal calcification in the cauterized remnant is prevented through suppression of secondary hyperparathyroidism and a reduction in calcium-phosphorus product. However, the striking protective effect of phosphorus restriction on the glomerular lesions of nephrotoxic serum nephritis suggests that mechanisms of renal damage other than calcification alone must be involved.

Glomerular Sclerosis and Aging

The occurrence of proteinuria in the aging male rat has long been recognized [53,54]. Although this proteinuria rarely gives rise to the nephrotic syndrome, renal lesions closely resembling focal and seg-

Table 5. Preservation of renal function in remnant kidney by phosphorus restriction.

	Urea Nitrogen				Creatinine (mg/dl)	
	Normal Diet		Phosphate Restriction			
Time	N	mg/dl	N	mg/dl	Normal Diet	Phosphate Restriction
Before nephrectomy	26	20 ± 0.5	12	18 ± 0.7	0.46 ± .02	0.60 ± .04
Day 28	24	107 ± 6	12	85 ± 6	1.43 ± 0.08	1.26 ± 0.07
Day 49	20	111 ± 6[a]	10	75 ± 4	1.46 ± 0.09[b]	1.12 ± 0.05
Day 70	15	118 ± 12[a]	10	67 ± 3	1.87 ± 0.16[b]	1.13 ± 0.05
Day 84	12	146 ± 15[a]	10	69 ± 10	2.87 ± 0.35[b]	1.11 ± 0.05
Day 105	7	186 ± 26[a]	10	69 ± 5	3.75 ± 0.57[b]	1.01 ± 0.02
Day 168	All dead		9	52 ± 3	All dead	0.76 ± .03

[a]$P < .01$ for differences between animals on normal diet and phosphate-restricted animals at same time.

Note: N, number of animals alive at that time.

Source: Reprinted, by permission of the *New England Journal of Medicine* 298:122–126, 1978 (Ref. 50).

mental glomerular sclerosis in humans are common in several species of aging male rats [45,55]. This phenomenon is of interest as a possible model for the investigation of the mechanisms responsible for progressive glomerular injury and sclerosis in human renal diseases. Protein loading accelerates the development of the lesion [42,43,45], whereas low sodium intake prevents both the increasing proteinuria and glomerular sclerosis [56]. Unilateral nephrectomy increases the incidence of glomerular sclerosis in the aging rat, especially when combined with increased dietary protein intake [57]. Recent ultrastructural and immunofluorescent observations have demonstrated increased IgM deposits in the mesangium as well as progressive glomerular basement membrane and epithelial cell damage associated with nonselective proteinuria [58–60].

These studies prompted the hypothesis that focal glomerular sclerosis in the aging rat might result from mesangial overload and dysfunction consequent to a persistent increase in glomerular permeability and proteinuria. By analogy, one can argue that mesangial functional overload and its consequences play a similar role in human glomerular diseases, especially when the hemodynamic consequences of reduced renal mass and hypertension are superimposed on damaged glomerular capillaries.

Age-related glomerular sclerosis also occurs as a phenomenon of aging in humans. Kaplan et al., in a postmortem study, found that the incidence of glomerular sclerosis did not exceed 10% in individuals under 40 years of age [61]. With increasing age, however, the frequency of sclerotic glomeruli reached almost 30%. Kappel and Olsen reported similar findings, i.e., a highly significant correlation between age and percentage of sclerotic glomeruli [62]. The weight of total renal and cortical mass decreases to about one-half between the ages of 40 and 80 to 90 years. During the same time span, renal hemodynamics and functional tubular mass decrease by 40 to 50% [63]. Although it is generally held that abiotrophic involutional sclerosis of glomeruli is secondary to vascular sclerosis, McLachlan et al. failed to find a significant correlation between vascular changes and glomerular sclerosis in the aging kidney [64]. An understanding of the mechanisms responsible for glomerular involution with aging might provide insights into disease progression.

Aminonucleoside Nephrotic Syndrome and Glomerular Sclerosis

A model of chronic renal disease utilizing repeated injections of aminonucleoside, an agent that usually produces a reversible renal lesion when given in a single course, was described by Wilson and associates in 1958 [65]. Others subsequently have investigated the presumed nonimmunologic pathogenesis of this form of renal injury [66]. Most recently, Glasser et al. reported that an apparent threshold level of protein excretion was essential for the development of focal glomerular sclerosis in this model [67]. Many groups have proposed that in this model of focal sclerosis, irreversible epithelial cell injury is the primary pathogenetic mechanism that leads to eventual glomerular sclerosis as a result of increased protein permeability, deposition of fibrin and related antigens, and protein-aggregate accumulation in the mesangium and subendothelium [68–72]. "Mesangial overload," the basis for glomerular injury and sclerosis hypothesized in this model, might prove to be one of the nonimmunologic mechanisms responsible for progression of renal disease in humans.

Glomerular Sclerosis in Reflux Nephropathy

Investigations into the progression of renal insufficiency after the surgical correction of reflux nephropathy have disclosed the occurrence of a focal, segmental, sclerosing glomerular lesion that often is associated with heavy proteinuria [73–77]. Immunopathologic studies suggest a possible immune mechanism of glomerular damage [78], but progressive parenchymal damage in this situation might represent still another example of the deleterious effects of adaptation to loss of renal mass on remaining intact nephrons.

Summary

Let me now summarize what these data have taught us. Our long-term observations in poststreptococcal glomerulonephritis and other glomerular diseases suggested that nonimmunologically mediated damage often was related to ischemia secondary to intrarenal vascular sclerosis which, in turn, could be attributed to hypertension. However, a new basis for glomerular obliteration has emerged from physiologic and morphologic studies of reduced renal mass, the aging kidney, post-salt or steroid-induced hypertension, and various forms of hypertension superimposed on experimental nephritis. It appears that nephron loss begets further glomerular damage through adaptive hemodynamic changes that take place in remaining nephrons and that expose the glomerular capillaries to increased flows and hydraulic pressures. When systemic hypertension occurs in conjunction with glomerulonephritis, glomerular damage is further increased, possibly through increased transmission of elevated pressures. One can hypothesize that elevated glomerular pressure and consequent hyperperfusion rather than ischemia is the mechanism by which hypertension aggravates glomerulonephritis: a failure of autoregulation in nephrons adapted to disease. The mechanism by which increments in glomerular capillary hydraulic pressure eventually result in sclerosis and obliteration of capillaries is not known, but epithelial cell damage with alterations in permselectivity and resultant mesangial overload and dysfunction might be responsible. The adverse effects of dietary protein and the protective role of phosphorus restriction might operate through similar mechanisms, in which altered glomerular hemodynamics play a key role.

Questions and Answers

Dr. John T. Harrington: Do you think that the fact that hypertension superimposed on nephrotoxic serum nephritis results in glomerular sclerosis gives us any insight into the pathogenesis of the focal sclerosis that occurs in patients with idiopathic nephrotic syndrome?

Dr. Baldwin: Insight into the pathogenesis of focal glomerulosclerosis may be gained from the work I cited by Michael and his associates on the model of this lesion that can be produced by chronic administration of aminonucleoside [67,68]. These studies and the observations on proteinuria and the development of glomerular sclerosis in the aging rat kidney [56–60] and in the remnant kidney [22] suggest that increased permeability to large molecules may be *responsible* for glomerular damage. In other words, proteinuria may not be only the passive result of abnormal glomerular capillary permeability; the increased passage of proteins may in itself cause further glomerular damage, possibly through "mesangial overload." This hypothesis revives the old argument as to whether minimal-change nephrotic syndrome can evolve into focal segmental glomerulosclerosis. Some patients seem to have minimal change as evidenced by biopsy and by the characteristic response to steroids, but they then become steroid resistant and progress to renal failure. This suggests that proteinuria itself may actually be damaging. Thus, in patients with minimal-change nephrotic syndrome, the goal of inducing a remission may be more important than simply raising serum albumin and ridding the patient of edema. By correcting the defect that allows the protein leak, one actually may be preventing the development of glomerular sclerosis.

Dr. Harrington: That is interesting because the data from both the Collaborative Study of the Adult Idiopathic Nephrotic Syndrome [79] and our combined Boston University–Tufts nephrotic syndrome study [80] show a very good correlation between the degree of proteinuria and renal function. Renal function remained normal in all patients with protein excretion of less than 2 g/day.

Dr. Jordan J. Cohen: I gather from your thesis that you would predict that further progression is inevitable once a patient with chronic glomerulonephritis reaches a certain critical level of renal insufficiency. Have you had the experience of seeing patients—as we thought we were seeing in today's first case—with serum creatinine levels of 4 or 5 mg/dl for many years who go on to live a normal lifetime and die from other causes?

Dr. Baldwin: Rarely, except in the elderly. A serious problem almost certainly exists if a patient with chronic renal disease loses function beyond a certain level, say 50%. We used to say that when glomerulonephritis goes into the hypertensive stage, you can count the years that patient will survive. I think what that really implied was that when the "magic number" of nephrons has been lost and the remaining ones have adapted to this loss, and hypertension is then added that is "unopposed," sclerosis of remaining arterioles and glomeruli is inevitable. The creatinine clearance seems to decrease arithmetically early in the patient's course. Then in the last 3 or 4 years it declines more rapidly. I think this change occurs because adapted nephrons and their arterioles are highly susceptible to the effects of hypertension. I don't wish to appear dogmatic in this regard. The reverse also occurs: loss of nephrons itself causes the hypertension. We may have to invoke the old "vicious cycle" here. Who can say which comes first? I think that the reason we were able to show what we did was because our model of experimental hypertension employed a renal artery clip, which does more than just produce hypertension. Clipping the kidney, and essentially ablating it functionally, increases the work of the remaining kidney: not only is the kidney nephritic and exposed to hypertension, but it also must adapt to having lost its mate. Thus, the perfect set-up for vascular and glomerular sclerosis is established.

Dr. Steven Zelman *(Renal Fellow, NEMC)*: Since the glomerular blood flow and glomerular pressures would be increased even if the systemic blood pressure were normal in patients who have a serum creatinine of 4 mg/dl, should we perhaps be lowering the blood pressure to subnormal levels so as to further reduce the glomerular pressure, and perhaps to protect these patients to some extent from this added adaptive hypertension?

Dr. Baldwin: That's an interesting theoretical consideration, but I don't know how much leeway you would have. If you lower the blood pressure in a patient with reduced nephron mass, the remaining nephrons, if not already maximally perfused, might undergo further vasodilation. When you reduce a normal individual's blood pressure, the renal arterioles constrict. Perhaps in the diseased kidney, adaptive mechanisms would continue to maintain flow even in the presence of reduced blood pressure. You are suggesting that in renal disease, we might maintain patients chronically under the stress of hypotension so that they might override their adaptive vasodilation. We thus would raise their creatinine and BUN levels but would spare their glomeruli the deleterious effects of increased pressures and hyperfusion. I'm not prepared to conjecture on the validity of this suggestion.

Dr. Michael Madaio *(Renal Service, NEMC)*: Do you think that the pathogenesis and subsequent course of the epidemic form of poststreptococcal glomerulonephritis is different than the sporadic form you are reporting? If the prognosis is better in the epidemic form of the disease, as many investigators claim, is it due simply to a difference in the way that patients have been studied?

Dr. Baldwin: Yes. I believe that patients with the epidemic form of acute PSGN do have a better prognosis. Some very good studies, such as those carried out in Trinidad, show that patients with epidemic PSGN do much better than patients with sporadic cases, at least over the first decade. Seven to 12 years was the period covered in the longest follow-up from Trinidad, which was published in 1979 [81]. Because this study included fewer patients with renal functional impairment or even proteinuria or hypertension, I think that epidemic nephritis (at least in Trinidad) is milder than is sporadic nephritis, and that many cases that would not be recognized sporadically are picked up during epidemics; possibly both theories are true. In general, it is acknowledged that during epidemics instances of mild nephritis are detected that otherwise would be missed. However, many of these children in Trinidad did not have mild disease. There must be some other explanation for the better prognosis of epidemic PSGN. For one thing, young people are primarily affected. We know, from our own sporadic cases [82] and the reports of others [83], that youngsters are affected less severely and that they do better at least over the first 10 to 15 years from onset than do adults. The fact that adults do worse may be related to the greater vulnerability of the aging kidney to glomerular sclerosis. To return to your question, I agree that there is a difference. I really don't know the reason for this difference except that more younger patients with milder disease may have been included in the studies of epidemics.

Dr. James Strom *(Renal Division, St. Elizabeth's Hospital, Boston, Massachusetts)*: Following your hypothesis, if you look at patients with progressive renal failure from interstitial disease but without hypertension, do you find progressive glomerular sclerosis in that instance as well?

Dr. Baldwin: Yes. But I still think that the observation that patients with tubulointerstitial diseases often progress more slowly than do those with primary glomerular disease is related to the fact that hypertension is less common or milder in interstitial nephritides, including pyelonephritis. We know that essential hypertension can last for 50 years and not lead to renal failure, but the presence or absence of hypertension makes a great difference in the rate of progression of intrinsic renal diseases, whether glomerular or tubulointerstitial.

Dr. Cohen: Kincaid-Smith and others have pointed out that patients with interstitial nephritis due to analgesic-abuse nephropathy, for example, may develop a very prominent glomerulosclerosis or focal sclerosis after many years [84]. Such occurrences may be relevant to your hypothesis.

Dr. Baldwin: That is a very pertinent comment. It is of particular interest, I believe, that these patients progress to renal failure even after they discontinue taking analgesics; this might be another example of sclerosis developing in remnant nephrons because of adaptation. Hypertension does occur, of course, in many of these patients and probably is responsible for additional vascular and glomerular damage to adapted nephrons.

Dr. David Clive *(Renal Unit, Beth Israel Hospital, Boston, Massachusetts)*: Can you apply this thesis to the natural history of diabetic glomerular disease, in which progression of renal failure occurs relentlessly following the appearance of proteinuria? Do you think there is any correlation? The development of heavy proteinuria, while obviously a sign of glomerular capillary wall disease, also may be responsible for accelerating glomerular mesangial sclerosis in diabetes mellitus.

Dr. Baldwin: Absolutely. The development of heavy proteinuria obviously is evidence of glomerular capillary wall disease. This same alteration in permselectivity of the capillary, however, may participate in the mechanism responsible for sclerosis in diabetes mellitus as well as other glomerular disease.

Dr. Nicolaos E. Madias *(Renal Service, NEMC)*: I have two questions. First, have you had the opportunity to observe the clinical course of patients with single kidneys who happened to get a form of glomerular disease that was identified? Second, have you followed patients with chronic nephritis who subsequently developed renovascular hypertension? Do such patients have an increase in proteinuria, a finding that would be in accord with your experimental observations?

Dr. Baldwin: I don't know of any patients with single kidneys who had morphologically documented acute glomerulonephritis. We would not hazard a renal biopsy in such patients. We have under observation patients with other forms of glomerular disease in whom it was deemed important to get a biopsy, and an open one was obtained because of unilateral renal agenesis. There are too few patients of this kind, however, to say whether they fare worse than do nephritics with two kidneys. I don't know of any of our patients with nephritis who have developed superimposed renovascular hypertension. A few individuals have been described who have renovascular hypertension and the nephrotic syndrome. I have often wondered if they did not perhaps have underlying glomerulonephritis.

References

1. Baldwin DS, Gluck MC, Schacht RG, Gallo G: The long-term course of poststreptococcal glomerulonephritis. Ann Intern Med 80:343–358, 1974
2. Schacht RE, Gluck MC, Gallo GR, Baldwin DS: Progression to uremia after remission of acute poststreptococcal glomerulonephritis. N Engl J Med 295:977–981, 1976
3. Baldwin DS: Poststreptococcal glomerulonephritis—A progressive disease? Am J Med 62:1–11, 1977
4. Fujise Y, Miyahara M: Comparison of the prognosis of hypertension associated with chronic glomerulonephritis with that of essential hypertension. Jpn Circ J 39:793–795, 1975
5. Hollenberg NK: The kidney in hypertension: Relevance to glomerulonephritis. In Yoshitoshi Y, Ueda Y (eds.): Glomerulonephritis. Baltimore, University Park Press, 1979, pp. 423–440
6. Kajiwara N: Therapy and prognosis of hypertension in chronic nephritis. Jpn Circ J 39:779–788, 1975
7. Kawaguchi Y, Mitarai T, Ueda Y: Clinical aspects of hypertension in advanced chronic glomerulonephritis. In Yoshitoshi Y, Ueda Y (eds.): Glomerulonephritis. Baltimore, University Park Press, 1979, pp. 473–482
8. Varga I, Beregi E: Clinical and histopathological studies of human renal disease. IV. Relationships of renal arterial fibroelastosis, glomerulonephritis and arterial hypertension. Acta Med Acad Sci Hung 30:165–175, 1973
9. Gallo GR, Feiner HD, Steele JM Jr, Schacht RG, Gluck MC, Baldwin DS: Role of intrarenal vascular sclerosis in progression of poststreptococcal glomerulonephritis. Clin Nephrol 13:49–57, 1978
10. Feiner JD, Cabili S, Schacht RG, Baldwin DS, Gallo GR: Intrarenal vascular disease in Berger's IgA nephropathy. Lab Invest 42:166, 1980
11. Kincaid-Smith P: The Kidney. Oxford, Blackwell Scientific, 1975, pp. 193–202
12. Morrison AB: Experimentally induced chronic renal insufficiency in the rat. Lab Invest 11:321–331, 1962
13. Chanutin A, Ferris EB Jr: Experimental renal insufficiency produced by partial nephrectomy. Arch Intern Med 49:767–787, 1932
14. Shimamura T, Morrison AB: A progressive glomerulosclerosis occurring in partial five-sixths nephrectomized rats. Am J Pathol 79:95–106, 1975
15. Purkerson ML, Hoffstein P, Klahr S: Pathogenesis of the glomerulopathy associated with renal infarction in rats. Kidney Int 19:407–417, 1976
16. Deen WM, Maddox DA, Robertson CR, Brenner BM: Dynamics of glomerular ultrafiltration in the rat. VII. Response to reduced renal mass. Am J Physiol 227:556–562, 1974
17. Hostetter TH, Olson JL, Rennke HG, Venkatachalam MA, Brenner BM: Increased glomerular pressure and flow: A potentially adverse adaptation to reduced renal mass. Clin Res 27:498A, 1979
18. Hostetter TH, Olson JL, Rennke RG, Venkatachalam MA, Brenner BM: Hyperfiltration in remnant nephrons: A potentially adverse response to renal ablation. Am J Physiol 10:F85–F93, 1981
19. Azar S, Johnson MA, Hertel B, Tobian L: Single-nephron pressures, flows,

and resistances in hypertensive kidneys with nephrosclerosis. Kidney Int 12:28–40, 1977
20. Maddox DA, Bennett CM, Deen WM, Glassock RJ, Knidsen D, Daugharty TM, Brenner BM: Determinants of glomerular filtration in experimental glomerulonephritis in the rat. J Clin Invest 55:305–318, 1975
21. Allison MEM, Wilson CB, Gottschalk CW: Pathophysiology of experimental glomerulonephritis in rats. J Clin Invest 53:1402–1423, 1974
22. Olson JL, Hostetter TH, Rennke HG, Brenner BM, Venkatachalam MA: Altered charge and size selective properties of the glomerular wall: A response to reduced renal mass. Proc Am Soc Nephrol, 1979, p. 87A
23. Shea SM, Raskova J, Morrison AB: Ultrastructure of the glomerular basement membrane of rats with proteinuria due to subtotal nephrectomy. Localization of anionic sites by cationic probe molecules. Am J Pathol 100:513–520, 1980
24. Wilson C, Byrom FB: The vicious cycle in chronic Bright's disease. Experimental evidence from the hypertensive rat. Q J Med 34:65–93, 1941
25. Knowlton AL, Stoerk H, Seegal BC, Loeb EN: Influence of adrenal cortical steroids upon the blood pressure and the rate of progression of experimental nephritis in rats. Endocrinology 38:315–324, 1946
26. Masuyama Y, Nishio I, Motoki K, Kusuyama Y, Tanaka S, Nagase M: Hypertension changes in experimental nephritis combined with experimental hypertension. Contrib Nephrol 6:13–22, 1977
27. Masuyama Y, Motoki K, Kusuyama Y, Nishio I, Tanaka S, Nagase M: Hypertension changes in experimental nephritis combined with experimental hypertension. In Yoshitoshi Y, Ueda Y (eds.): Glomerulonephritis. Baltimore, University Park Press, 1979, pp. 441–454
28. Motoki K, Kusuyama Y, Ueno Y, Miyamoto Y, Nishio I, Masuyama Y: Chronic nephrotoxic nephritis in spontaneously hypertensive rats. Jpn Heart J 19:662–664, 1978
29. Motoki K, Kusuyama Y, Jimbo S, Nishimura T, Nishio I, Masuyama Y: Nephrotoxic serum nephritis in DOCA-salt hypertension and SHR. Jpn Heart J 20:714, 1979
30. Teodoru CV, Saifer A, Frankel H: Conditioning factors influencing evolution of experimental glomerulonephritis in rabbits. Am J Physiol 196:457–460, 1959
31. Tikkanen I, Fyrquist F, Miettinen A, Tornroth T: Autologous immune complex nephritis and DOCA-NaCl load: A new model of hypertension. Acta Pathol Microbiol Scand 88:241–250, 1980
32. Iversen BM, Ofstad J: Influence of hypertension on the course of experimental hypertension in rats. Kidney Int 18:142, 1980
33. Hill GS, Heptinstall RH: Steroid-induced hypertension in the rat. Am J Pathol 52:1–20, 1968
34. Still WJS, Dennison SM: The pathogenesis of the glomerular changes in steroid-induced hypertension. Lab Invest 20:249–260, 1969
35. Azar S, Johnson MA, Iwai J, Bruno L, Tobian L: Single-nephron dynamics in"post-salt" rats with chronic hypertension. J Lab Clin Med 91:156–166, 1978
36. Mauer SM, Steffes MW, Azar S, Sandberg SK, Brown DS: The effects of Goldblatt hypertension on development of the glomerular lesions of diabetes mellitus in the rat. Diabetes 27:738–744, 1979

37. Azar S: Increased glomerular capillary pressure (PGC) in pancreatectomized rats with short-term diabetes. Clin Res 26:725A, 1978
38. Hostetter TH, Troy JL, Brenner BM: Glomerular hemodynamics in experimental diabetes mellitus. Kidney Int 19:410–415, 1981
39. Neugarten J, Feiner HD, Schacht RG, Gallo GR, Baldwin DS: Aggravation of experimental glomerulonephritis by superimposed clip hypertension. Proc Am Soc Nephrol, 1980, p. 81A
40. Farr LE, Smadel JE: The effect of dietary protein on the course of nephrotoxic nephritis in rats. J Exp Med 70:615–627, 1939
41. Smadel JE, Farr LE: The effect of diet on the pathological changes in rats with nephrotoxic serum nephritis. Am J Pathol 15:199–216, 1939
42. Medlar EM, Blatherwick NR: The pathogenesis of dietary nephritis in the rat. Am J Pathol 13:881–895, 1937
43. Blatherwick NR, Medlar EM: Chronic nephritis in rats fed high-protein diets. Arch Intern Med 59:572–596, 1937
44. Kennedy GC: Effects of old age and overnutrition on the kidneys. Br Med Bull 13:67–70, 1957
45. Lalich JJ, Allen JR: Protein overload nephropathy in rats with unilateral nephrectomy. II. Ultrastructural study. Arch Pathol 91:372–382, 1971
46. Kleinknecht C, Salusky I, Broyer M, Gubler M: Effect of various protein diets on growth, renal function and survival of uremic rats. Kidney Int 15:534–541, 1979
47. Shannon JA, Jolliffe N, Smith HW: The excretion of urine in the dog. IV. The effect of maintenance diet, feeding, etc., upon the quantity of glomerular filtrate. Am J Physiol 101:625–638, 1932
48. Van Slyke DD, Rhoads CP, Hiller A, Alving A: The relationship of the urea clearance to the renal blood flow. Am J Physiol 110:387–391, 1934
49. Pitts RF: The effect of protein and amino acid metabolism on the urea and xylose clearance. J Nutrition 9:657–666, 1935
50. Ibels LS, Alfrey AC, Haut L, Huffer WE: Preservation of function in experimental renal disease by dietary restriction of phosphate. N Engl J Med 298:122–126, 1978
51. Karlinsky ML, Haut L, Buddington B, Schrier NA, Alfrey AC: Preservation of renal function in experimental glomerulonephritis. Kidney Int 17:293–302, 1980
52. Hyperphosphatemia and renal function (letter). Lancet 1:753–754, 1978
53. Linkswiler H, Reynolds MS, Bauman CA: Factors affecting proteinuria in the rat. Am J Physiol 168:504–508, 1952
54. Sellers AL, Goodman HC, Marmorston J, Smith M: Sex difference in proteinuria in the rat. Am J Physiol 163:662–667, 1950
55. Guttman PH, Kohn HI: Progressive intercapillary glomerulosclerosis in the mouse, rat and chinese hamster, associated with aging and X-ray exposure. Am J Pathol 37:293–307, 1960
56. Elema JD, Arends A: Focal and segmental glomerular hyalinosis and sclerosis in the rat. Lab Invest 33:554–561, 1975
57. Striker GE, Nagle RB, Kohnen PW, Smuckler EA: Response to unilateral nephrectomy in old rats. Arch Pathol 87:439–442, 1969
58. Bolton WK, Benton FR, Maclay JG, Sturgill BC: Spontaneous glomerular sclerosis in aging Sprague-Dawley rats. I. Lesions associated with mesangial IgM deposits. Am J Pathol 85:277–300, 1976

59. Bolton WK, Sturgill BC: Spontaneous glomerular sclerosis in aging Sprague-Dawley rats. II. Ultrastructural studies. Am J Pathol 98:339–350, 1980
60. Couser WG, Stilmant MM: Mesangial lesions and focal glomerular sclerosis in the aging rat. Lab Invest 33:491–501, 1975
61. Kaplan C, Pasternack B, Shah H, Gallo GR: Age-related incidence of sclerotic glomeruli in human kidneys. Am J Pathol 80:227–234, 1975
62. Kappel B, Olsen S: Cortical interstitial tissue and sclerosed glomeruli in the normal human kidney, related to age and sex. A quantitative study. Virchow's Arch (Pathol Anat) 387:271–277, 1980
63. Davies DF, Shock NW: Age changes in glomerular filtration rate, effective renal plasma flow, and tubular excretory capacity in adult males. J Clin Invest 29:496–507, 1950
64. McLachlan MSF, Guthrie JC, Anderson CK, Fulker MJ: Vascular and glomerular changes in the aging kidney. J Pathol 121:65–78, 1977
65. Wilson SGF, Hackel DB, Horwood S, Nash G, Heymann W: Aminonucleoside nephrosis in rats. Pediatrics 20:963–973, 1958
66. Shimizu F: Histopathologic and immunologic studies on chronic renal lesions in rats induced by aminonucleoside of puromycin. Jpn J Exp Med 40:227–242, 1970
67. Glasser RJ, Velosa JA, Michael AF: Experimental model of focal sclerosis. I. Relationship to protein excretion in aminonucleoside nephrosis. Lab Invest 36:519–526, 1977
68. Velosa JA, Glasser RJ, Nevins TE, Michael AF: Experimental model of focal sclerosis. II. Correlation with immunopathologic changes, macromolecular kinetics, and polyanion loss. Lab Invest 36:527–534, 1977
69. Caulfield JP, Farquhar MG: Loss of anionic sites from the glomerular basement membrane in aminonucleoside nephrosis. Lab Invest 39:505–512, 1978
70. Ericsson JLE, Andres GA: Electron microscopic studies on the development of the glomerular lesions in aminonucleoside nephrosis. Am J Pathol 39:643–654, 1961
71. Lannigan R: The production of chronic renal disease in rats by a single intravenous injection of aminonucleoside of puromycin and the effect of low dosage continuous hydrocortisone. Br J Exp Pathol 44:326–333, 1963
72. Michael AF, Blau E, Vernier RL: Glomerular polyanion. Alteration in aminonucleoside nephrosis. Lab Invest 23:649–657, 1979
73. Bhathena DB, Weiss JH, Holland NH, McMorrow RG, Curtis JJ, Lucas BA, Luke RG: Focal and segmental glomerular sclerosis in reflux nephropathy. Am J Med 68:886–892, 1980
74. Kincaid-Smith P: Glomerular and vascular lesions in chronic atrophic pyelonephritis and reflux nephropathy. Adv Nephrol 5:3–17, 1975
75. Kincaid-Smith P: Glomerular lesions in atrophic pyelonephritis and reflux nephropathy. Kidney Int 8:S81–S83, 1975
76. Senekjian HO, Stinebaugh BJ, Mattioli CA, Suki WN: Irreversible, renal failure following vesicoureteral reflux. JAMA 241:160–162, 1979
77. Torres VE, Velosa JA, Holley KE, Lelalis PP, Stickler GB, Kurtz SB: The progression of vesicoureteral reflux nephropathy. Ann Intern Med 92:776–784, 1980
78. Zimmerman SW, Uehling DT, Burkholder PM: Vesicoureteral reflux

nephropathy. Evidence for immunologically mediated glomerular injury. Urology 11:534–538, 1973

79. Collaborative Study of the Adult Idiopathic Nephrotic Syndrome: A controlled study of short-term prednisone treatment in adults with membranous nephropathy. N Engl J Med 301:1301–1306, 1979
80. Idelson BA, Smithline N, Smith GW, Harrington JT: Prognosis in steroid-treated idiopathic nephrotic syndrome in adults. Analysis of major predictive factors after ten-year follow-up. Arch Intern Med 137:891–896, 1977
81. Nissenson AR, Mayon-White R, Potter EV, Mayon-White V, Abidh S, Poon-King T, Earle DP: Continued absence of clinical renal disease seven to 12 years after poststreptococcal acute glomerulonephritis in Trinidad. Am J Med 67:255–262, 1979
82. Schacht RG, Gallo GR, Gluck MC, Iqbal MS, Baldwin DS: Irreversible disease following acute poststreptococcal glomerulonephritis in children. J Chronic Dis 32:515–524, 1979
83. Dodge WF, Spargo BH, Travis LB, Srivastava RN, Caravajal HF, DeBeukelaer MM, Longley MP, Menchaca JA: Poststreptococcal glomerulonephritis. A prospective study in children. N Engl J Med 286:273–278, 1972
84. Kincaid-Smith P: Nephrology forum: Analgesic abuse and the kidney. Kidney Int 17:250–260, 1980

Acute Renal Failure

Principal Discussant
Robert W. Schrier

Case Presentation

An 85-year-old woman was transferred to New England Medical Center (NEMC) for management of acute renal failure (ARF). The patient was in apparent good health until 3.5 weeks earlier when she had a uterine prolapse and was admitted to another hospital. Her blood urea nitrogen (BUN) concentration, serum creatinine concentration, and results of urinalyses were normal. An electrocardiogram (EKG) revealed an old inferolateral myocardial infarction. The patient underwent a vaginal hysterectomy; in the immediate postoperative period she complained of chest pain. Over the week following the operation, EKG changes revealed the evolution of a new anterior myocardial infarction. During this same interval, several blood transfusions were required because of persistent vaginal bleeding. During one of these transfusions approximately 10 days prior to transfer to NEMC, the patient developed a fever (41 °C), shaking chills, and hemoglobinuria. She was treated with Benadryl and Solu-medrol. EKG revealed new Q waves in the inferior leads. Clindamycin, gentamicin, and nafcillin were also administered at this time. Over the next 10 days, urine output decreased, and the serum creatinine concentration increased. A Giovanetti diet and fluid restriction were instituted; the antibiotics were continued but in reduced dosage. Urine output remained in the range of 200–300 ml/day. At the time of transfer to NEMC, the serum creatinine concentration was 12 mg and the BUN concentration was 130 mg/100 ml.

On admission to NEMC, physical examination revealed the following: blood pressure, 170/80 mmHg; temperature, 38.5 °C; pulse, 68/min; respirations, 20/min; the skin had an erythematous maculopapular rash over the trunk; head, ears, eyes, nose, and throat were within normal limits; no jugular venous distention; the lungs had bibasilar dry rales and decreased breath sounds bilaterally with diffuse expiratory wheezes. Cardiac examination revealed a diffuse point of maximal impulse in the midclavicular line with no heave; normal S1 and S2; a grade II/VI systolic ejection murmur along the lower left sternal border; and no thrills, rubs, or gallops. Abdominal and neurologic examinations were unre-

markable. Pelvic examination revealed no masses or tenderness. There was no peripheral edema. Laboratory findings disclosed the following data: hemoglobin, 10.5 g/100 ml; hematocrit, 30%; white blood cell (WBC) count, 7200/mm^3 with a normal differential; serum sodium, 129 mEq; serum potassium, 5.6 mEq; serum chloride, 95 mEq; total carbon dioxide, 14 mEq/liter; BUN, 132 mg; serum creatinine, 12.9 mg; serum calcium, 7.8 mg; serum glucose, 82 mg/100 ml; arterial oxygen tension, 81 mmHg; arterial carbon dioxide tension, 28 mmHg; arterial pH, 7.29. EKG revealed a normal sinus rhythm at the rate of 70/min; a prominent Q wave in lead 3; and biphasic Q waves in AVL, V3, and V4. Results of urinalyses revealed the following: pH, 5; many red blood cells (RBC); a few WBC; and a few tubular epithelial cells. A radiograph of the chest revealed the trachea to be deviated slightly to the right and a few old calcified granulomas. Renal scan and abdominal echogram revealed bilateral kidneys of normal size and no evidence of obstruction.

For the first 36 of hospitalization, the patient underwent peritoneal dialysis (approximately 30 exchanges) during which the BUN concentration decreased to 59 mg and the serum creatinine concentration to 9.4 mg/100 ml. Following dialysis, the patient's serum creatinine concentration increased slightly to 10.1 mg/100 ml; it then decreased over the next 2 weeks to 1.9 mg/100 ml. The patient was discharged 17 days following admission.

Discussion

Dr. R. W. Schrier *(Chairman, Department of Medicine, University of Colorado Medical Center, Denver, Colorado)*: This 85-year-old patient underwent a vaginal hysterectomy complicated by an anterior myocardial infarction and some postoperative bleeding, which required blood transfusions. One of these transfusions was accompanied by fever, chills, hemoglobinuria, and possibly another myocardial infarction. In addition to treatment of the presumed transfusion reaction with Benadryl and Solu-medrol, several antibiotics (clindamycin, gentamicin, and nafcillin) were started. Immediately after this transfusion episode, the patient's serum creatinine concentration began to rise progressively, as her urine output remained in an oliguric range ($<$400 ml/24 h). Ten days after the transfusion reaction, the patient was transferred to NEMC with a serum creatinine concentration of 12 mg/100 ml and a BUN concentration of 130 mg/100 ml. The positive findings of the physical examination were a maculopapular rash of the trunk, bibasilar dry rales, and a systolic murmur. The laboratory findings were compatible with uremic metabolic acidosis and also revealed hypocalcemia, hyponatremia, and hyperkalemia. Results of urinalysis demonstrated hematuria and pyuria.

Predisposing Factors

This patient was predisposed to develop ARF for several reasons: (1) advanced age; (2) persistent bleeding with probable hypovolemia; (3) recent myocardial infarction; and (4) recent anesthesia.

It is known that ARF occurs more frequently in older individuals, and that the mortality rate associated with ARF is higher than in other age groups [1]. Renal function is known to deteriorate with age, so that an 85-year-old person is normally expected to have a creatinine clearance of only some 45 ml/min [2]. It also is possible that advancing age impairs the protective mechanisms of renal autoregulation and renal prostaglandin release, which are evoked during vasoconstrictive insults, but this speculation remains to be studied. Moreover, it is important to recall that the presence of inhibitors of prostaglandin synthesis (e.g., aspirin, indomethacin, phenylbutazone, ibuprofen, and naproxen), which are widely used for treatment of arthritis in the aged, may predispose the kidney to more severe ischemia whenever a hemodynamic insult occurs [3,4].

The patient described here had continued bleeding prior to the episode of hemoglobinemia and hemoglobinuria. Experimental evidence in ARF models indicates that fluid deprivation and volume depletion potentiate the development of pigment-induced (hemoglobin, myoglobin) ARF [5].

The postoperative complication of myocardial infarction must be considered in this patient's course toward ARF. A myocardial infarction can result in renal ischemia if the degree of myocardial dysfunction and decrease in cardiac output is sufficiently great. If cardiac failure occurs, however, the concomitant increase in left atrial pressure may exert an early protective effect on renal function. An increase in left atrial pressure initiates a reflex that decreases renal sympathetic tone and tends to vasodilate the kidney [6]. This phenomenon may account for the clinical aphorism that patients with an acute myocardial infarction do not develop ARF. This is of course not an absolute dictum; it is true, however, that for a given decrement in blood pressure, the degree of renal ischemia is less during cardiac failure (increase in left atrial pressure) than it is during hemorrhage (decrease in left atrial pressure) [7]. Finally, the occurrence of hematuria and renal functional deterioration in association with a recent myocardial infarction should always alert the clinician to the possibility of a mural thrombus with emboli to the kidney. Cardiac ultrasound and a renal scan are valuable tools for the detection of this disorder.

Whenever renal failure follows a recent operative procedure, it is important to discern whether the anesthetic used might be contributing to renal difficulty. Halothane and methoxyflurane are the anesthetics most frequently mentioned as potential etiologic factors in causing renal deterioration [8,9]. The renal toxicity of halothane is generally associated with hepatic damage and with the consequent release of tissue thromboplastin, which is then followed by intravascular coagulation and renal cortical necrosis. The renal toxicity of methoxyflurane appears to relate more closely to the resulting increase in plasma fluoride concentration than to the increase in oxalate excretion [9]. If microsomal enzymes in the liver have been induced by previous use of the anesthetic or by phenobarbital administration, then repeat exposure to methoxyflurane may result in more rapid metabolism of the drug and a higher concentration of plasma fluoride. Enflurane, a fluoride-containing anesthetic, releases less fluoride on metabolism than methoxyflurane; this probably explains the agent's lower renal toxicity [10]. It is interesting, however, that renal toxicity with enflurane has been described in the setting of prior use of the anesthetic and a high plasma fluoride concentration [11]. In the patient we are discussing here, although we are not told the nature of the anesthetic used, the length of time between the operation and the onset of renal failure would dismiss the anesthetic as a primary cause of renal failure. If reoperation for continued vaginal bleeding had become necessary, however, it would be important to know if a fluoride-containing anesthetic had been used in the earlier operation. An elevated serum fluoride concentration may persist for a week after methoxyflurane administration [10]; whether such elevation predisposes the kidney to toxicity with other nephrotoxic agents remains to be studied.

Etiologic Factors

As is often the case, this patient not only had several factors predisposing her to develop ARF, she also encountered multiple agents and conditions of potential importance in the etiology of ARF; these include (1) nephrotoxic aminoglycosides; (2) penicillin homologs capable of triggering acute interstitial nephritis; (3) recurrent acute myocardial infarction; (4) septicemia; and (5) transfusion reaction with hemoglobinuria.

The aminoglycosides have become the most relied on antibiotics in the treatment of gram-negative bacterial infections. The aminoglycoside introduced first, neomycin, has been restricted to oral or topical use because of its nephrotoxic potential. The aminoglycosides now used are less nephrotoxic but all of them, including kanamycin, gentamicin, amikacin, sisomicin, and tobramycin, can cause impairment in renal function. One of the newest aminoglycosides, netilmicin, may offer the hope of a comparable antimicrobial spectrum with less nephrotoxicity [12]. The nephrotoxicity of the aminoglycosides probably relates to tissue-binding of the drug in the renal cortex [13], and the degree of tissue-binding appears to correlate with the number of free amino groups contained in a given agent [14]. Strikingly, the most nephrotoxic aminoglycoside, neomycin, has six free amino groups, and the least nephrotoxic, streptomycin, has only two free amino groups. Aminoglycosides remain bound to renal tissue long after the antibiotic has disappeared from the circulation; the half-life of aminoglycosides in serum is 30 min, but in renal tissue it is 109 h [15]. Four weeks after a single injection of gentamicin in the rat, a therapeutic tissue concentration of 6 μg/g of tissue may persist [16]. This long tissue half-life no doubt explains why the onset of renal failure secondary to aminoglycosides has been reported to occur as late as several days after administration of the antibiotics has been discontinued. Cytosomes containing altered cell organelles (lysosomal cytosegrosomes) and lysosomal ingestion of phospholipid membranes (myeloid bodies) are characteristically found in the proximal tubular epithelium of patients treated with aminoglycosides; these anatomic changes, however, do not necessarily correlate with the degree of renal functional impairment [17].

Several factors are known to predispose patients to the development of aminoglycoside nephrotoxicity: (1) advancing age; (2) preexistent renal dysfunction; (3) volume depletion; and (4) recent exposure to aminoglycoside or another nephrotoxic agent. The older the patient is, the greater the likelihood that aminoglycoside toxicity will occur [18]. This effect may be partially explained by the failure of clinicians to decrease the drug dosage in proportion to the decrease in glomerular filtration rate (GFR) that occurs with age. Preexisting renal dysfunction is another factor that predisposes patients to aminoglycoside nephrotoxicity [18]. Sodium restriction and volume depletion increase the incidence of aminoglycoside nephrotoxicity presumably because they serve to increase the cortical concentrations of the drug [19]. In one study, the incidence of aminoglycoside nephrotoxicity increased from 7 to 22% in patients who had recent exposure either to aminoglycosides or to other potentially nephrotoxic agents [18]. The patient described here was elderly, probably was somewhat volume depleted because of continued bleeding, may have been recently exposed to a nephrotoxic anesthetic, and was treated with the combination of gentamicin and clindamycin. It has been suggested that the latter agent may increase the nephrotoxic effect of aminoglycosides [20]. Furosemide administration frequently potentiates aminoglycoside nephrotoxicity probably because of the diuretic's potent volume-depleting effect [21]. The ability of cephalosporins to increase aminoglycoside renal toxicity is not as well established; in fact, the results of one experimental study even suggest that cephalosporins decrease renal cortical tissue concentrations of aminoglycosides and thus protect against nephrotoxicity [22].

The clinical course of aminoglycoside nephrotoxicity is, however, quite different from that observed in this patient. The nephrotoxic effect of aminoglycosides is generally gradual in onset and related to the dose and duration of drug administration [23]. A nonoliguric self-limited form of ARF with a low mortality is most common with aminoglycoside nephrotoxicity [24]. It would be extremely rare for one to two doses of the drug to cause acute onset of oliguria and azotemia, as was observed in the patient presented here. In general, proteinuria, lysozymuria, and a renal concentrating defect with polyuria precede any decrease in GFR with aminoglycoside toxicity [13]; azotemia and glucosuria are later consequences of toxicity [25]. Since aminoglycosides are eliminated primarily by glomerular filtration, whenever serum creatinine concentration increases, the "trough" concentration of the antibiotic will also increase unless the dose has been altered. Thus, the serum creatinine concentration can be used to gauge the "trough" concentration of serum aminoglycoside when the latter measurement is unavailable.

Acute interstitial nephritis has become a more frequently recognized cause of ARF. The drugs associated with this renal hypersensitivity reaction include sulfonamides, sulfonamide diuretics, furosemide, diphenylhydantoin, cephalosporins, phenylbutazone, allopurinol, phenindione, rifampin, penicillin, and penicillin-homologs [26–32]. These reactions are generally associated with increased eosinophils in blood and urine: A Wright's stain of the urine is useful in detecting the eosinophiluria. Fever and skin rash are also frequent findings. This elderly woman received nafcillin and had a skin rash, thus suggesting the possibility of interstitial nephritis. The patient's fever, however, preceded the occurrence of the ARF. The immediate onset of the oliguria on the first day of penicillin homolog administration would be rare unless an amnestic reaction had occurred. No previous history of penicillin allergy, however, was noted. The patient's pyuria and hematuria are compatible with the diagnosis of acute interstitial nephritis.

The possible occurrence of another myocardial infarction, as evidenced by the finding of new Q waves, and septicemia also may have contributed to the ARF. Although fever and shaking chills occurred during the administration of a blood transfusion, other causes of fever must be considered. Culture of both the patient's blood and the transfused blood would have been helpful. ARF associated with septicemia is more common in the older age group. Immune complex glomerular disease associated with bacterial endocarditis [33] and abdominal abscesses [34] also might be considered, but again the rapidity of the onset of ARF in this patient makes both of these possibilities unlikely. A decrease in serum complement concentration, RBC casts in the urine, and positive blood cultures are important diagnostic features of diffuse proliferative glomerulonephritis associated with bacterial endocarditis [33]; none of these were noted in this patient. In patients with abdominal abscesses, however, neither positive blood cultures nor decreased serum complement concentrations are consistent findings [34].

Despite the profusion of potential predisposing and etiologic factors, the temporal association between the transfusion reaction with hemoglobinuria and the onset of oliguria provides the most likely explanation for the ARF in this patient. It is noteworthy that hemoglobin infusion alone has not provided a reproducible model of ARF; it appears that the addition of RBC stroma, or prior volume depletion, or both may play a critical role [35]. It is also important to emphasize that the presence of a benzidine-positive pigment in the RBC-free supernatant of the urine does not distinguish between hemoglobinuria and myoglobinuria. Myoglobinuria has come to be recognized more frequently as a cause of ARF [36]; as with hemoglobinuria, however, predisposing factors are important. Since myoglobin (mol wt, 17,000 daltons) is much smaller than hemoglobin (mol wt, 69,000 daltons) and since only hemoglobin has a plasma-binding protein (haptoglobin), the plasma is generally pink with hemoglobinemia and its normal straw color with myoglobinemia. Muscle damage secondary to pressure or trauma, viral infections (e.g., influenza), acute hypophosphatemia, hypokalemia, alcoholism, and heroin abuse are examples of important clinical settings in which myoglobinuria may occur. A substantial elevation in the activity of the muscle enzymes (aldolase, creatinine phosphokinase) is a hallmark of this condition. Unless a sensitive immunologic test is available, it may be very difficult to establish the presence of myoglobinuria with certainty; therefore, the diagnosis is generally inferred by the presence of a benzidine-positive pigment in the urine in the face of normal-appearing serum, elevated muscle enzyme activity in the plasma, and a proper clinical setting.

Pathophysiology of ARF

In keeping with the many predisposing and etiologic factors in ARF, the pathophysiology of this condition also appears to be multifactorial. This may be the reason why the pathophysiology of ARF has escaped clear delineation despite vigorous investigative efforts by many researchers over the past two decades. Some advances in our understanding of ARF, however, have been made. As implied, it now seems unlikely that any single pathogenetic sequence will account for all varieties of ARF. In addition, it is important to distinguish between initiating and maintenance factors in considering the pathogenesis of ARF. Until recently, the apparent absence of elevated intratubular pressures in a variety of experimental models of ARF and the presence of decreased renal blood flow (RBF) led many investigators to use the term "vasomotor nephropathy" to highlight the vascular role in the pathogenesis of ARF [37]. While vascular events are no doubt involved in the initiation of ARF, the maintenance of ARF probably cannot be explained solely by ischemic events. This tentative conclusion is based primarily on the finding that neither spontaneous nor pharmacologic restoration of normal RBF in man [38] or experimental animals [39,40] is capable of reversing the ARF. It is possible, however, that persistent afferent arteriolar constriction and efferent arteriolar dilatation obviate restoration of glomerular filtration pressure despite such restoration of RBF, and thus maintain the near absence of GFR.

Two recent findings have breathed new life into the theory that ARF is dependent on intratubular obstruction. First, the experimental model of ARF produced by renal artery-clamping in the rat has been found to be associated consistently with elevated intratubular pressures [41,42]. Second, and perhaps most important, when RBF is restored in experimental model of ARF, elevations in intratubular pressures are uncovered that were not detectable in the presence of continued renal ischemia [43,44]. These findings are compatible with the notion that relative tubular obstruction is an important factor in the maintenance of ARF.

The possibility that a decrease in glomerular permeability may contribute to the pathogenesis of ARF has been raised by the finding on scanning electron microscopy of "smudging" of glomerular epithelial podocytes in a model of ARF produced by high-dose norepinephrine [45]. The high doses of norepinephrine used in these studies, however, caused *irreversible* renal failure. When the dose of norepinephrine is decreased to produce a reversible form of ARF, there are no detectable changes in the ultrastructural appearance of the glomerular epithelium [46,47]. Recent studies by scanning electron microscopy of kidneys from patients with ARF have also failed to demonstrate any consistent glomerular abnormalities [48]. Although some direct micropuncture studies have found modest changes in glomerular permeability in experimental ARF [44,49], it seems unlikely that this factor is of primary importance in the pathogenesis of ARF.

It has become common practice to use the histologic term, acute tubular necrosis (ATN), and the clinical term, ARF, synonymously. Histologic studies, however, suggest that actual necrosis of tubular cells may, in fact, be present in only 10 to 20% of patients with clinical ARF [50]. The assumption that tubular necrosis was more common may have prompted the suggestion that excessive "back-leak" of glomerular filtrate across damaged tubular epithelium contributes importantly to the pathogenesis of the oliguria of ARF. Such "back-leak" has been documented in a few instances in experimental models of ARF, but generally only when severe tubular necrosis is produced [51–53]. Such a degree of tubular necrosis, however, does not occur in clinical ARF in man even when caused by nephrotoxic agents. Moreover, chronic saline loading [54] and the administration of mannitol [46] or furosemide [55] respectively can prevent the experimental ARF ordinarily induced by either mercuric chloride or norepinephrine, but do not prevent the associated tubular necrosis.

In summary, an interaction between vascular and tubular factors seems likely to be involved in the pathogenesis of ARF. An initial vascular insult may lead to events that cause relative tubular obstruction, perhaps secondary to impacted cytoplasmic blebs [56], and thereby maintain ARF. Changes in glomerular permeability and excessive "back-leak" across damaged tubular epithelium also may be contributing mechanisms, particularly when accompanied by severe ischemic insults. In this regard, the degree of involvement of any of these potential pathogenetic factors of ARF varies depending on the nature, severity, and duration of the initial insult.

Clinical Diagnosis of ARF

The clinical approach to the diagnosis of ARF must focus primarily on the exclusion of immediately reversible prerenal or postrenal factors [57]. Thus, ARF is a diagnosis of exclusion. Volume depletion, cardiac failure, and peripheral vasodilatation are the principal factors that may cause renal hypoperfusion and thus prerenal azotemia. Prolonged prerenal azotemia is probably the most common cause of ARF. Next, postrenal or obstructive factors must be excluded as a cause of azotemia. A postvoid urethral catheterization to assess residual bladder urine volume is used to exclude bladder neck or urethral obstruction. A flat plate radiograph of the abdomen can detect the 90% of renal calculi that are radiopaque. As used in the patient described here, renal ultrasonography and renal scan are noninvasive procedures which are useful in assessing the presence of upper urinary tract obstruction. Since the infusion of radiopaque contrast media has been reported with increasing frequency to cause or worsen ARF, high-dose i.v. pyelography must be used with caution to exclude urinary tract obstruction [58]. Patients with diabetes [59] and those with hyperuricemia or multiple myeloma [60] are particularly prone to develop ARF following administration of radiographic contrast media. The factors that predispose the diabetic patient to ARF following the use of radiocontrast media are (1) age greater than 55 years; (2) presence of renal insufficiency; (3) the presence of diabetes for more than 10 years with vascular complications, neuropathy, and retinopathy; (4) proteinuria; (5) dehydration; and (6) recent administration of nephrotoxic drugs. Many of these factors are similar to those that predispose patients to aminoglycoside nephrotoxicity. It should also be emphasized that nondiabetic patients without myeloma or hyperuricemia may be predisposed to ARF from contrast media studies [61]. Preexisting renal disease and advanced age are probably the most important factors in these patients. Contrast media-induced ARF is characterized by a rapid onset of oliguria, with a peak serum creatinine concentration reached within 3 to 6 days, followed by gradual recovery. Those patients with markedly elevated serum creatinine concentrations (> 3 to 6 mg/100 ml), however, may develop irreversible ARF [62].

Careful examination of the urine sediment and analysis of the biochemical composition of the urine are very important in the diagnosis of ARF. As already emphasized, urinary eosinophils suggest interstitial nephritis, whereas RBC casts suggest vasculitis or glomerulonephritis. A normal urine sediment suggests the presence of prerenal or postrenal azotemia.

In a recent prospective study from our laboratory, several urinary findings were evaluated to assess their diagnostic value in patients with azotemia [63]. The results of this study are shown in Table 1. In those patients whose azotemia was reversible by correction of a prerenal factor (e.g., volume depletion) within 24 h, the urinary indexes were generally as follows: urinary osmolality, > 500 mOsm/kgH_2O; urinary sodium, <20mEq/liter; urine to plasma ruea nitrogen ratio, > 8; and urine to plasma creatinine ratio, > 40. By contrast, in those patients who followed a course of oliguric renal failure the urinary indexes were generally as follows: urinary osmolality, < 350 mOsm/kgH_2O; urinary sodium, > 40 mEq/liter; urine to plasma urea nitrogen ratio, < 3; and urine to plasma creatinine ratio, < 20. In general, patients with acute glomerulonephritis had urinary indexes similar to those observed with prerenal azotemia, and patients with azotemia secondary to urinary tract obstruction had urinary indexes similar to oliguric ARF. The urinary indexes of patients with nonoliguric (> 800 ml/day) renal failure were similar to oliguric renal failure except the mean urinary sodium concentration was somewhat lower. Urinary sodium concentrations (< 20 mEq/liter) in our nonoliguric patients were, however, not as low as those observed by Vertel and Knochel [64] in burn patients; perhaps the large volumes of crystalloid-free solutions administered to burn patients with nonoliguric renal failure account for their much lower urinary sodium concentrations. Although these urinary indexes were discriminating in 80% of patients, approximately 20% of patients had indexes in an intermediate, nondiagnostic zone (e.g., urinary osmolality, 350–500 mOsm/kgH_2O; urinary sodium, 20–40 mEq/liter; urine to plasma urea nitrogen ratio, 3 to 8; and urine to plasma creatinine ratio, 20 to 40). This nondiagnostic zone could be narrowed, however, by the use of such derived indexes as the "renal failure index" [(urinary sodium, mEq/liter)/(urine to plasma creatinine ratio)] and the fractional sodium excretion index [(urine to plasma sodium ratio)/(urine to plasma creatinine ratio) × 100]. These two measures tended to be < 1 in prerenal azotemia and > 1 in patients with oliguric or nonoliguric renal failure.

Those patients whose urinary indexes fell within the nondiagnostic zone may well have been progressing from prerenal azotemia to ARF.

Table 1. Urinary diagnostic indexes for prerenal azotemia (PA), acute oliguric renal failure (AORF), acute nonoliguric renal failure (ANRF), acute obstructive uropathy (AOU), and acute glomerulonephritis (AG)

	PA	AORF	ANRF	AOU	AG
Urine osmolality (mOsm/kg H_2O)	518 ± 35	369 ± 20	343 ± 17	393 ± 39	385 ± 61
Urine sodium (mEq/liter)	18 ± 3	68 ± 5	50 ± 5	68 ± 10	22 ± 6
Urine/plasma urea nitrogen ratio	18 ± 7	3.0 ± 0.5	7 ± 1	8 ± 4	11 ± 4
Urine/plasma creatinine ratio	45 ± 6	17 ± 2	17 ± 2	16 ± 4	43 ± 7
Renal failure index (see text)	0.6 ± 0.1	10 ± 2	4 ± 0.6	8 ± 3	0.4 ± 0.1
Fractional excretion of filtered sodium (%)	0.4 ± 0.1	7.0 ± 1.4	3.0 ± 0.5	6 ± 2	0.6 ± 0.2

Note: Values are expressed as mean ± 1 SEM.

Source: Data from Ref. 63 and reproduced with permission of Annals of Internal Medicine.

It is tempting to suggest that it is this group of patients, in fact, who might benefit from prophylactic measures designed to prevent the development of ARF. In this regard, there is recent evidence suggesting that the efficacy of prophylactic measures relates to their ability to increase the rate of solute excretion; increased solute excretion, in turn, may exert its effect by attenuating secondary tubular obstruction [46,65]. Although the renin-angiotensin system [66] and cell swelling [67] have been proposed as vascular mediators in the pathogenesis of ARF, prophylaxis in experimental ARF can be dissociated from renal tissue renin [68] and extracellular fluid osmolality [46]. Administration of isotonic or hypertonic mannitol or furosemide with prompt replacement of urinary losses is most effective in increasing solute excretion rate and attenuating the ARF induced by low doses of norephinephrine [46,55].

Those measures that increase solute excretion may also have the capacity to convert oliguric to nonoliguric renal failure. This effect on urine flow may be quite important in view of a recent study in patients with azotemia that demonstrated a lower mortality in nonoliguric versus oliguric renal failure (26% versus 50%; $P < 0.05$) [24]. Morbidity (e.g., infection, gastrointestinal bleeding, fluid overload) was also lower in patients with nonoliguric ARF, and only 28% of these patients required dialysis as compared to 84% of patients with oliguric ARF [244]. These beneficial effects associated with increased urine flow occurred whether the nonoliguric ARF was spontaneous or whether it had been converted from an oliguric ARF by furosemide administration. The results also provide some clues about which patients are more likely to convert from oliguric to nonoliguric ARF in response to furosemide therapy. Those patients who responded to furosemide by converting from oliguric to nonoliguric ARF had significantly lower mean serum creatinine concentrations (3.8 mg vs. 5.0 mg/100 ml), lower urinary sodium concentrations (47 mEq vs. 67 mEq/liter), and lower fractional sodium excretions (2.9 vs. 6.9) as compared to those who remained oliguric [24]. These results suggest that early diagnosis through appropriate assessment of urinary indexes will be essential if furosemide is to improve morbidity and mortality in patients with ARF by inducing a nonoliguric state. As already suggested, it is conceivable that evolution to ARF may be prevented by furosemide or mannitol in those patients whose urinary indexes are in the nondiagnostic transition zone between prerenal azotemia and ARF. Of course, the use of these agents for this purpose is no substitute for and should only follow correction of any prerenal factor that may be present, such as hypovolemia or congestive heart failure. Moreover, a prospective, randomized study remains to be performed to document the efficacy of furosemide or mannitol in preventing or attenuating ARF in man. In this regard, past failures to demonstrate any efficacy for furosemide in man [69] or in experimental animals [70] may reflect administration of the agent too late in the course of the ARF [69] or inadequate replacement of urinary water and electrolyte losses with consequent volume depletion [70]. In the patient discussed today, early assessment of urinary indexes, restoration of blood volume, and a trial with furosemide might have converted an oliguric to a nonoliguric ARF.

Treatment

The use of hemodialysis in the Korean War diminished mortality of ARF from 95% to approximately 50 to 75% [71]; since then, however, the mortality among patients with traumatic ARF has not diminished further [72]. Certainly, much of the mortality in ARF is due to a complicating illness or illnesses. Nevertheless, since infection still remains the primary cause of death, it is possible that the uremic state predisposes to these infections [73] Thus, more efficient and earlier dialysis might further diminish the mortality rate in ARF. In this regard, some studies suggest that early dialysis, prior to the onset of uremic symptoms, may decrease mortality in ARF. This prophylactic approach involves using dialysis to maintain the serum creatinine concentration below 8 to 10 mg/100 ml and the BUN concentration below 100 mg/100 ml. This method, however, may still not be adequate to avoid some complications of uremia, such as the increased frequency and severity of infections.

Some evidence in support of this possibility is derived from a small series of military casualties in Viet Nam [74]. Two groups of comparably traumatized casualties were studied. In one group in which the BUN concentration was maintained below 50 mg/100 ml and the serum creatinine concentration below 5 mg/100 ml, the mortality was 37% (three of eight patients died); in another group in which the BUN concentration was maintained only below 120 mg/100 ml and the serum creatinine concentration below 10 mg/100 ml, the mortality was 80% (eight of ten patients died). Based on these limited findings, it would seem reasonable to explore further the possibility that a dialysis schedule more aggressive than presently used for "prophylaxis" might further decrease the mortality of ARF. With respect to the patient discussed here, arrangements to transfer her for dialysis at a time when the serum creatinine and BUN concentration had already reached 12 mg and 130 mg/100 ml, respectively, were made somewhat late in her course. An earlier transfer would have allowed for earlier evaluation and dialysis.

Fluid restriction, as undertaken in this patient, is appropriate in patients with oliguric ARF. It should be remembered, however, that patients with nonoliguric renal failure must receive adequate fluid and electrolytes to replace urinary and insensible losses. Failure to provide such fluid and electrolyte replacement in this setting may convert nonoliguric ARF to oliguric ARF with its attendant higher morbidity and mortality. The elderly woman was treated with a low-protein Giovanetti diet prior to institution of hemodialysis. Although this diet may be of value in chronic renal failure, its use in ARF is probably not appropriate. Restriction of protein, albeit of high quality, may indeed retard the rate of development of azotemia and delay the need for hemodialysis. On the other hand, Abel et al. [75] have demonstrated that hyperalimentation with glucose and amino acids—the so-called renal failure fluid—is associated with more rapid recovery of patients with ARF as well as with a lower mortality in those patients who required dialysis. Although this prospective study awaits confirmation, it seems appropriate, particularly in patients who are hypercatabolic because of fever, trauma, or rhabdomyolysis, to institute hyperalimentation using a similar type of parenteral fluid. Further support for this approach is provided by the observation that amino acid supplementation enhances recovery from experimental ARF [76].

The choice of either peritoneal dialysis or hemodialysis depends on a number of factors including the availability of equipment and trained personnel for hemodialysis. Although hemodialysis has certain disadvantages, such as greater hemodynamic stress, the requirement for anticoagulation, a need for vascular access, and a higher incidence of the dysequilibrium syndrome, it is much more efficient and clearly the method of choice in the hypercatabolic patient. The state of catabolism in the patient with ARF is often apparent from the clinical history and can be gauged by the rate of biochemical changes. General biochemical guidelines for determining whether a patient is catabolic or noncatabolic are listed in Table 2. Peritoneal dialysis is a simpler and more economic means of dialysis and is quite acceptable in the noncatabolic patient, barring recent intraabdominal surgery or the presence of abdominal adhesions. A major disadvantage is the elevation of the dia-

Table 2. Biochemical parameters suggesting hypercatabolism in patients with acute renal failure.

BUN	> 30 mg/100 ml/day increase
Serum creatinine	> 1 mg/100 ml/day increase
Serum potassium	> 1 mEq/liter/day increase
Serum uric acid	> 15 mg/100 ml[a]
Serum phosphate	> 8–10 mg/100 ml, frequently with severe hypocalcemia, < 6 mg/100 ml
Serum bicarbonate	> 2 mEq/liter/day decrease

[a]Urine uric acid to creatinine ratio > 1 suggests hyperuricemia was cause rather than consequence of acute renal failure.

Source: Data from Ref. 77.

phragm produced by the fluid in the peritoneal cavity; diaphragmatic immobility may lead to pulmonary complications such as atelectasis and pneumonia and worsen chronic obstructuve pulmonary disease, if present.

In closing, it is well to remember the quote by Smith [78], which highlights the importance of normal renal function in man: "Bones can break, muscles can atrophy, glands can loaf, even the brain can go to sleep, without immediately endangering our survival; but should the kidneys fail . . . not bone, muscle, gland, nor brain could carry on."

Questions and Answers

Dr. John T. Harrington: What was the time course over which intratubular pressures were measured in the experimental model of ARF evoked by clamping of the renal artery [41,43]?

Dr. Schrier: At approximately 2 to 4 h, intratubular pressures were increased, but at 24 h they were normal. At 24 h, however, if sufficient saline solution was administered to restore RBF to normal, intratubular pressures were found to be increased. Other studies using the experimental model of ARF produced by norepinephrine in low doses [44,46] also have demonstrated that intratubular pressures are higher than normal when the RBF is returned to control levels.

Dr. Harrington: Do intratubular pressures in the low-dose norepinephrine model of ARF fall back to normal after a few days even though normal renal hemodynamics are maintained? If intratubular pressures are elevated sufficiently by tubular obstruction, filtration might well cease, allowing tubular pressure to return to normal.

Dr. Schrier: To my knowledge there are insufficient data to answer your question, but your proposal seems likely. For example, complete ureteral ligation will increase intratubular pressures, which will eventually return to normal through one or more mechanisms that are not well understood such as tubular compliance, and reflex pathways. Thus, an element of tubular obstruction is difficult to exclude at almost every stage of ARF even though the absolute intratubular pressures are not found to be elevated at all times.

Dr. F. John Gennari *(Renal Service, NEMC)*: I would like to sound a note of caution in the use of a single overall mortality figure of 50 to 60% for ARF. It is well recognized that ARF can be divided into subgroups with widely divergent mortality rates. For example, mortality may be near zero in young patients with ARF induced by a nephrotoxin or an incompatible blood transfusion; by contrast, patients with ARF and severe trauma or extensive burns may have a mortality rate of 80 to 100%. In order for a prospective study to provide truly useful information concerning the value of a particular treatment in patients with ARF, the patients in each study group should be paired according to the illness on which the ARF is superimposed.

Dr. Schrier: These are good points. A related question is whether the failure to reduce the mortality in ARF over the last 30-odd years is explained by the fact that we are dealing with sicker patients. That is to say, if we could go back 2 to 3 decades and apply our modern techniques, could we bring the mortality rate down to 20%? This contention can be neither proved nor disproved. It could be argued that some of the changes in the mix of patients with ARF over the past 30 years should actually have improved the mortality figures. For example, the mortality rate of patients with aminoglycoside-induced ARF may be as low as 18% [24]. There is no question that any study of a randomized large group of patients with ATN, containing comparable numbers of good-risk and poor-risk subgroups, would be most helpful. Granted, to pair patients may be even better, but it is very hard to obtain adequate numbers of patients using this approach.

Dr. Jerome P. Kassirer: How do you interpret the recent micropuncture study of ARF by Baylis et al. [79] on glomerular permeability with aminoglycosides? As I recall, these investigators suggested that the reduction in filtration coefficient (Kf) might be responsible for the decrease in glomerular function, at least in their particular rat model.

Dr. Schrier: That study demonstrated that rats given 4 mg/kg of gentamicin had a measurable reduction in GFR, which could be explained largely on the basis of a diminished Kf. The magnitude of the fall in GFR was not sufficient to cause azotemia, but it certainly could be a potential contributing pathogenetic mechanism.

Dr. Kassirer: Might a larger dose of an aminoglycoside produce a greater diminution in Kf and GFR?

Dr. Schrier: In the study by Baylis et al. [79] the decrease in Kf in the group of rats receiving 40 mg/kg was not greater than that in a group of rats receiving 4 mg/kg. The decrease in GFR was greater in the group receiving 40 mg of gentamicin, thus demonstrating the importance of other glomerular factors. Of course, it is always possible that results obtained using these very large doses of aminoglycosides in rats may not be directly applicable to man.

Dr. Jordan J. Cohen: Your comments suggested that gentamicin-induced ATN may be slowly progressive and may continue to worsen after administration of the agent is discontinued. In your experience, how long can the serum creatinine concentration continue to increase once the drug is stopped?

Dr. Schrier: Because aminoglycosides accumulate and persist in the renal cortex, discontinuation of the drug will not rapidly reverse the azotemia and improvement may take several days to weeks.

Dr. Jeffrey Krant *(Renal Fellow, NEMC)*: In evaluating a patient suspected of having ATN, do you think it is necessary to obtain a urine to plasma creatinine ratio as well as a urinary sodium concentration?

Dr. Schrier: As mentioned earlier, I think there is some evidence for a nondiagnostic zone in which patients who are evolving from prerenal failure to ATN may fall [63]. This area of overlap between prerenal failure and ATN seems to be smaller when the renal failure index (urinary sodium/urine to plasma creatinine) is used. Before we performed our study, my bias was that the urine to plasma creatinine ratio would be more valuable than the urinary sodium concentration; this possibility was not substantiated. We had a 20% overlap of patients whether the urinary sodium concentration or urine to plasma creatinine concentration was used. Combining this information in the renal failure index was helpful, however. Even so, a significant percentage of patients still fall into a nondiagnostic zone.

Dr. Cohen: In your study [24], what criteria were used to assign patients into the ATN group?

Dr. Schrier: This categorization was done by correcting all prerenal factors that could be identified; those patients in whom azotemia was reversed within 24 h by correction of prerenal factors were considered to have had prerenal failure. We also excluded urinary tract obstruction, which occurred in 8% of the patients with azotemia. This latter exclusion was important, since the urinary indexes with obstruction were similar to those in ATN. Thus, a diagnosis of ATN was made by excluding prerenal and postrenal (obstructive) causes of azotemia.

Dr. Nicolaos E. Madias *(Renal Service, NEMC)*: What constitutes an adequate trial with furosemide?

Dr. Schrier: It is known that furosemide may induce a significant diuresis when the GFR is less than 10 ml/min. A dose of 300–600 mg of furosemide may be necessary, however, to induce a diuresis in the presence of either advanced acute or chronic renal impairment.

Dr. Cohen: Some have argued that administration of mannitol is a useful prophylactic maneuver, e.g., in patients undergoing abdominal aortic aneurysm surgery. Considering the information you now have, do you think pretreatment of high-risk patients with furosemide would be worthwhile?

Dr. Schrier: On the basis of our experimental studies in low-dose norepinephrine-induced ARF [46,47,55,65], the common parameter of prophylaxis seemed to be increased solute excretion, not the particular agent used. Thus, furosemide administration should theoretically be as effective as mannitol if volume depletion is avoided. In the absence of volume depletion, the large volumes of administered saline necessary to achieve solute excretion rates comparable to those obtained following mannitol or furosemide administration makes saline a less desirable prophylactic agent.

References

1. McMurray SD, Luft FC, Maxwell, DR, Hamburger RJ, Futty D, Szwed JJ, Lavelle, KJ, Kleit SA: Prevailing patterns and predictor variables in patients with acute tubular necrosis. Arch Int Med 138:950–951, 1978
2. Robson AM: Glomerular filtration rate, other clearances, and tubular maxima values. In Altman PH, Katz DD (eds.): Human Health and Disease. Bethesda, Federation of American Societies for Experimental Biology, 1977, pp. 194–199
3. Henrich WL, Berl T, McDonald KM, Anderson RJ, Schrier RW: Role of angiotensin II, renal nerves and prostaglandins in renal hemodynamics during hypotensive hemorrhage. Am J Physiol 235:F46–F51, 1978
4. Henrich WL, Anderson RJ, Berns AS, McDonald KM, Paulsen PJ, Berl T, Schrier RW: The role of renal nerves and prostaglandins in control of renal hemodynamics and plasma renin activity during hypotensive hemorrhage. J Clin Invest 61:744–750, 1978
5. Jaenike JR: The renal lesion associated with hemoglobinemia: a study of the pathogenesis of the excretory defect in the rat. J Clin Invest 46:378–386, 1967
6. Weaver LC: Cardiopulmonary sympathetic afferent influences on renal nerve activity. Am J Physiol 233(5):H592–9, 1977
7. Gorfinkel JH, Szidon JP, Hirsch LJ, Fishman AP: Renal performance in experimental cardiogenic shock. Am J Physiol 222:1260, 1972
8. Mazze RI, Shue GL, Jackson SH: Renal dysfunction associated with methoxyflurane anesthesia: A randomized, prospective clinical evaluation. JAMA 216:278–288, 1971
9. Cousins MJ, Mazze RI: Methoxyflurane nephrotoxicity: A study of dose-response in man. JAMA 225:1611–1616, 1973
10. Cousins MJ, Greenstein LR, Hitt BA, Mazze RI: Metabolism and renal effects of enflurane in man. Anesthesiology 44:44–53, 1976
11. Eichhorn JH, Hedley-White J, Steinman TI, Kaufmann JM, Laasberg LG: Renal failure following enflurane anesthesia. Anesthesiology 45:557– 560, 1976
12. Luft FC, Yum, MN, Kleit SA: Comparative nephrotoxicities of netilmicin and gentamicin in rats. Antimicrob Agents Chemother 10:845–849, 1976
13. Luft FC, Patei V, Yum MN, Patei B, Kleit SA: Experimental aminoglycoside nephrotoxicity. J Lab Clin Med 86:213–220, 1975
14. Kunin CM: Binding of antibiotics to tissue hemogenates. J Infect Dis 121:55–64, 1970

15. Luft FC, Kleit SA: Renal parenchymal accumulation of aminoglycoside antibiotics in rats. J Infect Dis 130:656–659, 1974
16. Fabre J, Rudhardt M, Blanchard P, Regamey C: Persistence of sisomicin and gentamicin in renal cortex and medulla compared with other organs and serum of rats. Kidney Int 10:444–449, 1976
17. Bennett WM, Plamp C, Porter GA: Drug-related syndromes in clinical nephrology. Ann Int Med 87:582–590, 1977
18. Lane AZ, Wright GE, Blair DC: Ototoxicity and nephrotoxicity of Amikacin. Proc U.S. Amikacin Symposium, Univ. of California Medical School, Los Angeles, November 9–10, 1976. Am J Med 62:911–918, 1977
19. Bennett WM, Hartnett MN, Gilbert D, Houghton D, Porter GA: Effect of sodium intake on gentamicin nephrotoxicity in the rat. Proc Soc Exp Biol Med 151:736–738, 1976
20. Butkus DE, De Torrente A, Terman DS: Renal failure following gentamicin in combination with clindamycin. Nephron 17:307, 1976
21. Lawson DH, Macadam RF, Singh H, Gavias H, Hartz S, Turnball D, Linton AL: Effect of furosemide on antibiotic-induced renal damage in rats. J Infect Dis 126:593–600, 1972
22. Dellinger P, Murphy T, Pinn V, Barza M, Weinstein L: The protective effect of cephalothin against gentamicin-induced nephrotoxicity in rats. Antimicrob Agents Chemother 9:172–178, 1976
23. Hewitt WL: Gentamicin: toxicity in perspective. Postgrad Med J 50(Suppl 7):55–59, 1974
24. Anderson RJ, Linas SL, Berns AS, Henrich WL, Miller TR, Gabow PA, Schrier RW: Nonoliguric acute renal failure. N Engl J Med 296:1134–1138, 1977
25. Ginsburg DS, Quintanilla AP, Levin M: Renal glycosuria due to gentamicin in rabbits. J Infec Dis 134:119–122, 1976
26. Appel GB, Neu HC: Nephrotoxicity of antimicrobial agents. I, II, and III. N Engl J Med 296:663–670, 722–728, 783–787, 1977
27. Agarwal BN, Cabebe FG, Hoffman BI: Diphenylhydantoin-induced acute renal failure. Nephron 18:249–251, 1977
28. Gelbart DR, Weinstein AB, Falardo LF: Allopurinol-induced interstitial nephritis. Ann Int Med 86:196–198, 1977
29. Fuller TJ, Barcenas CG, White MG: Diuretic-induced interstitial nephritis. JAMA 235:1998–1999, 1976
30. Lyons H, Pinn VW, Cortell S, Cohen JJ, Harrington JT: Allergic interstitial nephritis causing reversible renal failure in four patients with idiopathic nephrotic syndrome. N Engl J Med 288:124–128, 1973
31. Richardson JH, Alderfer HH: Acute renal failure caused by phenylbutazone, N Engl J Med 268: 809, 1963
32. Wright JS: Phenindione sensitivity with leukaemoid reaction and hepatorenal damage. Postgrad Med J 46:452, 1970
33. Gutman, RA, Striker GE, Gilliland BC, Cutler RE: The immune complex glomerulonephritis of bacterial endocarditis. Medicine 51:1–25, 1972
34. Beaufils M, Morel-Maroger L, Sraer JD, Kanfer A, Kourilsky O, Richet G: Acute renal failure of glomerular origin during visceral abscesses. N Engl J Med 295:185–189, 1976
35. Mason AD, Alexander JW, Teschan PE: Studies in acute renal failure. I.

Development of a reproducible lesion in experimental animals. J Surg Res 3:430–441, 1963
36. Murray T, Goldberg M: Chronic interstitial nephritis. Etiologic factors. Ann Int Med 82:453–459, 1975
37. Stein JH, Lifschitz MD, Barnes LD: Current concepts on the pathophysiology of acute renal failure. Am J Physiol 234(3):F171–F181, 1978
38. Reubi FC, Vorburger C, Tuckman J: Renal distribution volume of indocyamine green, ^{51}chromium EDTA and ^{24}sodium in man during acute renal failure after shock. J Clin Invest 52:223–235, 1973
39. Hsu CH, Kurtz TW, Rosenzweig J, Weller JM: Renal hemodynamics in $HgCl_2$-induced acute renal failure. Nephron 18:326–332, 1977
40. Mauk, RH, Patak RV, Fadem SZ, Lifschitz MD, Stein JH: Effect of prostaglandin E administration in a nephrotoxic and a vasoconstrictor model of acute renal failure. Kidney Int 12:122–130, 1977
41. Arendshorst WJ, Finn WF, Gottschalk CW: A micropuncture study of acute renal failure following temporary renal ischemia in the rat. Kidney Int 10:S100, S105, 1976
42. Tanner, GA, Steinhausen M: Tubular obstruction in ischemia-induced acute renal failure in the rat. Kidney Int 10:S65, S73, 1976
43. Arendshorst WJ, Finn WF, Gottschalk CW: Pathogenesis of acute renal failure following renal ischemia in the rat. Circ Res 37:558–568, 1975
44. Conger JD, Robinette JB, Falk SA: Post-ischemic acute renal failure (ARF): Pathogenic events at 24 and 48 hours. Proc Am Soc Nephrol, Washington, D.C., 1977, p. 70A
45. Cox JW, Bahler RW, Sharma H, O'Dorisio T, Osgood RW, Stein JH, Ferris TF: Studies on the mechanism of oliguria in a model of unilateral acute renal failure. J Clin Invest 53:1546–1558, 1974
46. Cronin RE, De Torrente A, Miller PD, Bulger RE, Schrier RW: Pathogenic mechanisms in early norepinephrine-induced acute renal failure: Functional and histological correlates of protection. Kidney Int 14:115–125, 1978
47. Cronin RE, Erickson AM, McDonald KM, Schrier RW: Norepinephrine-induced acute renal failure: A reversible ischemic model of acute renal failure. Kidney Int 14:187–190, 1978
48. Langlinais P, Merrill RH: Glomerular alterations by scanning electron microscopy in acute renal insufficiency in man. Proc Mtg Am Soc Nephrol, Washington, D.C., 1977, Abstr p. 79A
49. Blantz RC: The mechanism of acute renal failure after uranyl nitrate. J Clin Invest 55:621–635, 1975
50. Olsen S: Renal histopathology in various forms of acute anuria in man. Kidney Int 10:S1, S8, 1976
51. Bank N, Mutz BF, Aynedjian HS: The role of "leakage" of tubular fluid in anuria due to mercury poisoning. J Clin Invest 46:695–701, 1967
52. Donohoe JF, Venkatachalam MA, Bernard DB, Levinsky NG: Tubular leakage and obstruction in acute ischemic renal failure. Kidney Int 10:567, 1976
53. Donohoe JF, Venkatachalam MA, Bernard DB, Levinsky NG: Tubular leakage and obstruction after renal ischemia: structural-functional correlations. Kidney Int 13:208–222, 1978

54. DiBona GF, McDonald FD, Flamenbaum W, Dammen GJ, Oken DE: Maintenance of renal function in salt-loaded rats despite severe tubular necrosis induced by $HgCl_2$. Nephron 8:205–220, 1971
55. De Torrente A, Miller PD, Cronin RE, Paulsen PE, Erickson AL, Schrier RW: Effects of furosemide and acetylcholine in norepinephrine-induced acute renal failure. Am J Physiol 235:F131–F136, 1978
56. Venkatachalam MA, Bernard DB, Donohoe JF, Levinsky NG: Ischemic damage and repair in the rat proximal tubule: differences among the S_1, S_2, and S_3 segments. Kidney Int 14:31–49, 1978
57. Schrier RW, Conger JD: Acute renal failure: Pathogenesis, diagnosis, and management. In Schrier RW (ed.): Renal and Electrolyte Disorders. Boston, Little, Brown, 1976, pp. 289–318.
58. Ansari Z, Baldwin DS: Acute renal failure due to radiocontrast agents. Nephron 17:28–40, 1976
59. Diaz-Buxo JA, Wagoner RD, Hatter RR, Palumbo PJ: Acute renal failure after excretory urography in diabetic patients. Ann Int Med 83:155–158, 1975
60. Myers GH, Witten DM: Acute renal failure after excretory urography in multiple myeloma. Am J Roentgenol 113:583–588, 1971
61. Van Zee BE, Hoy WE, Talley TE, Jaenike JR: Renal injury associated with intravenous pyelography in nondiabetic and diabetic patients. Ann Int Med 89:51–54, 1978
62. Kamdar A, Weidmann P, Makoff DL, Massry SG: Acute renal failure following intravenous use of radiographic contrast dyes in patients with diabetes mellitus. Diabetes 26:643–49, 1977
63. Miller TR, Anderson RJ, Linas SL, Henrich WL, Berns AS, Gabow PA, Schrier RW: Urinary diagnostic indices in acute renal failure. A prospective study. Ann Int Med 89:47–50, 1978
64. Vertel RM, Knockel JP: Non-oliguric acute renal failure. JAMA 200:598–602, 1967
65. Schrier RW, Cronin RE, Miller P, De Torrente A, Burke T, Bulger R: Role of solute excretion in prevention of norepinephrine (NE)-induced acute renal failure. Symposium on Renal Adaptation, Montreaux, Switzerland. Yale J Biol Med (In press)
66. Flamenbaum W, Hamberger R: Juxtaglomerular apparatus renin activity: Role of the renin-angiotensin system in acute renal failure. Circulation 50(Suppl.3):134, 1974
67. Flores J, DiBona DR, Beck CH, Leaf A: The role of cell swelling in ischemic renal damage and the protective effect of hypertonic solute. J Clin Invest 51:118–126, 1972
68. Thiel G, McDonald FD, Oken DE: Micropuncture studies of the basis for protection of rat kidneys against $HgCl_2$-induced acute renal failure by induction of high urine flow without renin suppression. Kidney Int 10:S191–S200, 1976
69. Epstein M, Scheider NS, Befeler B: Effect of intrarenal furosemide on renal function and intrarenal hemodynamics in acute renal failure. Am J Med 58:510–516, 1975
70. Greven J, Klein H: Renal effects of furosemide in glycerol-induced renal failure of the rat. Pflugers Arch 365:81–87, 1976

71. Teschan PE, Lawson NL: Studies in acute renal failure. Prevention by osmotic diuresis and observations on the effect of plasma and extracellular volume expansion. Nephron 3:1–16, 1966
72. Eliahou HE, Boichis H, Bott-Kanner G, Barell V, Barnoach N, Modan B: An epidemiologic study of renal failure. Am J Epidemiol 101:281–286, 1975
73. Kleinknecht D, Jungers P, Chanard J, Barbanel C, Ganeval D: Uremic and non-uremic complications in acute renal failure: evaluation of early and frequent dialysis on prognosis. Kidney Int 1:190–196, 1972
74. Conger JD: A controlled evaluation of prophylactic dialysis in post-traumatic acute renal failure. J Trauma 15:1056–1063, 1975
75. Abel RM, Beck CH, Abbott WM, Ryan JA, Barnett GO, Fisher JE: Improved survival from acute renal failure after treatment with intravenous essential 1-amino acids and glucose. N Engl J Med 288:695–699, 1973
76. Toback FG: Amino acid enhancement of renal regeneration after acute tubular necrosis. Kidney Int 12:193–198, 1977
77. Kelton J, Kelley WN, Holmes EW: A rapid method for the diagnosis of acute uric acid nephropathy. Arch Int Med 138:612–615, 1978
78. Smith HW: From Fish to Philosopher: The Story of Our Internal Environment. Summit, N.J., Ciba Pharmaceuticals, 1959
79. Baylis C, Rennke HR, Brenner, BM: Mechanisms of the defect in glomerular ultrafiltration associated with gentamicin administration. Kidney Int 12:344–353, 1977

Acute Oliguric Interstitial Nephritis

Principal Discussant
Charles van Ypersele de Strihou

Case Presentation

A 58-year-old woman was admitted to the Cliniques Universitaires St-Luc for fever of 4 days duration. The patient, a laboratory technician in a medical research unit, uses methylcholanthrene at regular intervals and without gloves handles rats as part of her duties. She had been bitten by rats on several occasions, most recently 8 days earlier. Seven days prior to admission while on holiday in France, the patient ate a spoiled pate. Six days prior to admission, she became anorectic. Three days prior to admission, she noticed herpetic vesicles on her lips. On the same day, she also developed acute right lumbar pain and her temperature rose to 38.7°C. She treated herself with one tablet of cotrimoxazole. During the next 2 days, her temperature remained between 39.5 and 40.4°C despite the continued use of cotrimoxazole and acetylsalicylic acid. Because of persistent fever and right lumbar pain, the patient returned to Belgium and was admitted the following evening.

The physical examination revealed the following data: temperature, 39.5°C; pulse, 100 beats/min; blood pressure (supine), 110/80 mmHg; chest, no rales; cardiac auscultation, grade I/VI early systolic murmur; the tip of the spleen was palpated as well as the lower pole of the right kidney; the liver was not increased in size; the remainder of the examination was unremarkable.

Laboratory findings revealed the following: blood urea, 43 mg; serum creatinine, 1.4 mg/dl; serum sodium, 131 mEq; serum potassium, 3.6 mEq; total carbon dioxide content, 23 mEq/liter; hemoglobin, 15.6 g/dl; white blood cell (WBC) count, 5200/mm^3; serum lactate dehydrogenase (LDH), 619 U (normal, 140–300 U); creatinine phosphokinase (CPK), 31.5 U (normal, 3–65 U); serum glutamic oxaloacetic transaminase (SGOT), 36 U (normal, 6–30U); serum glutamic pyruvic transaminase (SGPT), 16 U/liter (normal, 4–40 U/liter); serum bilirubin, 0.5 mg/dl. Results of urinalysis revealed the following: specific gravity, 1.015; pH, 5; no proteinuria, glucosuria, or sediment abnormalities. Several blood cultures and urine cultures, obtained during the first 24 h, were sterile. ASLO titers were within normal limits. Paul-Bunnell, Widal, and Wright reactions were negative. Serologic studies for the following agents were within *normal limits or negative: 16 different serotypes of leptospirosis; toxoplasma; influenza A and B; parainfluenza I, II, and III; adenovirus; Q fever; Eaton agent; Coxsackie B_1 through B_5; herpes; cytomegalovirus; EB virus; and hepatitis B.*

During the first two hospital days, right lumbar and abdominal pain persisted and the patient vomited once. She was treated with acetylsalicylic acid administered intravenously, but she remained febrile. Several blood cultures obtained were sterile. In the evening of the second hospital day, her temperature fell to 37.8 °C and remained below 37 °C throughout the rest of her hospital course. The patient continued to be anorectic and vomited several times; persistent right lumbar and abdominal pain required the administration of pentazosin (Fortal). Twelve hours after admission, a second urinalysis disclosed slight proteinuria (0.2 g/liter), 2 to 4 WBC per high-power field (HPF), and a few hyaline and granular casts. Urine culture was sterile. During the first 24 h, urine volume was 1050 ml. The urine contained sodium, 3 mEq; urea, 13.3 g; and creatinine, 1185 mg/liter. On the morning of the third hospital day, blood analysis revealed the following: urea, 113 mg; creatinine, 3.6 mg; hemoglobin, 17 g/dl; WBC count, 14,100/mm^3 with 83% neutrophils and no eosinophils. A morning urine sample contained protein, 19 g; glucose, 0.4 g/liter; 1 to 3 WBC and 10 to 15 red blood cells (RBC)/HPF. The 24-h urine volume at that time was only 180 ml and it contained sodium, 89 mEq; urea, 2.75 g; and creatinine, 485 mg/liter; 24-h urine protein excretion was 1.9 g. The patient appeared to be slightly dehydrated, and 4 liters of saline were administered. On the fourth day, however, the patient remained oliguric (24-h urine volume, 110 ml). Blood urea concentration increased to 180 mg, and serum creatinine concentration increased to 6.1 mg/dl. Echography revealed kidneys of normal size without evidence of obstruction.

Six days after admission, anuria persisted; blood urea concentration was 228 mg, and serum creatinine concentration was 8.8 mg/dl. Intravenous urography revealed a slight but persistent nephrogram and a normal pelvicalyceal system visible on late films. A percutaneous renal biopsy was obtained immediately thereafter, and the results will be described later. One week after admission, IgA and IgM levels were elevated at 165 and 321%, respectively. IgE and IgG levels were normal. Serum complement was at the lower limit of normal. Ten days later, the same observations were made but in addition IgG levels had increased to 138%. No specific treatment was given. Two weeks after admission, the urine volume exceeded 400 ml/day for the first time and increased to normal levels thereafter. The patient underwent hemodialysis three times in the interim. Results of urinalysis 12 days after admission revealed protein content of 5 g/liter, 50 WBC/HPF, and 10 RBC/HPF. Sixteen days after admission, the 24-h urine volume exceeded 1 liter, and protein and sediment abnormalities disappeared from the urine.

Twenty days after admission, serum creatinine concentration was 1 mg and blood urea concentration was 33 mg/dl. Results of urinalysis were normal.

Discussion

Dr. Charles van Ypersele de Strihou (*Professor of Medicine, Head, Renal Service, University of Louvain Medical School, Cliniques Universitaires St-Luc, Louvain en Woluwe, Brussels*): I should like first to discuss the patient's presentation and the initial physical and laboratory findings. In brief, she suffered for 4 days prior to admission from intense right lumbar pain and elevated temperature, while not responding to cotrimoxazole therapy. Although deterioration of her general condition was the immediate problem on admission, renal failure soon appeared and progressed to oliguria and anuria. On admission, the patient appeared to be slightly dehydrated. Urinary sediment was normal and the urinary concentration of sodium was low, whereas the urinary concentrations of urea and creatinine were elevated. Infusion of several liters of saline, however, failed to restore renal function. Dehydration can thus be eliminated as the sole cause of renal failure. Urinary tract obstruction, suggested by the right lumbar pain and the lack of urinary sediment abnormalities, can be ruled out as well because neither echographic examination nor i.v. urography demonstrated any evidence for obstruction.

The diagnostic process thus inevitably leads to primary renal disease as the cause of the severe oliguria in this patient. Acute or subacute glomerulonephritis is unlikely because she did not initially have hypertension, edema, proteinuria, or any urinary sediment abnormalities, in particular hematuria and red cell casts. It is noteworthy, however, that 3 days after admission, a second urinalysis disclosed a high protein content and red blood cells, but not red blood cell casts. Acute ascending pyelonephritis is also unlikely because (1) the patient did not have chills or pyuria; (2) her temperature remained constant after the second hospital day; and (3) urine cultures were sterile. The findings of the urine cultures, however, should be interpreted cautiously because the patient received cotrimoxazole prior to admission.

The sudden onset of oligoanuric renal failure in a patient with symmetric, slightly enlarged kidneys certainly suggests acute tubular necrosis (ATN); the dense, persisting nephrogram observed on i.v. urography also supports this diagnosis, although in one series of 20 patients both signs were absent in 20% of the patients [1]. Several features in this patient, however, are not common in ATN. A causal factor could not be identified: despite a detailed history, no toxic factors were discovered, and although an increase in temperature was seen early in her course, there was no evidence for septic shock. Slight lumbar pain may be present in ATN, but intense pain, which required potent analgesics in this patient, is not a usual finding. Lumbar pain is seen rarely, however, in toxic nephropathies such as that induced by carbon tetrachloride inhalation. Serum analysis failed to disclose any sign of hepatic dysfunction, rhabdomyolysis, or intravascular hemolysis. Finally, chemical analysis of the urine argues against a diagnosis of ATN on admission because the urinary sodium concentration was low, and the urine-to-plasma ratios for urea and creatinine were high. In a recent prospective study, Miller et al. observed a urinary sodium concentration below 20 mEq/liter in less than 10% of the patients with nonoliguric ATN [2]. Similarly, a urine-to-plasma ratio for creatinine above 40 was observed in less than 10% of these patients. A combination of these two indexes, the "renal failure index" [(urinary sodium, mEq/liter)/(urine-to-plasma creatinine ratio)], was below 1 in only 6% of the patients with nonoliguric ATN, whereas in our patient this index reached 0.6. Taken together, these observations lead us to suspect another cause of acute renal failure, namely, acute interstitial nephritis (AIN).

Acute interstitial nephritis is probably less rare than is believed currently. In a recent series of 976 patients with acute renal failure, Richet et al. performed renal biopsy in 218 patients in whom the diagnosis was not clear-cut [3]. Pure AIN was observed in 29 patients—i.e., 14%. An almost identical proportion has been reported by Wilson et al. [4]. Over the last few years, we have been more aggressive in performing renal biopsy in acute renal failure because the biopsy results provide clues not only to AIN but also to other unsuspected glomerular or vascular diseases. Richet argues that renal biopsy is indicated in all patients with acute renal failure under the following conditions: (1) when accompanied by systemic manifestations such as a cutaneous rash, arthralgias, unexplained temperature, raised level of blood eosinophils; (2) when the expected diuresis does not occur within the usual time limits; and (3) when renal failure is subacute and associated with atypical urinary features [3]. In his series of biopsies, Richet reported only a few perirenal hematomas [5]. They were encountered only in vascular renal diseases and led to nephrectomy in three patients. The frequency of this complication, though low, justifies a cautious approach to renal biopsy in acute renal failure and requires rigorous control of the hemorrhagic tendency and hypertension commonly associated with acute renal failure. Dr. Cosyns, would you report the findings of the renal biopsy?

Dr. Jean-Pierre Cosyns *(Department of Pathology, Cliniques Universitaires St-Luc, Louvain en Woluwe, Brussels)*: The renal tissue obtained by needle biopsy was composed of 25 glomeruli and a large portion of medulla. Except for one hyalinized glomerulus, the glomeruli showed only minimal abnormalities—i.e., a few polymorphonuclear neutrophils in some capillary lumina and some swelling of the epithelial cells. The vessels were normal. There was considerable congestion of the intertubular capillaries with areas of interstitial hemorrhage and there were nucleated cells in the vasa recta. There was no interstitial fibrosis. There was, however, diffuse interstitial edema and cellular infiltration predominantly in a large subcapsular area, in the boundary zone, and in the medulla (Fig. 1). The infiltrating cells were mainly lymphocytes, mononuclear cells, a few plasma cells, and rare polymorphonuclear neutrophils. There were no eosinophils. The tubular architecture was normal except for spotty tubular loss without atrophy and some dilatation in the cortex. Some epithelial linings were flattened and showed increased cytoplasmic acidophilia and nuclear density. These findings were obvious in the upper medulla, in the midportion of the cortex where a few mitoses were seen, and in the severely infiltrated subcapsular area where there was some tubular loss and rare atrophic tubules. In this area, the staining of the tubular basement membranes by PAS and PASM was very weak (Fig. 2). No overt rupture was seen. The inflammatory cells were in close relation with the altered basement membranes. A few inflammatory cells were visible between tubular

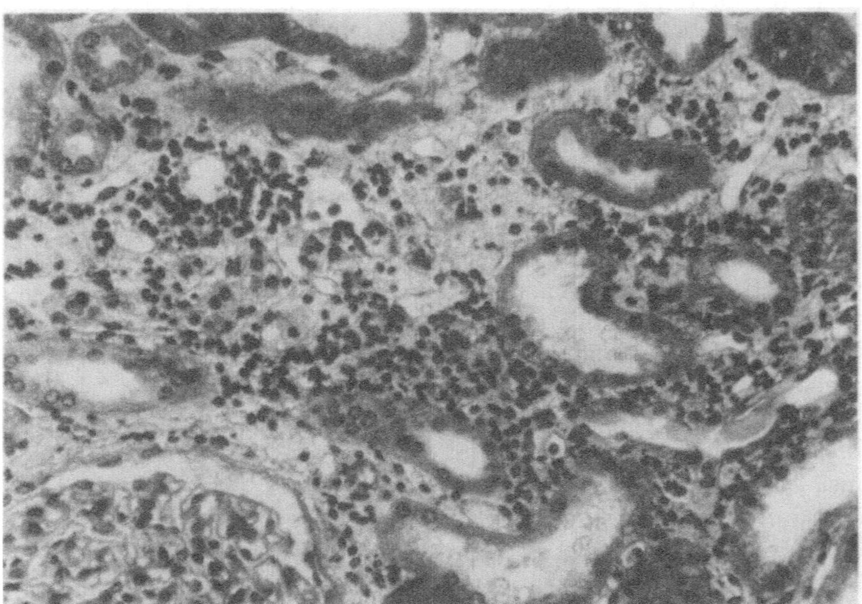

Fig.1. Subcapsular area with considerable degree of interstitial edema and cellular infiltration. There is some tubular loss but no glomerular abnormalities (trichrome, × 390).

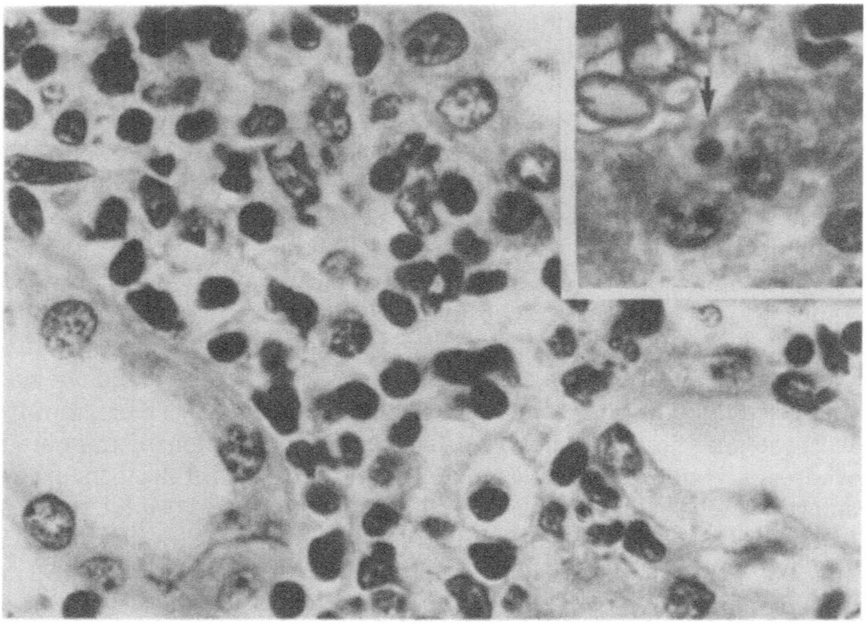

Fig. 2. Weakly stained tubular basement membranes in the interstitial areas infiltrated by chronic inflammatory cells, chiefly by polymorphonuclear leukocytes (trichrome; × 6251). Insert shows inflammatory cells (*arrow*) infiltrating between the tubular epithelial cells and the tubular basement membrane (trichome, × 1560).

epithelial cells but not in the tubular lumen. Rare eosinophilic proteinaceous casts but no granular or pigmented casts were seen. Finally, rare crystalline deposits resembling calcium oxalate were present in the lumen of cortical tubules. Direct immunofluorescent staining failed to reveal IgG, IgA, IgE, fibrinogen, or the third component of complement (C3). A few plasma cells fixed the anti-IgM antiserum. The electron microscopic examination revealed a normal glomerulus, interstitial edema, and well-differentiated tubules.

The microscopic study allows us to exclude glomerular or vascular disease. We are dealing either with ATN or AIN. This differential diagnosis is not always easy for the pathologist since shock-induced ATN with a prominent cellular interstitial reaction and AIN may be histologically similar [6]. Ooi et al. [7] have described a tubular lesion named "tubulitis" defined as the infiltration of acute or chronic inflammatory cells, or both, in the peritubular regions or between the lining epithelial cells, with or without disruption of the tubular basement membrane. This lesion is not specific to AIN since it has also been observed by the same group in a patient with ATN following abortion. Furthermore, agents such as cephalothin [6,8] or gentamicin [9] may produce either ATN or AIN. It is noteworthy that the lesions observed as a consequence of adverse reaction to certain drugs such as glafenin have been termed acute tubulointerstitial lesions [10]. These lesions seem to be representative of an "intermediate phase" between ATN, following an episode of shock, and AIN. In light of current data, observers are questioning whether these lesions should be classified as ATN with prominent interstitial cellular infiltration, or more properly as true AIN [3]. Nevertheless, in view of the clear findings of interstitial cellular infiltration, particularly in the important subcapsular area, I believe this patient has AIN. We should remain cognizant, however, both of the lack of well-defined histopathologic criteria in AIN and of the small sample of renal tissue obtained by needle biopsy, which is not necessarily representative of the whole renal parenchyma [11].

Dr. van Ypersele: We and Dr. Cosyns thus conclude that this patient has AIN. I should like to comment further on a few unusual aspects of this patient's course, and then proceed to a discussion of the possible cause of AIN in this patient.

Intense lumbar pain has been reported in several patients with AIN [12–15]. It is probably due to the distention of the renal capsule by interstitial edema, evidenced sometimes by an increase in renal size [16,17]. Interestingly, in two patients with antibiotic-induced interstitial nephritis [16,18] the lumbar pain was unilateral, as it was in our patient. A dense immediate nephrogram has also been observed in another patient with antibiotic-induced interstitial nephritis [19]. These cases viewed together suggest that i.v. urography does not help in distinguishing between ATN and AIN.

The "prerenal" characteristics of the urine observed at the onset of renal failure in our patient continue to be puzzling. Indeed, the limited data available suggest that the results of chemical urine analysis in AIN are identical with those seen in ATN. It is possible, however, that at its earliest stage AIN behaves differently. In acute ureteral obstruction, it has been demonstrated that the urine sodium concentration decreases, whereas the concentrating power of the kidney is preserved [20]. Two patients with obstructive renal failure in whom the sodium concentration was initially low have been observed [21]. It is thus possible that the results in our patient indicate an incipient intrarenal obstruction. Whatever the interpretation, it should be remembered that when the patient became oliguric, the results of urine chemistries were compatible with ATN.

What are the possible causes of AIN in our patient? Acute interstitial nephritis is a very heterogeneous condition but two major causes have been identified: drugs and infection. Our patient had not taken any drugs save acetylsalicylic acid and cotrimoxazole. Acute interstitial nephritis has been attributed to sulfonamide toxicity [22], and cotrimoxazole does contain a sulfonamide derivative. Further, acute reversible deterioration of renal function after administration of cotrimoxazole has been reported in 20 patients [23,24]; in two of those patients renal biopsy showed ATN with an interstitial reaction [23]. Two instances of cotrimoxazole-induced AIN have been reported; one patient had an increased serum concentration of IgE, and another patient had many eosinophils in the urine [18,25]. In our patient, however, cotrimoxazole toxicity does not seem to be the cause of the disease. Indeed, the amount taken was much lower than that in reported observations of acute renal failure from this agent. Furthermore, the symptoms of fever and lumbar pain antedated intake of the drug.

The presence of an infection responsible for the fever is suggested by the history, the elevated WBC count, and the evolution of serum protein changes, i.e., the early increase of IgM and IgA followed 10 days later by an increase in IgG concentration. The fact that the serum complement concentration remained at the lower limit of normal during this inflammatory reaction suggests that complement was consumed by circulating immune complexes. The concentration of immune complexes, as measured by the Cambiaso method [26], was initially at the upper limit of normal but fell subsequently. These findings should be interpreted with caution as the detection of immune complexes depends very much on the technique used; results may be negative with some techniques and positive with others. Although our observations are suggestive of an infectious disease, we must acknowledge that no causal agent could be identified. Blood and urine cultures were consistently sterile, antistreptolysin titers were normal, and the antibodies against a multitude of microbial species were normal. The spontaneous decrease in temperature suggests a viral infection. This hypothesis is further supported by the striking occurrence of acute renal failure in two additional patients, both working in the same laboratory and manipulating rats, within the 3 months preceding this patient's illness. Similarities can be seen among all three patients. Dr. Vandenbroucke, would you present briefly the history of these other two patients?

Dr. Jean M. Vandenbroucke *(Physician, Renal Service, Cliniques Universitaires St-Luc, Louvain en Woluwe, Brussels)*: As Dr. van Ypersele mentioned, a few weeks prior to admission of the patient under discussion today, we observed an identical clinical picture in two people working in the same laboratory as this patient. The first patient, a 37-year-old man, works with rats and pigeons. He suffered, a few days after his wife, with an influenza-like syndrome and was treated with phenacetin and doxacycline. Three days later he had an episode of vomiting, and 2 days later he had chills and a temperature of 39°C. At that time, the patient complained of heavy lumbar pain, predominantly on the right side, and urine volume decreased. His physician found proteinuria; the next day urinalysis disclosed the protein content to be 17 g/liter with moderate leukocyturia. Serum creatinine concentration reached 6.5 mg/dl and the patient was admitted to the hospital. Physical examination revealed hypertension (200/120 mmHg) and bilateral flank pain. Blood analysis disclosed an accelerated erythrocyte sedimentation rate (ESR) and an increased concentration of fibrinogen: creatinine concentration was 9.2 mg; blood urea was 135 mg/dl; enzymes were normal; WBC count was normal without eosinophils. Results of urinalysis revealed protein content, 0.4 g/liter; sediment, 3 to 6 WBC/HPF, 2 to 4 RBC/HPF; urine culture, sterile. An i.v. urogram showed kidneys of increased size with parenchymatous edema; excretion was symmetric but slight; there was no evidence of obstruction. During the hospital course, daily urine volume remained above 1.5 liters; there was no fever, and renal function returned rapidly to normal with no specific treatment.

Two weeks later, the second patient was referred to us for treatment of acute renal failure with massive proteinuria. The clinical history was similar: intense lumbar pain, predominantly on the right, at the beginning; a few days later, development of fever and vomiting; and proteinuria accompanied by hematuria. On admission, the patient was febrile, normotensive without symptoms of hypervolemia, but had hepatosplenomegaly and an enlarged, tender right kidney. Laboratory examination revealed an accelerated ESR and increased concentration of fibrinogen in the blood; serum creatinine, 3.4 mg; blood urea, 104 mg/dl; LDH, 764 U; SGOT, 93 U; SGPT, 74 U. Hemogram was normal: WBC count, 9200/mm^3 with monocytosis (15%) but with no eosinophils. Urinary protein was 7.3 g/liter initially but rapidly decreased; microhematuria also disappeared rapidly. During the first two hospital days the patient was oliguric; subsequently the daily urine volume increased, exceeding 1.5 liters, with a simultaneous decrease in serum creatinine concentration to normal.

In neither of these two patients did we find an etiologic factor for the acute renal failure: toxicologic research was negative and serology was negative for leptospirosis and toxoplasmosis. Only in the first patient did we observe a rise in titer for Coxsackie B_4 antibodies of questionable significance—1/128 to 1/512 and later 1/128. Immunoglobulin studies showed a transient increase in IgA concentration.

Dr. van Ypersele: The striking similarity in the courses of these three patients indeed suggests the presence of an infectious agent which to date we have not been able to identify.

I should now like to turn to a more in-depth discussion of the pathogenesis of AIN. Heptinstall defines AIN as an acute inflammatory lesion of the interstitium occasionally associated with tubular lesions but without glomerular involvement [6]. This pathologic picture is observed in a great variety of clinical renal disturbances, ranging from simple proteinuria with only slight alterations of the urinary sediment to acute renal failure. It may have various immunologic manifestations and may occur in a variety of circumstances, which suggests that AIN is the common endpoint of diverse diseases acting through different mechanisms. To the restrictively defined AIN of Heptinstall, one should add the acute interstitial lesions that may accompany glomerular or vascular diseases. It is probable that AIN, like glomerulonephritis, will be divided into a variety of subgroups in the future.

Experimental Acute Interstitial Nephritis

I plan to review the various clinical conditions associated with AIN, but first I will summarize the experimental immunologic manipulations that may induce AIN. Three different mechanisms have been identified: the first relies on immune complexes, the second on antitubular membrane antibodies, and the third on the induction of delayed hypersensitivity.

Two models of AIN demonstrate the first mechanism: The repeated injection of homologous cytoplasmic tubular (HCT) antigens [27] or the repeated administration of heterologous bovine albumin (HBA) [28] in the rabbit result in the development of interstitial nephritis characterized by mononuclear infiltration and tubular lesions. In the HCT antigen model, the glomeruli are spared, whereas in the HBA model they are involved. On immunofluorescence, granular IgG and C3 deposits are seen along the tubular membrane. In the HBA model deposits are also located along the glomerular basement membrane. The lesions in the HCT antigen model result apparently from the in situ combination of cytoplasmic tubular antigens slowly diffusing from tubular cells with circulating antibody brought by blood flow to the basal membrane. In the HBA model, immune complexes of bovine albumin and antibovine albumin antibodies are carried through the circulation into the glomeruli and along the tubular basement membrane. From these models, we may conclude that immune complexes may provoke acute interstitial reaction whether they are formed within the interstitium or are located there secondarily.

The second mechanism is demonstrated by experiments in which purified rabbit tubular membranes are injected into the guinea pig [29]. Acute interstitial nephritis develops subsequently and is characterized by cellular infiltration of plasmacytes, mononuclear cells, macrophages, and giant cells, which provoke tubular lesions. On immunofluorescent examination, linear deposits of IgG and C3 are observed along the tubular basement membrane. This model of AIN is due to the development of circulating antitubular basement membrane (anti-

TBM) antibodies, which have been identified in the circulation. Furthermore, injection of guinea pig serum induces the disease in nonimmunized recipients [30]. This reaction requires the activation of complement, at least through the alternate pathway [31–33], and probably also requires the presence of intact bone marrow cells in the recipient [34]. When the disease is transferred to a nonimmunized recipient, the injected antibody initiates the tubular lesion, but subsequently the recipient develops autoantibodies, thus amplifying the initial reaction [35]. From this model, we conclude that anti-TBM antibodies may provoke interstitial nephritis mediated by complement activation and marrow cells, which might suggest cellular immunization as well. These anti-TBM antibodies may be generated either by the injection of heterologous TBM or by the liberation of autologous hidden tubular membrane antigens. The third mechanism relies on delayed hypersensitivity. Guinea pigs or rats are injected with bovine gamma globulin (BGG) at a rate appropriate to stimulate delayed hypersensitivity [36]. Aggregated BGG is then injected into the subcortical region of the kidney. Immediately, there is an intense mononuclear cell infiltration, which destroys the tubular components. This type of interstitial reaction is certainly due to delayed hypersensitivity because it is transferable by lymphocytes but not by the serum of the donor. Furthermore, no circulating anti-BGG antibodies are demonstrated and no immunoglobulins are present in the kidney [37]. This model demonstrates therefore that delayed hypersensitivity may result in AIN if the stimulating antigen is located within the kidney.

Clinical Acute Interstitial Nephritis

How can these mechanisms intervene in human disease? I will comment only briefly on the interstitial lesions associated with glomerular diseases. Immune complexes, probably DNA and anti-DNA, are observed along the tubular basement membrane in more than half the patients with lupus nephritis [38]. Other immune complexes along the tubular basement membrane have been reported in cryoglobulinemia [38] and renal transplants [39,40]. Linear anti-TBM antibody deposits have been observed in rapidly progressive glomerulonephritis with antiglomerular basement membrane (anti-GBM) antibodies [38,40] and in renal transplants [41,42]. These observations illustrate the pathogenic role of humoral immunity in the genesis of AIN. It is noteworthy that in renal transplants the same immune challenge may result in two different types of lesions. A detailed analysis suggests that in addition to these two antibody-mediated lesions some cellular-mediated lesions—delayed hypersensitivity—are also involved.

In order to review AIN that is unaccompanied by glomerular lesions, I will follow Richet's classification [43]. This classification is based on the type of cells infiltrating the kidney: polymorphonuclear or mononuclear cells.

Acute interstitial nephritis with massive infiltration of polymorphonuclear cells and formation of microabscesses is induced by septicemias, occasionally of urinary origin. Urinary protein excretion reaches 2 to 3 g/liter and is accompanied by pyuria. Renal insufficiency is usually progressive, may be severe, and is only slowly and partially reversible. No immunoglobulins are seen in the kidney, and circulating anti-TBM antibodies have not been detected. Resolution of this type of AIN requires a careful search for the cause of the septicemia and its prompt treatment [44]. This variety of AIN was observed in 6% of the 218 patients with acute renal insufficiency biopsied by Richet [3].

Acute interstitial nephritis with mononuclear cell infiltration is more heterogeneous and may be provoked either by drugs or infection. A drug may be toxic by itself, as demonstrated by the dose dependency of the lesions. This mechanism has been invoked to account for the important interstitial lesions occasionally observed after administration of polymyxin E, cephaloridine, cephalothin, and glafenin [13,17,45–47]. Interestingly, the acute renal failure provoked by these substances may be accompanied solely by minimal tubular lesions without cellular interstitial infiltration, a picture identical to that of ATN.

In other instances, drugs act apparently through immune mechanisms: AIN is evoked by a normal dose of the drug, sometimes simultaneously with extrarenal manifestations of an immunologic conflict. The list of incriminated drugs is very long, but the most frequently mentioned are methicillin, phenytoin, phenindione, rifampin, sulfonamides, and less frequently, cephalothin, glafenin, and diuretics (Table 1) [8,48]. The delay between the administration of the drug and the onset of renal lesions varies from a few hours to several weeks.

The clinical picture is heterogeneous. Frequently, the onset of renal failure is acute and associated with hematuria, which is sometimes macroscopic, whereas a few series reveal consistent pyuria with a large number of eosinophils. Occasionally, however, renal failure develops slowly without urinary manifestations: the kidney may be increased in size with associated severe lumbar pain, or in some patients, the kidneys may be normal in size or only slightly enlarged. Renal failure is variable in severity and may require hemodialysis. Withdrawal of the offending drug is usually accompanied by improvement in renal function, providing further evidence for a cause-and-effect relationship. Readministration of the drug can lead to another episode of renal insufficiency [13,48]. Total healing is frequent, but occasionally persistent chronic renal failure has been reported [8,18,49–51].

The existence of an immunologic conflict is suggested by systemic clinical manifestations such as fever, cutaneous rash, and arthralgias.

Table 1. Prevalence of drug-induced acute interstitial nephritis.

Frequent	Rare
Methicillin	Oxacillin
Penicillin	Nafcillin
Ampicillin	Carbenicillin
Rifampin	Cephalothin
Glafenin	Tetracycline
Sulfonamides and cotrimoxazole	Thiazide
Phenindione	Furosemide
Phenytoin	Phenylbutazone
	Aminophenazone
	PAS acid
	Gold and bismuth salts
	Azathioprine
	Allopurinol
	Phenobarbital
	Cephalexin

Source: Data from Refs. 8 and 59.

These are by no means always present. An increased number of circulating eosinophils is often observed after administration of methicillin [18,52,53] or diuretics [48,54,55], in sporadic cases [56,57], and rarely after administration of drugs such as rifampin [8], glafenin [13], or cephalothin [58]. On biopsy, lymphocytes, plasmacytes, and mononuclear cells are present in abundance, often but not always accompanied by eosinophils. In a few patients, epithelioid cell granulomas with giant cells were observed [59–61]. The existence of a humoral immune reaction is also suggested by the finding on renal biopsy of linear IgG and occasionally of C3 deposits along the tubular basement membrane. This has been reported, however, only in a few instances of methicillin-, penicillin-, or phenytoin-induced AIN [52,53,59,62]. In these patients, circulating anti-TBM antibodies were also demonstrated [52,59,62]. It should be pointed out, however, that these abnormalities are exceptional: indeed, immunoglobulins were absent in the renal biopsy of the six patients with methicillin-induced AIN reported by Galpin et al. [18]. In a few patients with methicillin-induced AIN and in one patient with cotrimoxazole-induced AIN, increased serum concentrations of IgE were observed [25,63]. In a single patient with phenobarbital-induced AIN, plasmacytes filled with IgE were observed in the interstitium [64]. Usually, however, all of these parameters are normal. Further evidence for an antibody-mediated immune reaction can be found in a positive Coombs reaction in a few instances of ampicillin-, rifampin-, or glafenin-induced AIN [8,65,66]. Lymphoblastic stimulation or inhibition of leukocyte migration has been occasionally reported in AIN due to methicillin, rifampin, glafenin, phenytoin, and phenindione [13,61,62,67,68]. But, as mentioned earlier, the tests are often negative. In summary, these data suggest that the same drugs may evoke AIN through a variety of immune mechanisms, either humoral or cellular, as well as produce toxic, dose-dependent renal lesions.

The following hypothetical scheme might integrate the different pathogenic mechanisms defined experimentally with the various immunologic disturbances observed in clinical AIN. Interstitial accumulation of the drug may result either from a direct toxic effect of the drug on tubular cells with subsequent diffusion through a ruptured tubular basement membrane, or from its concentration within peritubular capillaries, or from its combination with the tubular membrane acting as a hapten. Once in the interstitium, the drug challenges immunity and induces either humoral immunization or cellular, delayed hypersensitivity immunization. Humoral reaction is either systemic, manifested in the formation of circulating antibodies directed against the drug or against the tubular membrane, or local with infiltration of monocytes, lymphocytes, and plasmacytes. These latter cells are able to synthesize immunoglobulins locally and form immune complexes in situ. Delayed hypersensitivity will bring about the invasion of the interstitium with macrophage-stimulating lymphocytes. Within this framework, it is conceivable that the same drug elicits the same tubular lesions through different immune mechanisms, the type of response being determined by the genetically determined immune responsiveness of the patient, the degree of stimulation of immunity, and the characteristics as well as the quantity of the offending agent.

Whatever the mechanisms involved, it is quite clear that it is extremely important, both in patients with acute renal failure and in those with chronic renal insufficiency who have an unexpected decline in function, to look for evidence of activation of the immune system and to suspect a deleterious role for any drug recently taken by the patient. Detection of increased amounts of eosinophils in the urine may be helpful. If there is any doubt, renal biopsy should be performed. Immunologic tests for the detection of anti-TBM, IgE, Coombs reaction, inhibition of lymphocyte migration, or lymphoblastic transformation are useful to support the hypothesis of drug-induced interstitial nephritis. This critical attitude allowed Lyons et al. [48] to modify the apparently inevitable degradation of renal function observed in some patients with glomerulonephritis simply by interrupting the administration of diuretics.

The role of infectious agents in the genesis of AIN with mononuclear infiltration has been demonstrated, although it is less extensively documented than drug-induced AIN. The streptococcus has been implicated in the context of a hyperergic reaction that is sometimes associated with eosinophilia [43,69,70] and is reminiscent of AIN following scarlet fever, described more than a century ago [71]. Leptospirosis may also produce AIN. Its mechanism has been delineated in studies performed in infected dogs [72]. The leptospires are initially found in the tubular lumen, but subsequently their antigenic material is found in the interstitium, either within macrophages or as discrete granular deposits combined with antileptospire antibodies, which are secreted locally by plasmacytes. An analogous lesion has been found in a lepromatous patient [43]: the Hansen bacillus or its antigenic component has not been identified, but plasmacytes that produce IgG have been found in the interstitium.

Toxoplasmosis [73], mononucleosis [74], and measles [4] have also been incriminated. No antibodies have been identified in situ but the viral antigens have been identified in the tubular cells. Virus-induced AIN is well documented in animals. In the fowl, infectious bronchitis virus is able to damage tubular cells and induce a mononuclear infiltration of the interstitium [75]. In the dog infected with canine adenovirus, the virus penetrates into tubular cells and destroys them. Focal necrotic material is then surrounded by lymphocytes, macrophages, and plasmacytes that are filled with IgG anticanine adenovirus antibodies [72]. Under those circumstances, however, anti-TBM antibodies have not been demonstrated.

The same scheme as used earlier for drugs can account for these observations: accumulation in the interstitium of bacterial or viral antigens, which arrive there either through tubular cells or by blood flow; formation in situ of antibodies secreted by plasmacytes; or arrival of delayed hypersensitivity lymphocytes, creating a general inflammatory reaction. Moreover, it has been demonstrated in a patient with leptospirosis that the infectious agent may elicit further the formation of anti-TBM antibodies, thus "amplifying" the initial renal lesion [76]. In addition to AIN generated by drugs or infectious agents, there are several reports in which it has not been possible to indict either of these agents because of the complexity of the situation [17,77,78].

At the end of this discussion of the causes of AIN, I should reiterate that renal biopsies of many patients with ATN do show conspicuous interstitial infiltration. This occurrence is not unusual; of the 69 patients with ATN reported by Richet [43], 15 had slight interstitial lesions and nine had severe ones. These lesions have also been described by Kimmelstiel [79], by Zollinger [80], and more recently by Pasternack [81] in patients with ATN. The origin of the infiltration has not been clearly defined: it may represent residue of hematogenous bacterial dissemination; it may be due to drug toxicity; or, as we suggested earlier, it may be attributable to autoimmune reactions.

As already stated, the course of AIN is usually favorable as soon as the offending drug is withdrawn or the infectious agent destroyed. In a few patients, however, the response was less favorable and prednisone has been administered with some success [16,18,48,54,77,78]. Recently, Galpin et al. evaluated the effectiveness of steroids in methicillin-induced AIN [18]. Of the eight patients who were treated with prednisone, serum creatinine returned to control values in six patients, and stable concentrations were obtained after an average of only 9 days. In contrast, in the six patients who did not receive prednisone, serum creatinine returned to control values in only two, and stable concentrations were obtained only after 54 days. Although these data suggest that prednisone may be effective in AIN, the incidence of residual renal functional impairment in the control group was higher than that reported elsewhere in the literature. In conclusion, I should like to point out that the more frequent use of renal biopsy in acute renal failure may be very helpful. This technique discloses unsuspected glomerular or vascular disease, allows the identification of AIN as in the patient discussed today, and should make it possible to institute appropriate treatment more promptly.

Questions and Answers

Dr. Norbert Lameire *(Instructor in Medicine, Renal Service, Akademische Ziekenhuis, University of Ghent)*: We discussed the first patient presented today earlier in Ghent, and our tentative diagnosis was salmonella food poisoning with dehydration and possible ATN. That diagnosis was based on the history of ingestion of the spoiled pate, the splenomegaly, the absence of lymphocytosis, and the pulse rate of only 100 beats/min despite a temperature of 40°C. Of course, now that the two other cases from the same laboratory have been presented, our original hypothesis must be dropped. Nonetheless, I would return to your comments on the urinary findings used to distinguish between ATN and AIN. The first urine tests revealed a low concentration of sodium and a high concentration of urea. During the first several days following admission, she received no saline and she was vomiting. That suggests to me that she had prerenal acute renal failure, which later evolved to ATN simply because of dehydration.

Dr. van Ypersele: On admission renal failure was already present as evidenced by a serum creatinine concentration of 1.9 mg/dl, but there were no clinical signs of dehydration and the patient was not yet oliguric. Therefore, I do not think that the patient initially had prerenal acute renal failure. As to the subsequent progression of renal failure, I have rarely seen prerenal failure from dehydration evolve to ATN without associated severe signs of hypovolemia, which this patient never had.

Dr. Paul Michielsen *(Professor of Medicine, Head, Renal Service, University of Leuven Medical School, Akademische Ziekenhuis, St-Rafaël,*

Leuven): With respect to Dr. Lameire's diagnosis in this patient, you dismissed the hypothesis that she had ATN secondary to dehydration. I believe we should recall that this patient took aspirin in addition to cotrimoxazole prior to admission, and that she received 1 g of acetylsalicylic acid intravenously just before the episode of dehydration. The recent work of Henrich suggests that prostaglandins seem to balance the vasoconstrictive action of angiotensin and renal nerves during hypovolemic or hemorrhagic hypotension [82]. It could be argued that the degree of dehydration seen in this patient, which would not have evoked ATN, did so here because of the earlier treatment with acetylsalicylic acid.

Dr. van Ypersele: That is an interesting idea, but I believe that hypothesis must remain speculative until sufficient data have been collected. Furthermore, this hypothesis does not fit with the interstitial infiltrate found on biopsy.

Dr. Michielsen: There is a study by Torres in which indomethacin has been shown to aggravate glycerol-induced ATN in rabbits [83]. At one time, we gave indomethacin to patients following transplantation, but we had to discontinue this practice because of the high incidence of ATN in this group [84]. Thus, these observations support my hypothesis.

Dr. van Ypersele: I think it is an alternative possibility. As Dr. Lameire already pointed out, the similar findings in the two other patients also argue against that explanation.

Dr. Jean-Pierre Godon *(Agrégé, University of Liege)*: To follow up the comments of Dr. Michielsen, we observed a case of aspirin-induced AIN several years ago in a woman who had absorbed 9 g of aspirin.

Dr. Michielsen: The clinical evolution of the two other patients was much more benign. They had an acute febrile evolution followed by rapid recovery of renal function. They did not have the protracted anuria characteristic of the first patient's course. She also had an i.v. urographic procedure before the biopsy; do you know when that took place?

Dr. van Ypersele: Yes, the i.v. urography was performed in preparation for the biopsy, which was done 2 h after urography; the patient had already been anuric for several days.

Dr. Michielsen: Are there any data that allow us to eliminate the iodine given on urography as the cause of some of the interstitial infiltration? The earliest report I know from the literature indicates that definite ATN lesions can appear 1 day after the procedure [85].

Dr. John T. Harrington: While I don't have any systematic data regarding this issue, we have performed many biopsies using fluoroscopy and

I don't believe we have seen an unanticipated degree of interstitial infiltration or edema.

Dr. Lameire: Performing i.v. urography in a dehydrated, anuric patient is certainly not without danger, and for this reason we never use this procedure preparatory to renal biopsy. Instead, we use echography prior to biopsy, which gives a very good visualization of the kidney even in a patient with anuria.

Dr. van Ypersele: I should point out that the patient was not dehydrated at the time of the urographic procedure. Dehydration had been corrected earlier.

Dr. Michielsen: Another question, if I may. Which kidney did you biopsy?

Dr. van Ypersele: The right kidney was biopsied.

Dr. Michielsen: I am somewhat puzzled by the occurrence of intense pain on the right side in this patient.

Dr. van Ypersele: As I mentioned earlier, Hamburger, who has enormous experience in this area, reports that diffuse lumbar pain in ATN may be a bit more characteristic on the right side for reasons that are not clear [86].

Dr. Lameire: If you suspect that the acute episodes of the three patients presented today have a similar etiology, you may have a slight clue to a possible cause in the rise in the antibody titer against Coxsackie virus in the second patient. As you know, Coxsackie virus has been associated with the lesions of glomerulonephritis, not interstitial nephritis [87]. May I have your comments on this possibility?

Dr. van Ypersele: First, our virologist believes that the small changes in the antibody titer against Coxsackie virus noted in our patient should not be viewed too rigorously. As I pointed out, I think AIN is a very heterogeneous condition in which most of the mechanisms that have been implicated in the development of the several types of glomerulonephritis are also involved. I quoted a report of AIN following measles, and measles has also been implicated in the development of glomerulonephritis. Thus, I don't think there is an incompatibility—as a matter of fact, it makes things more interesting.

Dr. Harrington: You mentioned earlier Richet's indications for kidney biopsy and stated that one was "prolonged" oliguria. What would you consider to be prolonged oliguria—2 weeks, 3 weeks?

Dr. van Ypersele: In our department we are slightly more conservative than Richet. I would consider oliguria that lasts beyond 1 month to be a prolonged episode.

Dr. Harrington: Earlier, you commented on the difficulty in distinguishing between ATN and AIN in the absence of a kidney biopsy. This is a specific example of a more general problem, that of making two different diagnoses affecting the same organ system. We had similar difficulties with that problem in the patients we described who had diuretic-induced interstitial nephritis [48]. All were patients who had known chronic glomerular disease and in whom renal failure slowly progressed over a matter of months. The major clue that superimposed disease was causing the renal failure was the persistence of normal kidney size. That was the primary reason for repeating the kidney biopsies. Only later, when we carefully perused the clinical records systematically, did we realize that mild intermittent eosinophilia and fleeting skin rashes had often occurred.

Dr. George Rorive *(Established Investigator, Fonds National de la Recherche Scientifique, Head, Renal Hypertension Unit, Hôpital de Bavière, University of Liege)*: I am somewhat surprised by the delay between the first symptom and renal failure. In my experience, the evolution of AIN is more rapid.

Dr. van Ypersele: The delay between drug ingestion and the onset of renal failure is highly variable—a few hours in the case of patients who have probably been presensitized, several weeks in other patients.

Dr. Rorive: I agree that the delay between drug absorption and the first symptoms varies considerably among patients. Once the clinical signs are present, however, the disease has an acute course, and the reduction in renal function is maximal within a few hours or days. The evolution of this patient was somewhat slower.

Dr. van Ypersele: The course of AIN is by no means always as acute as you suggest; in diuretic-induced AIN, for instance, the evolution observed by Dr. Harrington in his patients [48] extended over a period of several months.

Dr. Rorive: In five cases of glafenin-induced AIN, I was struck by the rapidity of the evolution, which lasted 3 or 4 days. One patient complained of lumbar pain and three had anuria; urine volume returned to normal rapidly and renal function became normal within 4 to 5 days.

Dr. van Ypersele: Your observations are in agreement with those of many others who have attributed these signs to an overdose of the drug, thus characterizing the effect as toxic, which is only part of the picture. The possible existence, documented in a few cases, of preformed antibodies should not be ignored in evaluating the clinical evolution of AIN. Once the concentration of glafenin is sufficient in the kidney, an interstitial reaction ensues.

Dr. Rorive: I should like to know if you can classify the drugs involved in AIN according to the type of immune reaction elicited by each agent.

Dr. van Ypersele: I do not believe that such a classification can be made. As a matter of fact, there is evidence that the same drug may be nephrotoxic through different mechanisms. For instance, in methicillin-induced AIN, anti-TBM antibodies have been present in a few patients. Clearly, another mechanism must be invoked in those patients in whom no anti-TBM antibodies have been demonstrated. This latter category includes the majority of patients with methicillin-induced AIN [18]. It is also possible that one mechanism, such as the development of anti-TBM antibodies, is only a secondary response that amplifies the interstitial lesions induced by another primary reaction.

Dr. Harrington: Dr. McCluskey has stated that in ten patients with drug-induced allergic interstitial nephritis they were unable to find circulating anti-TBM antibodies in any patients, yet all had similar histologic findings and clinical histories [88]. That observation would relegate anti-TBM antibodies to secondary importance.

Dr. Yves Pirson *(Physician, Renal Service, Cliniques Universitaires St-Luc, Louvain en Woluwe, Brussels)*: Dr. Masson, what is the specificity of the different types of immunologic tests that have been mentioned in identifying humoral and cellular immune reactions and delayed hypersensitivity?

Dr. Pierre Masson *(Professor of Experimental Medicine, University of Louvain Medical School, Louvain en Woluwe, Brussels)*: It is impossible, in fact, to get an immune reaction if there is no lymphoblastic transformation. Each time an immune response occurs there is a lymphoblastic transformation. Thus, it is impossible on the basis of this test to say whether the immune response is either humoral or cellular. When the antibody is detected in the blood, then of course it is a humoral response, but on the basis of just a lymphoblastic transformation I would not dare to say that it was just a cellular one. The lymphocyte incorporation of thymidine, which is used in this test, will be due not only to T lymphocytes but also to the B lymphocytes and other cells that could be involved. So I would be very careful in interpreting it.

Dr. Rorive: Would you say the reverse? Would you say that if you have lymphoblastic transformation, this means that the drug could produce such an effect?

Dr. Masson: That means that the body is mounting an immune response against this drug, but it doesn't mean that the mechanism is necessarily involved in the pathogenesis of the disease.

Dr. Lameire: Patients with AIN often take one or more drugs. In one case we have seen, the patient took approximately 20 drugs. In such a patient, it is difficult to determine whether the reaction is drug related and which drug is responsible. Couldn't you then perform a lymphoblastic transformation test in which all 20 drugs would be tested, eliminate some of them, and conclude that one or another drug may be responsible?

Dr. Masson: Statistically, you increase your chances. If you have a lymphoblastic transformation with a given drug, of course you have more chance that this drug is involved. I would ask a question myself. Is AIN very often associated with other disorders? You mentioned a positive Coombs test. What I mean is, for example, is there hemolysis or thrombocytopenic purpura, or is the disorder restricted to the kidney?

Dr. van Ypersele: Hemolytic anemia has been occasionally reported, for instance in association with glafenin-induced AIN.

Dr. Rorive: Perhaps the most usual hematologic disorder is eosinophilia. Isn't it?

Dr. van Ypersele: Yes. If I may go back to the question which was put to Dr. Masson. You said that the lymphoblastic transformation test merely shows that some immune stimulation has occurred. Whether it reacts in the kidney or not is another matter. What is your feeling on the specificity of the leukocyte migration inhibition test?

Dr. Masson: Exactly the same. The specificity is certainly not better than the lymphoblastic transformation test and personally I would trust the lymphoblastic transformation more than the so-called MIF test, which is measuring the migration inhibiting factor.

Dr. van Ypersele: Why?

Dr. Masson: Oh, just for technical reasons; the lymphoblastic transformation test is easier to perform. Personally, I would recommend obtaining an intradermal reaction as soon as you suspect a drug; a simple scratch test or an intradermal injection of a small amount of this could be useful and perhaps be more informative than all of these sophisticated tests, which are somewhat fashionable. I think that sometimes a skin test can give as much information as a laboratory test.

Note Added by the Author, July 1982 The etiology of the acute interstitial nephritis in the patients described in this edition of *Nephrology Forum* remained unknown for approximately 2 years. Serum samples were saved on all the patients in case a particular etiologic agent was suspected later. In July 1981, Dr. J. Desmyter, Professor of Virology at Katholieke Universiteit Leuven (Belgium), suggested the possibility that the etiologic agent might be the virus of Korean hemorrhagic fever (KHF; or hemorrhagic fever with renal syndrome, HFRS), which has recently been renamed Hantaan virus. He sent a serum sample of the patient discussed in this forum that had been obtained in September 1979 (15 months after her discharge) to Dr. K. M. Johnson, director of the hazardous viruses program at the U.S. Army Medical Research Institute of Infectious Diseases, Fort Detrick, Maryland, for assessment of KHF antibody by indirect immunofluorescence. The substrate used was the A-459 cell line infected with KHF virus strain 76-118 (*Science* 211:1046, 1981). An anti-KHF titer of 1024 was found. Sera of the two other patients reported briefly in the discussion also were assayed at Fort Detrick. In patient 2, a titer of 1024 was found in a sample taken 3 years after the acute episode. In patient 3, a titer of 256 was found in a sample taken 2 years after acute renal failure. These values are highly specific for KHF, and KHF-reactive antibody was virtually absent in the general population.

These results strongly suggest that the acute interstitial nephritis observed in these patients was due to Korean hemorrhagic fever virus. It was subsequently demonstrated that the source of the agent was infected rats, as suggested in the discussion. The three cases represent the first known instances of human illness due to rat-borne Hantaan virus that have been documented outside the Far East.

References

1. Vandenbroucke JM, Gilbeaux JP, van Ypersele de Strihou C: Excretion urography in acute renal failure. Br Med J 3:291–292, 1973
2. Miller TR, Anderson RJ, Linas SL, Henrich WL, Berns AS, Gabow PA, Schrier RW: Urinary diagnostic indices in acute renal failure. A prospective study. Ann Intern Med 89:47–50, 1978
3. Richet G, Sraer JD, Kourilsky O, Kanfer A, Mignon F, Whitworth J, Morel-Maroger L: La ponction biopsie rénale dans les insuffisances rénales aiguës. Ann Méd Int 129:445–447, 1978
4. Wilson DM, Turner DR, Cameron JS, Ogg CS, Brown CB, Chantler C: Value of renal biopsy in acute intrinsic renal failure. Br Med J 2:459–461, 1976
5. Richet G, Sraer JD, Kourilsky O, Morel-Maroger L: La ponction biopsie rénale au cours des insuffisances rénales aiguës. Rev Prat 28:3769–3773, 1978
6. Heptinstall RH: Pathology of the Kidney, 2nd ed. Boston, Little, Brown, 1974
7. Ooi BS, Jao W, Frist MR, Mancilla R, Pollak VE: Acute interstitial nephritis. A clinical and pathologic study based on renal biopsies. Am J Med 59:614–629, 1975
8. Kleinknecht D, Kanfer A, Morel-Maroger L, Mery JP: Immunologically mediated drug-induced acute renal failure. Contr Nephrol 10:42–52, 1978

9. Solez K, Morel-Maroger L, Sraer JD: The morphology of "acute tubular necrosis" in man. Analysis of 57 renal biopsies and a comparison with the glycerol model. Medicine (Baltimore) 58:362–376,1979
10. Gaultier M, Bismuth C, Efthymiou ML, Morel-Maroger L, Romion A: Nephropathie tubulo-interstitielle aiguë au cours d'une intoxication par la glafenine. Nouv Presse Méd 46:3125–3128, 1972
11. McCluskey RT, Colvin RB: Immunological aspects of renal tubular and interstitial diseases. Ann Rev Med 29:191–203, 1978
12. Campese VM, Marzullo F, Schena FP, Coratelli P: Acute renal failure during intermittent rifampicin therapy. Nephron 10:256–261, 1973
13. Dequiedt P, Vanhille P, Devulder B, Furon D, Tacquet A: Insuffisance rénale aiguë à la glafenine. Lille Méd 20:708–714, 1975
14. Dobrin RS, Vernier RL, Fisch AJ: Acute eosinophilic interstitial nephritis and renal failure with bone marrow-lymph node granulomas and anterior uveitis. Am J Med 59:325–333, 1975
15. Kuhlmann U, Fontana A, Briner J, Steinemann U, Siegenthaler W: Akute interstitielle Nephritis mit oligurischem Nierenversagen nach Phenylbutazon-Medikation. Schweiz Med Wochenschr 108:494–499, 1978
16. Simenhoff ML, Guild WR, Dammin GJ: Acute diffuse interstitial nephritis. Review of literature and case report. Am J Med 44:618–625, 1968
17. Richet G, Fillastre JP, Ulmann A: Néphropathies interstitielles. In: Encyclopédie médico-chirurgicale, 18052 A10, 1978, pp. 11–50
18. Galpin JE, Shinaberger JH, Stanley TM, Blumenkrantz MJ, Bayer AS, Friedman GS, Montgomerie JZ, Guze LB, Coburn JW, Glassock RJ: Acute interstitial nephritis due to Methicillin. Am J Med 65:756–765, 1978.
19. Shapiro R, Kundargi R: Antibiotic nephrotoxicity: a cause of persistent bilateral nephrogram. J Urol 106:823–827, 1971
20. Suki WN, Guthrie AG, Martinez-Maldonado M, Eknoyan G: Effects of ureteral pressure elevation on renal hemodynamics and urine concentration. Am J Physiol 220:38–43, 1971
21. Hoffman LM, Suki WN: Obstructive uropathy mimicking volume depletion. JAMA 236:2096–2099, 1976
22. Robson M, Levi J, Dolberg L, Rosenfeld JB: Acute tubulo-interstitial nephritis following sulfadiazine therapy. Isr J Med Sci 6:561–566, 1970
23. Kalowski S, Nanra RS, Mathew TH, Kincaid-Smith P: Deterioration in renal function in association with cotrimoxazole therapy. Lancet I:394–397, 1973
24. Bailey RR, Little PJ: Deterioration in renal function in association with cotrimoxazole therapy. Med J Aust 1:914–916, 1976
25. Dry J, Leynadier F, Herman D, Pradalier A: L'association sulfaméthoxazole-triméthoprime (cotrimoxazole). Réaction immuno-allergique inhabituelle. Nouv Presse Méd 4:36, 1975
26. Cambiaso CL, Riccomi H, Sindic C, Masson PL: Particle counting immunoassay (PACIA). II. Automated determination of circulating immune complexes by inhibition of the agglutinating activity of rheumatoid sera. J Immunol Meth 23:29–50, 1978
27. Klassen J, McCluskey RT, Milgrom F: Nonglomerular renal disease produced in rabbits by immunization with homologous kidney. Am J Pathol 63:333–358, 1971

28. Brentjens JF, O'Connell DW, Pawlowski IB, Andres GA: Extraglomerular lesions associated with deposition of circulating antigen-antibody complexes in kidneys of rabbits with chronic serum sickness. Clin Immunol Immunopathol 3:112–122, 1974
29. Steblay RW, Rudofsky UH: Renal tubular disease and autoantibodies against tubular basement membrane induced in guinea pigs. J Immunol 107:589–594, 1971
30. Steblay RW, Rudofsky UH: Transfer of experimental autoimmune renal cortical tubular and interstitial disease in guinea pigs by serum. Science 180:966–968, 1973
31. Rudofsky UH, McMaster PRB, Ma WS, Steblay RW, Pollara B: Experimental autoimmune renal cortical tubulointerstitial disease in guinea pigs lacking the fourth component of complement (C4). J Immunol 112:1387–1393, 1974
32. Rudofsky UH, Steblay RW, Pollara B: Inhibition of experimental autoimmune renal tubulointerstitial disease in guinea pigs by depletion of complement with cobra venom factor. Clin Immunol Immunopathol 3:396–407, 1975
33. Rudofsky UH, Esposito LL, Dilwith RL, Pollara B: Studies on the pathogenesis of experimental autoimmune renal tubulointerstitial disease in guinea pigs. V. Deposition of C3PA on the tubular basement membranes. Clin Immunol Immunopathol 8:467–474, 1977
34. Rudofsky UH, Pollara B: Studies on the pathogenesis of experimental autoimmune renal tubulointerstitial disease in guinea pigs. II. Passive transfer of renal lesions by antitubular basement membrane autoantibody and nonimmune bone marrow cells to leukocyte-depleted recipients. Clin Immunol Immunopathol 6:107–114, 1976
35. Hall CL, Colvin RB, Carey K, McCluskey RT: Passive transfer of autoimmune disease with isologous IgG_1 and IgG_2 antibodies to the tubular basement membrane in strain XIII guinea pigs. J Exp Med 146:1246–1260, 1977
36. Van Zwieten MJ, Leber PD, Bhan AK, McCluskey RT: Experimental cell-mediated interstitial nephritis induced with exogenous antigens. J Immunol 118:589–593, 1977
37. Baldamus CA, Schoeppe W: Cellular immunity as a possible cause of interstitial nephritis (IN). Abst Int Congr Nephrol, Montreal, 1978, p. G13
38. Lehman DH, Wilson CB, Dixon FJ: Extraglomerular immunoglobulin deposits in human nephritis. Am J Med 58:765–786, 1975
39. McCluskey RT, Klassen J: Immunologically mediated glomerular, tubular and interstitial renal disease. N Engl J Med 288:564–570, 1973
40. Andres G, Brentjens J, Kohli R, Anthone R, Anthone S, Ballah T, Montes M, Mookerjee BS, Prezyna A, Sepulveda M, Venuto R, Elwood C: Histology of human tubulo-interstitial nephritis associated with antibodies to renal basement membranes. Kidney Int 13:480–491, 1978
41. Andres GA, Accinni L, Hsu KC, Penn I, Porter KA, Rendall JM, Seegal BC, Starzl TE: Human renal transplants. III. Immunopathologic studies. Lab Invest 22:588–604, 1970
42. Wilson CB, Lehman DH, McCoy RC, Gunnells JC Jr, Stickel DL: Antitubular basement membrane antibodies after renal transplantation. Transplantation 18:447–452, 1974

43. Richet G: Néphrites interstitielles aiguës avec insuffisance rénale. Abst Int Congr Nephrol, Montreal, 1978, pp. 707–713
44. Richet G, Mayaud C: The course of acute renal failure in pyelonephritis and other types of interstitial nephritis. Nephron 22:124–127, 1978
45. Fillastre JP, Laumonier R, Humbert G, Dubois D, Metayer J, Delpech A, Leroy J, Robert M: Acute renal failure associated with combined gentamicin and cephalothin therapy. Br Med J 2:396–397, 1973
46. Lechat P, Levillain R, Dechezlepretre S, Cluzan R: Mise en évidence de la néphrotoxicité aiguë de la glafénine chez le rat. Thérapie 29:567–573, 1974
47. Walker RG, Thomson NM, Dowling JP, Ogg CS: Minocycline-induced acute interstitial nephritis. Br Med J 1:524, 1979
48. Lyons H, Pinn VW, Cortell S, Cohen JJ, Harrington JT: Allergic interstitial nephritis causing reversible renal failure in four patients with idiopathic nephrotic syndrome. N Engl J Med 288:124–128, 1973
49. Jensen HA, Halveg AB, Saunamaki KI: Permanent impairment of renal function after methicillin nephropathy. Br Med J 4:406, 1971
50. Sraer JD, Beaufils PH, Morel-Maroger L, Richet G: Néphrite interstitielle chronique due à la phénylindanedione. Nouv Presse Méd 1:193–196, 1972
51. Mayaud C, Kourilsky O, Kanfer A, Sraer JD: Interstitial nephritis after methicillin. N Engl J Med 292:1132–1133, 1975
52. Border WA, Lehman DH, Egan JD, Sass HJ, Glode JE, Wilson CB: Antitubular basement-membrane antibodies in methicillin-associated interstitial nephritis. N Engl J Med 291:381–384, 1974
53. Baldwin DS, Levine BB, McCluskey RT, Gallo GR: Renal failure and interstitial nephritis due to penicillin and methicillin. N Engl J Med 279:1245–1252, 1968
54. Fuller TJ, Barcenas CG, White MG: Diuretic-induced interstitial nephritis. Occurrence in a patient with membranous glomerulonephritis. JAMA 235:1998–1999, 1976
55. Fialk MA, Romankiewicz J, Perrone F, Sherman RL: Allergic interstitial nephritis with diuretics. Ann Intern Med 81:403–404, 1974
56. Ooi BS, First MR, Pesce AJ, Pollak VE: IgE levels in interstitial nephritis. Lancet 1:1254–1256, 1974
57. Olsen S: Renal histopathology in various forms of acute anuria in man. Kidney Int 10:S2–S8, 1976
58. Burton JR, Lichtenstein NS, Colvin RB, Hyslop NE Jr.: Acute renal failure during cephalothin therapy. JAMA 229:679–682, 1974
59. Mery JP, Morel-Maroger L: Acute interstitial nephritis. A hypersensitivity reaction to drugs. Proc Int Congr Nephrol, Florence. Basel, Karger, 1976, pp. 524–529
60. Maher JF: Toxic nephropathy. In Brenner BM, Rector FC Jr (eds.): The Kidney, Vol. 2. Philadelphia, Saunders, 1976, pp. 1355–1395
61. Kanfer A, Kleinknecht D, Morel-Maroger L, Mery JP, Richet G: Les néphropathies aiguës immuno-allergiques d'origine médicamenteuse (NAIM). Abst Int Congr Nephrol, Montreal, 1978, p. L13
62. Hyman LR, Ballow M, Knieser MR: Diphenylhydantoin interstitial nephritis. Roles of cellular and humoral immunologic injury. J Pediatr 92:915–920, 1978

63. Ooi BS, Ooi YM, Mohini R, Pollak VE: Humoral mechanisms in drug-induced acute interstitial nephritis. Clin Immunol Immunopathol 10:330-334, 1978
64. Faarup P, Christensen E: IgE containing plasma cells in acute tubulo-interstitial nephropathy. Lancet 2:178, 1974
65. Tannenberg AM, Wicher KJ, Rose NR: Ampicillin nephropathy. JAMA 218:449, 1971
66. Kleinknecht D, Homberg JC, Decroix G: Acute renal failure after rifampicin. Lancet 1:1238-1239, 1972
67. Sheth KJ, Casper JT, Good TA: Interstitial nephritis due to phenytoin hypersensitivity. J Pediatr 91:438-441, 1977
68. Chevet D, Garre M, Thomas R, Ramee MP, Goasguen J, Alquier P: Néphropathies induites par la phényl-indanedione. Intérêt du test d'inhibition de migration des leucocytes. Nouv Presse Méd 5:588, 1976
69. Knepshield JH, Carsten PHB, Gentile DE: Recovery from renal failure due to acute diffuse interstitial nephritis. Pediatrics 43:533-539, 1969
70. Webster ADB, Hall GH: Acute post-streptococcal toxaemic renal failure. Br Med J 4:665-666, 1969
71. Councilman WT: Acute interstitial nephritis. J Exp Med 3:393-420, 1898
72. Morrison WI, Wright NG: Canine leptospirosis: an immunopathological study of interstitial nephritis due to *Leptospira canicola*. J Pathol 120:83-89, 1976
73. Guignard JP, Torrado A: Interstitial nephritis and toxoplasmosis in a 10-year-old child. J Pediatr 85:381-382, 1974
74. Woodroffe AJ, Row PG, Meadows R, Lawrence JR: Nephritis in infectious mononucleosis. Q J Med 43:451-460, 1974
75. Siller WG, Cumming RB: The histopathology of an interstitial nephritis in the fowl produced experimentally with infectious bronchitis virus. J Pathol 114:163-173, 1974
76. Daoudal P, Mahieu P, Bloch B, Barale F: Leptospirose avec immunisation anti-membrane basale glomérulaire. Nouv Presse Méd 7:3535-3537, 1978
77. Chazan J, Garella S, Esparza A: Acute interstitial nephritis. A distinct clinico-pathological entity? Nephron 9:10-26, 1972
78. Brass H, Lapp H, Heinz R: Akute interstitielle Nephritis—mögliche Ursache eines akuten Nierenversagens. Dtsch Med Wochenschr 99:2335-2340, 1974
79. Kimmelstiel P: Acute hematogenous interstitial nephritis. Am J Pathol 14:737-761, 1938
80. Zollinger HU: Interstitial nephritis. In Mostofi FK, Smith DE (eds.): The Kidney. Baltimore, Williams & Wilkins, 1966, pp. 269-281
81. Pasternack A, Tallqvist G, Kuhlback B: Occurrence of interstitial nephritis in acute renal failure. Acta Med Scand 187:27-31, 1970
82. Henrich WL, Anderson RJ, Berns AS, McDonald KM, Paulsen PJ, Berl T, Schrier RW: The role of renal nerves and prostaglandins in control of renal hemodynamics and plasma renin activity during hypotensive hemorrhage in the dog. J Clin Invest 61:744-750, 1978
83. Torres VE, Strong CJ, Romero JC, Wilson DM: Indomethacin enhancement of glycerol-induced acute renal failure in rabbits. Kidney Int 7:170-178, 1975

84. Michielsen P, Roels L: Antiinflammatoires et transplantation rénale. In Touraine JL, Traeger J, Triau E (eds.): Transplantation and Clinical Immunology. Villeurbannes, Simep Ed, 1977, pp. 180–188
85. Van Zee B, Hoy WE, Talley TE, Jaenike JR: Renal injury associated with intravenous pyelography in nondiabetic and diabetic patients. Ann Intern Med 89:51–54, 1978
86. Hamburger J, Richet G, Crosnier J, Funck-Brentano JL, Antoine B, Ducrot H, Mery JP, De Montera H, Royer P: Néphrologie. Editions Méd Flammarion, 1966, p. 682
87. Bayatpour M, Zbitnew A, Dempster G, Miller KR: The role of coxsackie virus B_4 in the pathogenesis of acute glomerulonephritis. Can Med Assoc J 109:873–875, 1973
88. Case Records of the Massachusetts General Hospital (Case 49-1975). N Engl J Med 293:1308–1316, 1975

Part II

Fluid and Electrolyte Disturbances

Introduction

The six Forums in this section deal with disorders of sodium and water conservation, with hyperkalemia, and with ketosis. The section commences with an elegant analysis by Dr. Neal Bricker of current concepts regarding sodium homeostasis in patients with chronic progressive renal disease. The focus for Dr. Bricker's discussion is a case of renal salt wasting in an azotemic man in whom renal sodium conservation was normalized by extremely gradual adaptation to a low salt intake. Dr. Bricker is Professor of Medicine and Director, Program in Kidney Diseases at UCLA School of Medicine. He uses this Forum to present a novel conceptual framework for understanding the formidable task faced by the diseased kidney in maintaining homeostasis and to explain the importance of what he has dubbed the "magnification phenomenon." He also summarizes the available data in support of the existence of a natriuretic hormone, thought to play a critical role in regulating sodium excretion in health and in advancing renal failure.

Dr. Norman Levinsky uses a case of refractory ascites in cirrhosis as a lead-off for his discussion of disordered renal sodium retention. Dr. Levinsky, Chairman of the Department of Medicine at the Boston University School of Medicine, summarizes the basic pathophysiology of salt and water retention in patients with advanced liver disease. He takes into account both the conventional view, which ascribes salt retention to a decrease in "effective" intravascular volume, as well as a provocative new hypothesis, which ascribes salt retention to a primary effect of disordered hepatic function on renal sodium reabsorption—the so-called overflow hypothesis. Dr. Levinsky brings his extensive investigative and clinical experience to bear on his analysis of the treatment of refractory ascites by well-accepted conservative measures as well as by the LaVeen peritoneal-jugular shunt.

Dr. Robert Berliner, currently Dean of Yale University School of Medicine, contributes a masterful, historical review of the development of our concepts of urine concentration. Dr. Berliner's own contributions, coupled with his personal familiarity with many of the major workers in this field, make this discussion especially insightful. As an example of the elegant coupling of form and function, the urine concentrating mechanism has few parallels in mammalian biology.

Dr. Alexander Leaf, Professor of Medicine at Harvard Medical School, discusses a case of central diabetes insipidus and examines the mechanisms and consequences of this major disorder of water conservation. He reviews the ways by which this condition can be differentiated from nephrogenic diabetes insipidus and from primary polydipsia. Dr. Leaf, who has had a longstanding interest in the mechanism of action of antidiuretic hormone, includes in his discussion of the experimental and clinical aspects of neurogenic diabetes insipidus an analysis of therapeutic alternatives. Special emphasis is given to the use of dDAVP, a potent synthetic analog of vasopressin.

A patient with sickle cell disease, persistent hyperkalemia, and hyporeninemic hypoaldosteronism affords Dr. Ralph DeFronzo an opportunity to review the normal mechanisms underlying potassium homeostasis as well as the pathophysiology of life-threatening hyperkalemia. He develops a useful classification scheme for the etiology of hyperkalemia. The increasing recognition of hyporeninemic hypoaldosteronism makes this installment of "Nephrology Forum" especially timely. Dr. DeFronzo, a well-known clinician-physiologist on the faculty of Yale University School of Medicine, assesses the experimental evidence bearing on the pathogenesis of this syndrome as a foundation for an extensive consideration of the therapy of hyperkalemia.

Dr. George F. Cahill, Jr., Professor of Medicine at Harvard Medical School, uses a case of ketosis in a diabetic patient suffering from starvation and alcohol abuse as an opening wedge in a most illuminating discussion of the biochemistry and cellular physiology of energy metabolism. One of the leading international authorities on disordered metabolism, Dr. Cahill places the processes responsible for ketosis in the general framework of intermediary metabolism, emphasizing the variety of ways in which normal regulation of ketone body production can give rise to serious clinical derangements.

Sodium Homeostasis in Chronic Renal Disease

Principal Discussant
Neal S. Bricker

Case Presentation

A 63-year-old man was admitted to the Wadsworth Veterans Administration Hospital for evaluation of azotemia and hypertension. The patient had been in apparent good health until one year earlier, when studies during a hospitalization elsewhere revealed a serum creatinine of 5.2 mg/dl, a BUN of 45 mg/dl, and 3+ proteinuria. An intravenous pyelogram was within normal limits. Hypertension was noted on admission and antihypertensive medications were given. The patient subsequently was lost to follow-up. Forty years previously the patient had been hospitalized because of transient gross hematuria of unknown cause.

On admission to Wadsworth, the patient's blood pressure was 170/100 mmHg and funduscopic examination revealed arteriolar narrowing. The cardiopulmonary and abdominal examinations were normal, the prostate was not enlarged, and no edema was present. The rest of the physical examination was within normal limits. Laboratory findings revealed serum creatinine, 10.6 mg/dl; BUN, 81 mg/dl; serum sodium, 139 mEq/liter; potassium, 5.3 mEq/liter; chloride, 107 mEq/liter; bicarbonate, 16 mM/liter; calcium, 7.2 mg/dl; and phosphorus, 4.5 mg/dl. The serum albumin, bilirubin, glucose, uric acid, and transaminase levels all were normal. Ultrasound examination revealed small kidneys bilaterally.

The patient was given a diet containing 46 mEq of sodium as part of his antihypertensive regimen. Within 36 he became progressively somnolent. The blood pressure fell to 90/60 mmHg in the recumbent position and 70 mmHg when the patient was standing.

The patient was transferred to the Metabolic Ward, where 2 liters of isotonic saline were administered and a dietary sodium intake of 150 mEq/day was instituted. Following stabilization on this diet, the patient's blood pressure returned to 150/100 mmHg, and he required propranolol for optimal blood pressure control.

As part of a protocol to determine the functional adaptation of surviving nephrons in advanced chronic renal failure, the patient was subjected to a water immersion study (Fig. 1). Control plasma volume, mea-

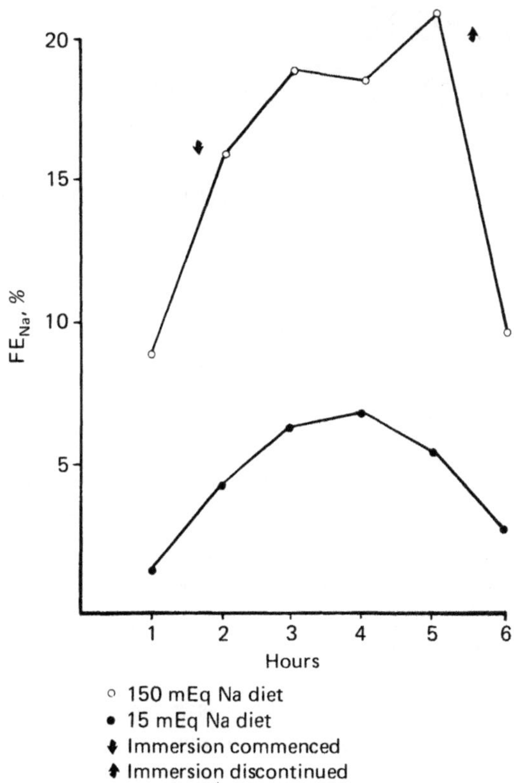

Fig. 1. The effect of water immersion on fractional excretion of sodium during two levels of dietary sodium intake. The upper curve represents the results of water immersion to the neck in an "adapted" uremic patient. The lower curve represents the results of water immersion in the same patient following "deadaptation." Details of the method of deadaptation are included in the text.

sured by dilution of radiolabeled albumin, was 1908 ml and the body weight was 71.4 kg. The patient was immersed for 4 h in the seated position in a tank of water (kept at a constant temperature of 35.4 ± 5 °C) up to his neck. Both sodium excretion and fractional excretion of sodium (FE_{Na}%) increased during immersion and returned to nearly baseline levels during the recovery period. Sodium excretion increased from 113.3 μEq/min in the 60-min prestudy period to 252 μEq/min during the third hour of immersion and returned to 101.3 μEq/min in the recovery (postimmersion) period. The FE_{Na}% rose from 9.1% in the prestudy period to 18.8% during the third hour of immersion and returned to 10.1% in the recovery period. Plasma renin activity decreased from 1.7 ng/ml/h in the prestudy period to 0.62 ng/ml/h by the fourth hour of immersion. The inulin clearance remained stable throughout the study at 9 ml/min. Following this study the sodium content of the patient's diet was reduced by 20 mEq per day at weekly intervals.

By the second week of the study, the patient was noted to be losing more sodium than was provided in the diet. He became hypotensive and again required intravenous saline to restore a euvolemic state. Dietary sodium content was returned temporarily to a higher level and subsequent decrements in sodium intake were carried out more gradually. After 3 weeks it was possible to discontinue the antihypertensive medication and, after 12 weeks, dietary sodium intake had been reduced to 15 mEq/day. At the end of this period, the patient's weight was 68 kg and his plasma volume was 2174 ml. He was excreting 13 to 20 mEq of sodium daily.

A second water immersion study revealed that sodium excretion and FE_{Na}% again increased during the period of immersion, but both control and immersion values were considerably lower than those observed during the initial study. Sodium excretion increased from 4 μEq/min in the prestudy period to 55 μEq/min by the third hour and returned to 29.6 μEq/min in the recovery period. Similarly, the FE_{Na}% increased from 1.49 to 6.9% by the third hour and returned to 3.1% in the recovery period. The plasma renin activity decreased from 3.2 to 1.9 ng/ml/h during the fourth hour of immersion. Measurement of natriuretic factor by rat bioassay, which had been negative during the first water immersion study, turned positive during the second. The inulin clearance was lower than before (6 ml/min) but remained stable during the study.

Following completion of this study, the patient was given a diet containing 80 mEq/day of sodium and was observed for 7 days, after which vascular access was created for subsequent dialysis. On discharge the patient had a serum creatinine of 10.8 mg/dl and a blood pressure of 130/85 mmHg.

Discussion

Dr. Neal S. Bricker *(Professor of Medicine, Director, Program in Kidney Diseases, UCLA School of Medicine, Los Angeles, California)*: If one could eliminate nephrons one at a time in 2 million consecutive steps while maintaining salt intake constant, the continued preservation of sodium balance would require resetting the rate of sodium excretion by all surviving nephrons 2 million times. Thus, each time another nephron is destroyed, the average rate of sodium excretion by each surviving nephron would have to increase to avoid permanent sodium retention, even though the mean increment might be as small as 5×10^{-14} mEq/min/nephron.

Although single-file destruction of nephrons does not occur in chronic renal disease, it is the rule rather than the exception that sodium balance is maintained until the vast majority of the original nephron population has been destroyed. How a system might operate to preserve sodium homeostasis in the presence of the relentless destruction of nephrons and a constant salt intake, effecting precise changes in the average rate of sodium excretion per nephron as small as those quoted above, constitutes a major area of current interest and inquiry.

Special Problems Created by Chronic Renal Disease

Variation in Excretory Rates Among Nephrons

Figure 2 depicts values for single-nephron sodium excretion rates in three hypothetical subjects ingesting the same amount of salt daily: (1) a normal person; (2) a patient with chronic renal disease secondary to chronic glomerulonephritis; and (3) a patient with chronic interstitial nephritis. The three bars for each subject refer to different subsets of nephrons, based on mean values for single-nephron GFR (SNGFR). The data, as will be discussed, provide a compelling case for the exis-

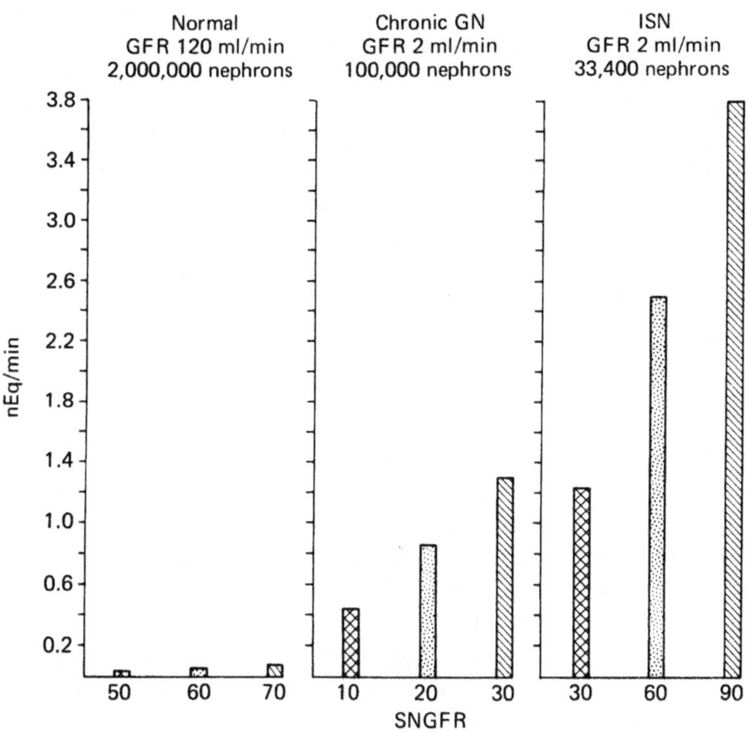

Fig. 2. Sodium excretion per nephron (nEq/min) when the intake is 120 mEq/day. Each bar represents one-third of the total nephron population for each of three hypothetical subjects based on mean values for single-nephron GFR. The values for single-nephron GFR for each of the subgroups are shown in Table 2. The basis for the calculations used to derive the values for sodium excretion rate per nephron is described in the text.

tence of a complex biologic control system for the regulation of sodium homeostasis. I will attempt to describe the biologic task confronting such a control system and to emphasize some of the obstacles that must be overcome if the task is to be accomplished. Finally, I will present a model for a control system that can operate in chronic renal disease as well as in health.

The data in Figure 2 are based on the following assumptions: All three subjects are the same size (70 kg), have the same extracellular fluid volume (14 liters), and have the same serum sodium concentration (140 mEq/liter). All three ingest the same amount of sodium daily (120 mEq/day), and all three excrete the same amount of sodium daily (120 mEq); hence all three maintain external sodium balance with equal precision.

Table 1 presents an estimate of the number of nephrons in each subject and of the mean value for SNGFR of these nephrons. The normal person has a GFR of 120 ml/min and 2 million nephrons. Both patients have GFRs of 2 ml/min. However, patient A, who has chronic glomerulonephritis, has 100,000 nephrons, whereas patient B, who has interstitial nephritis, has approximately 33,000 nephrons. The reason for the threefold difference in the number of nephrons in two patients with *equal whole-kidney GFRs* is that the average value for single-nephron GFR is three times as great in patient B as in patient A.

In each subject, as already noted, the nephrons have been divided into three subgroups, each having a different mean value for SNGFR. These data are shown in Table 2. To simplify the calculations, each subgroup is assumed to have one-third of the total number of functioning nephrons. I should point out here that the values assigned for SNGFR represent extrapolations from studies in experimental animals with normal kidneys, kidneys with severe glomerular lesions, and kidneys with interstitial lesions [1–12].

Table 1. Details of adaptation in sodium excretion: Total number of nephrons and mean SNGFR value.

Subject	Diagnosis	GFR (ml/min)	Number of Nephrons	Mean SNGFR (nl/min)
1	Normal	120	2 million	60
2	Patient A (chronic GN)	2	100,000	20
3	Patient B (interstitial nephritis)	2	33,400	60

Note: SNGFR refers to single-nephron glomerular filtration rate.

Table 2. Details of adaptation in sodium excretion: Nephron subgroups.

Subject	Diagnosis	Nephron Subgroups	Mean Value SNGFR/Nephron (nl/min)
1	Normal	A	50
		B	60
		C	70
2	Patient A (chronic GN)	A	10
		B	20
		C	30
3	Patient B (interstitial nephritis)	A	30
		B	60
		C	90

Figure 2 clearly shows that the values for sodium excretion rates per nephron in the normal subject differ to an astonishing degree from the values in both patients. Remarkable differences also are evident between patient A and patient B. Finally, in the normal subject, the values for *each* subgroup are somewhat different from one another, and in the two patients the variation among subgroups is striking. *Yet in all three subjects, the single-nephron sodium excretion rates occur in response to the ingestion of the same amount of salt, and, at the end of each 24-h period, each subject excretes the same total amount of sodium into the urine.*

Table 3. Details of adaptation in sodium excretion: Proximal tubular sodium reabsorption.

			(nEq/min/nephron)	
Subject	Nephron Subgroup	SNGFR (nl/min)	Proximal Reabsorption	Sodium Excretion
Normal	A	50	3.5	0.035
	B	60	4.2	0.042
	C	70	4.9	0.049
Patient A (chronic GN)	A	10	0.7	0.43
	B	20	1.4	0.86
	C	30	2.1	1.29
Patient B (interstitial nephritis)	A	30	2.1	1.25
	B	60	4.2	2.49
	C	90	6.3	3.74

Note: 50% of the filtered sodium is assumed to be reabsorbed proximally in all groups.

Variation in Proximal Tubular Sodium Reabsorptive Rates

The potential problems confronting a biologic control system charged with maintaining sodium homeostasis become even more complex when the calculated values for net sodium *reabsorption* in different nephron segments of the individual subgroups of each of the subjects are examined. Values for proximal reabsorption are shown in Table 3. We can assume that homogeneity of glomerulotubular (G-T) balance is maintained in all three subjects [13] and that by the end of the accessible portion of the proximal tubule, all nephrons, irrespective of their subgroup, have reabsorbed 50% of the filtered sodium. Despite the equal values for *fractional* reabsorption, however, there are seven different values for *absolute* sodium reabsorption for the nine nephron subgroups. These values range from 0.7 to 6.3 nEq/min/nephron. Underscoring the seemingly random quality of the mechanism we are attempting to analyze, the subgroup of nephrons with the *highest* rate of sodium *excretion* per nephron (patient B, subgroup C) simultaneously has the *greatest* rate of proximal *reabsorption* of any of the nine groups.

Variation in Distal Sodium Reabsorptive Rates

Values for single-nephron sodium reabsorption for the segment of the nephron beyond the accessible portion of the pars convoluta of the proximal tubule are shown in Figure 3. The subjects and subgroups are the same as those in Figure 2. For each subgroup, the per-nephron rate of distal reabsorption is compared with the calculated value for sodium excretion. In all three subjects, tubulotubular (T-T) balance, as well as G-T balance, is assumed to remain homogeneous throughout the entire nephron population. Based on the calculated rates of distal sodium delivery (50% of the filtered load) and sodium excretion, 90% of the distal sodium load is reabsorbed by the nephrons of the normal subject, 38% by the nephrons of patient A (with chronic glomerulonephritis), and 40% by the nephrons of patient B (with interstitial nephritis). If lower values for fractional reabsorption in the proximal tubule are used in one or both patients, the values for absolute distal reabsorption will increase, but the dispersion of values among the different subgroups will be qualitatively the same.

In the normal subject, the degree of variation in reabsorption rates among the three subgroups is moderate. Within the six subgroups of the two patients, however, *distal reabsorption rates vary over a range of almost tenfold.* Moreover, (1) the mean value is different in each of the six subgroups; (2) the overall mean value (i.e., for the three subgroups combined) in patient B is three times the comparable value in patient A; and (3) in all six subgroups, the values for distal reabsorption are less than the *lowest* value in any of the subgroups in the normal subject. I

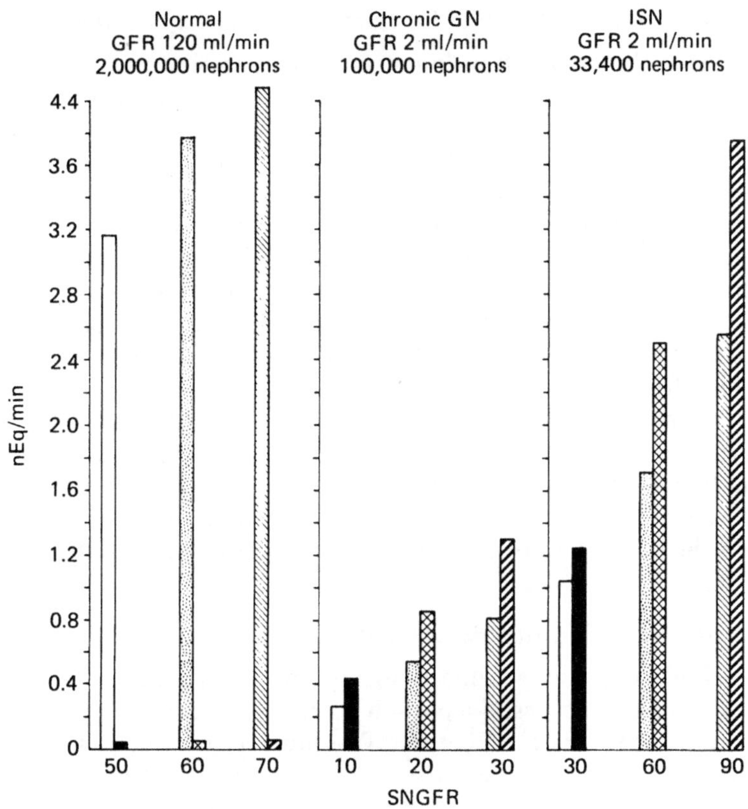

Fig. 3. Distal sodium reabsorption compared with sodium excretion per nephron (nEq/min). Six bars are shown for each of the three subjects. For each set of two bars, the one on the right represents sodium excretion per minute per nephron and the values are the same as those shown in Fig. 2. The left-hand bars represent the calculated values for net sodium reabsorption beyond the last point of the "proximal tubule" accessible to micropuncture. The assumption is made that 50% of the filtered sodium was reabsorbed proximally in each of the three subsets of all three subjects. The effects of using different values for fractional reabsorption in the two uremic patients are commented on in the text.

will come back to the last observation later when considering the possible role of aldosterone in the control of sodium excretion in chronic renal disease.

The Effect of a Change in Sodium Intake

The physiologic response to a change in salt intake adds further to our difficulty in interpreting the characteristics of the control system. Table 4 depicts the effects of a modest increase in sodium intake (from 60 to

Table 4. Details of adaptation in sodium excretion: The effects of increasing sodium intake from 60 to 120 mEq/day on single-nephron sodium excretion.

Subject	Total GFR (ml/min)	Nephrons	SNGFR (nl/min)	Sodium Excretion (nEq/min/nephron) 60 mEq Diet[a]	120 mEq Diet[a]	
Normal[b]	120	2,000,000	50	0.018	0.035	0.018
Patient B[c] (interstitial nephritis)	2	33,400	90	1.87	3.74	1.87

[a]The values for sodium intake are for 24-h periods.
[b]The data for the normal person are from subgroup A (Table 2 and Fig. 2).
[c]The data for patient B are from subgroup C (Table 2 and Fig. 2).

120 mEq/day) on single-nephron sodium excretion rates. To simplify the presentation, data are shown for only two nephron subgroups, group A in the normal subject and group C in patient B. In response to an identical change in salt intake, equal to 3.5 g of sodium chloride per day, the increase in sodium excretion per nephron is 100 times greater in the patient's nephron than in that of the normal person. It might be noted that if all 2 million nephrons in the normal subject responded as did the group C nephrons in patient B, the 24-h sodium excretion would greatly exceed the total amount of sodium in the extracellular fluid. Obviously, life would terminate long before the 24 h passed. On the other hand, life persists in the patient *because of* the magnified natriuretic response.

Let me reemphasize that (1) a wide range of values exists for proximal sodium reabsorption; (2) there is a wide range of values for distal sodium reabsorption; and (3) *an especially wide range of values* is found for overall sodium excretion per nephron. These differences obtain when one compares one patient with the other, and they obtain when one compares an individual nephron subgroup with another. Yet all three subjects excrete identical amounts of sodium in their urine daily. The system that subserves the maintenance of sodium balance would seem to possess remarkable, if not mysterious, qualities.

Adaptation

For sodium homeostasis to be maintained in advancing chronic renal disease, the addition of any given amount of sodium to the extracellular fluid must progressively raise the average rate of sodium excretion per nephron as GFR falls. We have termed this central feature of the adaptation in sodium excretion in chronic renal disease the "magnification phenomenon"[14].

Of the many examples of the magnification phenomenon, perhaps the most graphic is the continued ability of patients with chronic renal disease to maintain external sodium balance on an unrestricted salt intake as GFR falls from normal to extremely low levels [15]. To accomplish this on a relatively constant sodium intake, $FE_{Na}\%$ must double with each 50% fall in GFR [16]. In Figure 4, values for whole-kidney $FE_{Na}\%$ are shown for the same three subjects described earlier (the $FE_{Na}\%$ values represent 24-h averages). On the identical sodium intake of 120 mEq/day, the normal person excretes 0.5% of the filtered sodium (i.e., one of 200 filtered sodium ions), whereas in each of the two patients, $FE_{Na}\%$ equals 32%. Presumably, these values for $FE_{Na}\%$ are the same for all the nephrons in the individual subjects regardless of SNGFR values.

Another example of the magnification phenomenon is seen when extracellular fluid is translocated from one portion of the body to another without changing total extracellular fluid volume. If a human

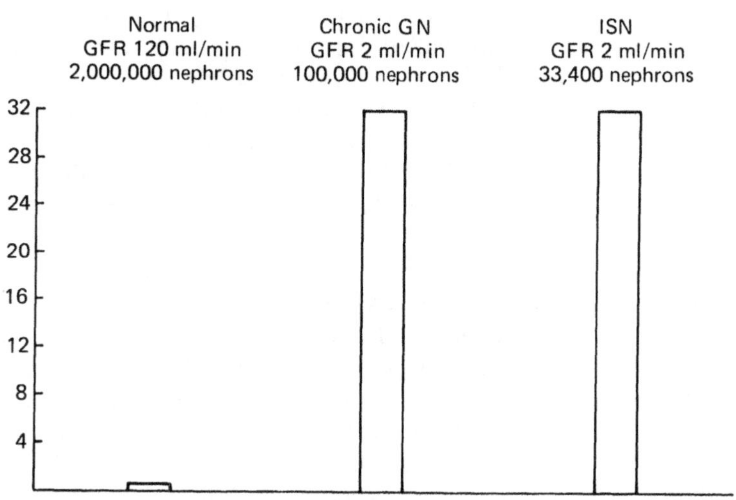

Fig. 4. Fractional excretion of sodium when the intake is 120 mEq/day. The value for fractional reabsorption of sodium in each subject represents the composite mean for all functioning nephrons (i.e., the values for the three subsets have been averaged). As discussed in the text, the preservation of homogeneity of G-T and T-T balances would make the values for *fractional* (but not absolute) excretion the same in all three nephron subsets of each subject. The calculated values are for a 24-h period and assume that the total amount of sodium excreted is equal to the total amount ingested (i.e., 120 mEq/day).

is immersed in a tank of water to the level of the neck, there is a shift of extracellular fluid from the legs into the upper portions of the body. In normal individuals, the increase in central and intrathoracic extracellular fluid volume is attended by a natriuresis [17]. When patients with chronic renal disease of varying severity are subjected to water immersion, not only does sodium excretion increase, but the lower the steady-state GFR, the greater is the rise in $FE_{Na}\%$ (Epstein M, Hoffman D, DeNunvio AG, unpublished observations). These patients are nonedematous, in external sodium balance, and presumably the volume of fluid translocated is closely comparable irrespective of the level of the GFR.

The Phenomenon of "Deadaptation"

The typical patient with chronic renal disease exhibits a salt-losing state when GFR falls below 30 ml/min. In most instances, this condition is characterized by the patient's inability to reduce the obligatory sodium excretion in the urine to less than approximately 30 mEq/24 h despite restriction of the dietary sodium intake to less than this level [18]. Rarely, the obligatory sodium loss can be much higher, exceeding 200 to 300 mEq/day [19,20]. If the sodium intake is diminished below the "floor" of sodium excretion, negative sodium balance will ensue, and a contraction of extracellular fluid volume necessarily will follow.

The general explanation for the salt-losing state of chronic renal disease has varied from the dictates of electric neutrality imposed by the excretion of unreabsorbable anions to a tubular defect in sodium reabsorption. It also has been thought that there is a limitation in the lower limit of sodium concentration achievable in the urine and thus that the magnitude of sodium loss varies with urine flow [18]. An entirely different explanation for the salt-losing has emerged from recent studies by Danovitch et al. [20]. Patients with chronic renal disease whose GFRs ranged from 5.2 to 16 ml/min were maintained in a metabolic balance ward from 4 to 14 weeks. The initial sodium intake, based on a detailed dietary history, varied from 58 to 342 mEq/day. In each subject, salt intake was reduced by small amounts at intervals of no less than 1 week. At the end of the study period, all the patients could maintain sodium balance on a diet containing 5.0 ± 2.9 (SD) mEq/day. Moreover, there was no reduction in GFR or in estimated plasma volume, nor were any adverse effects noted. The salt-losing state in these patients thus was reversed by slow and gradual "weaning" of sodium intake. The explanation proposed was that the adaptation in sodium excretion in chronic renal disease that results in the high rates of sodium excretion per nephron at low GFRs is not rapidly suppressible, but that "deadaptation" can be induced if sodium withdrawal is accomplished slowly over a long period. The patient under discussion today is a good example of this deadaptive response.

Certain of the effects of deadaptation on the magnification phenomenon recently have been studied by Rever, Licht, and Bricker (unpublished observations). Using the same salt-weaning technique just described, we subjected patients with chronic renal disease to water immersion before and after the sodium-losing state was reversed. The resulting data clearly demonstrate that the magnified natriuretic response to water immersion in adapted patients with chronic renal disease is blunted following the deadaptation process (Fig. 1). Measurements of plasma volume before and after deadaptation showed no change. Our present interpretation is that the magnification phenomenon for sodium depends on the preexistence of an adaptive natriuresis per nephron, but further documentation of this thesis is necessary.

General Design of the Sodium Control System

I already have emphasized the view that a sophisticated biologic control system seems to be required for the maintenance of sodium balance. I also believe that although qualitative changes in the mode of operation of this system occur continuously as GFR falls, the basic components of the system must be the same in a patient with advancing chronic renal disease as in a normal person. If these views are correct, it follows that each person not only is born with a sodium control system, but that the system is designed so as to alter its patterns of function progressively in any individual who becomes afflicted with a nephron-destroying process.

The control system is believed to contain a minimum of three component parts [15]. The first is a *detector element* capable of sensing an alteration in body fluids produced by the addition or loss of sodium chloride. The second is a *transmitting element* capable of relaying information about the perturbation of the extracellular fluid to the nephrons and altering their rate of sodium transport. The third is the *end organ*, which consists of the total pool of functioning nephrons whether the number be 2 million or 30,000. There also is a possibility that an *integrator element* may exist if there is not a single detector element, but rather widely dispersed detector elements. The integrator, presumably located in the central nervous system, would receive the input from all detector elements, collate the data, and determine whether the message sent to the kidneys via the transmitter is to increase or to decrease the rate of sodium excretion. An integrator would be of special value in the presence of internal translocations of volume such as water immersion wherein there is a decrease in the effective extracellular fluid volume in the legs and a simultaneous increase in the thorax.

The Detector Element

Neither the location nor the nature of the detector element is yet known. It seems most likely, however, that the perturbation that is monitored is a change in extracellular fluid volume or a hemodynamic alteration induced by a volume change, rather than a change in the extracellular fluid sodium concentration per se. Thus, the sodium control system in fact is probably a volume control system, and sodium balance is maintained by virtue of the usually close coupling between changes in extracellular fluid sodium content and extracellular fluid volume.

Several lines of evidence suggest that the detector element is located in the upper half of the body, possibly within the thorax, perhaps in the brain. In addition to the water immersion studies, space flight is associated with an early natriuretic response; the change from the 1-g environment of earth to the 0-g environment of space is attended by the movement of approximately 2 liters of fluid from the lower extremities into the more cephalad portions of the body [21]. Prolonged bedrest also leads to a cephalad shift of extracellular fluid and typically produces a natriuresis. Movement of extracellular fluid volume from the upper to the lower portions of the body, such as is induced by quiet standing and application of thigh tourniquets, also changes sodium excretion, but in the opposite direction [22].

The Integrator Element

The basis for considering the existence of a centrally located "computer"-type mechanism that would monitor simultaneous, and in some instances opposing, changes in regional ECF volumes already has been alluded to. If such an integrator element exists, however, its location and mechanism of action remain unknown.

The Transmitting Element

There is an extensive and growing list of factors known to influence sodium excretion. Among these are (1) changes in GFR throughout the nephron population; (2) changes and/or redistribution of GFR values in cortical versus juxtamedullary glomeruli; (3) changes in medullary blood flow with an alteration of sodium concentration gradients between the medullary interstitium and the vasa recta and loop of Henle; (4) changes in sympathetic nervous activity; and (5) alterations in the activity of one or more of a number of humoral substances including aldosterone, prostaglandins, vasopressin, oxytocin, the kallikrein-kinin system, parathyroid hormone, calcitonin, and finally the putative natriuretic hormone.

For any one of the foregoing factors to be established as the key modulator of sodium excretion, its activity must be shown to correlate closely and consistently with both short- and long-term changes in sodium excretion under many different circumstances, including chronic renal disease. None of the factors listed has yet been examined under enough circumstances to establish which, if any, is the principal modulator of sodium excretion. It does appear, however, that most of the factors listed can be excluded on the basis of negative correlations. The evidence in regard to aldosterone and natriuretic hormone will be considered later.

The End Organ: The Nephron

A vast amount of data relating to the manner in which sodium is handled by the nephron has been accumulated, and most of this information falls beyond the scope of this discussion. But I would like to comment a little later about the possibility that intrinsic changes in nephron function might contribute to the magnification phenomenon.

Special Comments About Aldosterone and Natriuretic Hormone

Aldosterone

Clear and incontrovertible evidence shows that aldosterone augments epithelial cell sodium transport capacity. However, the biologic role of aldosterone in regulating tubular reabsorption of sodium seems to involve the induction of the synthesis of proteins concerned with sodium transport rather than the modulation of the minute-to-minute rate of sodium transport and excretion [23]. In chronic renal disease, the pattern of change in aldosterone levels is not consistent as GFR falls from normal to low levels. Elevated levels have been reported, yet in the data shown in Fig. 3, values for distal tubular reabsorption in the two patients were *lower* in all nephron subgroups than in any of the three subgroups in the normal subject. The values were particularly low in the patient with glomerulonephritis. A number of experimental observations also fail to support the view that aldosterone is the primary "transmitter" in the sodium control system in chronic renal disease [16,24,25].

Natriuretic Hormone

Although natriuretic hormone has not yet been isolated and synthesized, the body of evidence supporting its existence is compelling. Much of this evidence has been reviewed in a recent monograph [26]. I will limit my comments about natriuretic hormone to a brief summary of certain of the more relevant data. The natriuretic factor, the term I generally prefer to use rather than natriuretic hormone, is a low-molecular-weight compound (approximately 500 daltons), which has been separated from the serum and urine of uremic patients who have high fractional sodium excretion rates [27,28]. Because natriuretic factor is present in increased amounts in both the serum and urine of uremic patients, one can assume that its rate of production is increased in uremia. Natriuretic factor is not detectable, however, in the urine or serum of patients with advanced chronic renal disease who are nephrotic and edematous and, hence, are not undergoing a natriuresis [28]. A sodium transport inhibitor, probably the same substance present in uremia, also has been found in (1) normal individuals ingesting a high-salt diet [29]; (2) healthy dogs ingesting 15 g of sodium chloride and 0.2 mg of fludrocortisol per day following escape [30]; (3) normal subjects during water immersion [31]; (4) patients with aldosterone-secreting tumors (sodium transport inhibition disappears following removal of the tumor) [32]; and (5) patients with head trauma who are manifesting a natriuresis [33].

As in nephrotic uremic patients, natriuretic activity was not demonstrable with standard bioassay techniques in uremic dogs in which the typical natriuresis per nephron was prevented by a reduction in dietary sodium intake in exact proportion to the reduction in GFR [34]. Activity also was absent in patients with head trauma in whom a natriuretic state did not develop [33]. We have studied two patients with chronic renal disease in whom assays for natriuretic activity in the urine were inexplicably negative; but in both the assays became positive during water immersion (Rever B, Licht A, Bricker NS, unpublished observations).

Natriuretic factor inhibits sodium transport by the isolated toad bladder [28], the isolated frog skin [28], the isolated perfused cortical collecting tubule of the rabbit [35], and two cell types grown in tissue culture (Licht A, Bricker NS, unpublished observations). One of these cell lines, the so-called "MDCK" strain, originally was derived from tubular epithelial cells of the dog. The other, the 3T6 strain, is a line of fibroblasts that actively transports sodium. Finally, natriuretic factor produces a sodium diuresis both in the normal water-loaded rat [36] and in the uremic rat fed a high-salt diet for 36 to 48 h before the material is administered [28].

In the isolated tubule preparation, toad bladder, and the frog skin, natriuretic factor is active only when added from the basolateral, or the "blood," surface [37]. It increases the intracellular sodium content of isolated toad bladder epithelial cells and decreases their rate of pyruvate oxidation [38]. Natriuretic factor inhibits sodium efflux in the isolated perfused tubule but does not affect sodium influx [35]. It inhibits sodium efflux by both the MDCK and the 3T6 cell systems and does not produce further inhibition of sodium efflux in the same cell types incubated in 10^{-3} M ouabain (Licht A, Bricker NS, unpublished observations). It inhibits rubidium influx in the 3T6 system (Licht A, Bricker NS, unpublished observations), but it is not kaliuretic in the rat [27,28].

Intensive efforts are in progress to isolate natriuretic factor, and a relatively high degree of purity has been obtained using high-performance liquid chromatography. The active fraction is water soluble, soluble in some organic solvents [36,39] but not in others, and presumably is polar in nature. Natriuretic factor appears in a chromatographic peak (using high-performance liquid chromatography) that contains an active amine group; it is inactivated by some proteolytic enzymes but not by others, and disagreement still exists as to whether it is a peptide. Many of its effects resemble those of ouabain, and it has been suggested that natriuretic factor might be an endogenous digitalis glycoside-like compound [40].

Operation of the Control System: A Hypothetical Model

The model to be presented fits within the classic framework of a "detector-transmitter-end organ" system that maintains sodium homeostasis by controlling the constancy of effective extracellular fluid volume. Given the changing circumstances inherent in advancing renal insufficiency, how does such a system continue to operate? In essence, how can a specific amount of sodium, an amount that can vary from meal to meal and day to day, be excreted with some precision by a population of nephrons that varies in number from 2 million to perhaps 30,000 and that can exhibit the spectrum of values for proximal and distal sodium reabsorption and sodium excretion per nephron, exemplified by Figs. 2 and 3 and Table 3. We can focus this question around two related issues: (1) is there a mechanism that serves as the "control center," overseeing the continuous operation of the system and overriding seemingly insurmountable obstacles; and (2) how can the magnification phenomenon be explained?

The "Control Center"

Theoretically, the system could be "effector oriented," i.e., have its control center located in the kidneys per se, or it could be "detector oriented," and have the control center located anywhere in the body. The first possibility would require that the kidneys possess a means of determining how much sodium is acquired daily and thus how much must be excreted. Following the addition of sodium to the extracellular fluid, excretion per nephron then would have to be increased, presumably by a reduction in distal sodium reabsorption [35]. The reabsorption of sodium might emit some biochemical signal and a feedback loop then might modulate the rate of release of a transmitter element and evoke a subsequent decrease (or increase) in distal sodium reabsorption. However, a model that places the control center in the kidneys leaves a major problem unsolved. For the end organ to monitor the rate of addition (or deletion) of sodium to the extracellular fluid, a sensing device would be required. Despite the intrarenal location of such a hypothetical sensor, it nevertheless would be monitoring a volume-related, presumably hemodynamic, change. In this sense, such a control system would be just as "detector oriented" as it would be if it resided in the chest rather than in the renal parenchyma. Thus, we believe the volume control system can be viewed as detector oriented with its "control center" probably residing in the detector element per se. Let us examine a working model of the system having the general design presented in Fig. 5.

The model control system is designed to maintain an optimal extracellular fluid volume. The upper portion of the figure depicts the basal state, wherein the volume of the extracellular fluid is normal. The detector element receives little input and sends out only minimal pulses to the site of synthesis of the major transmitter element, which we will

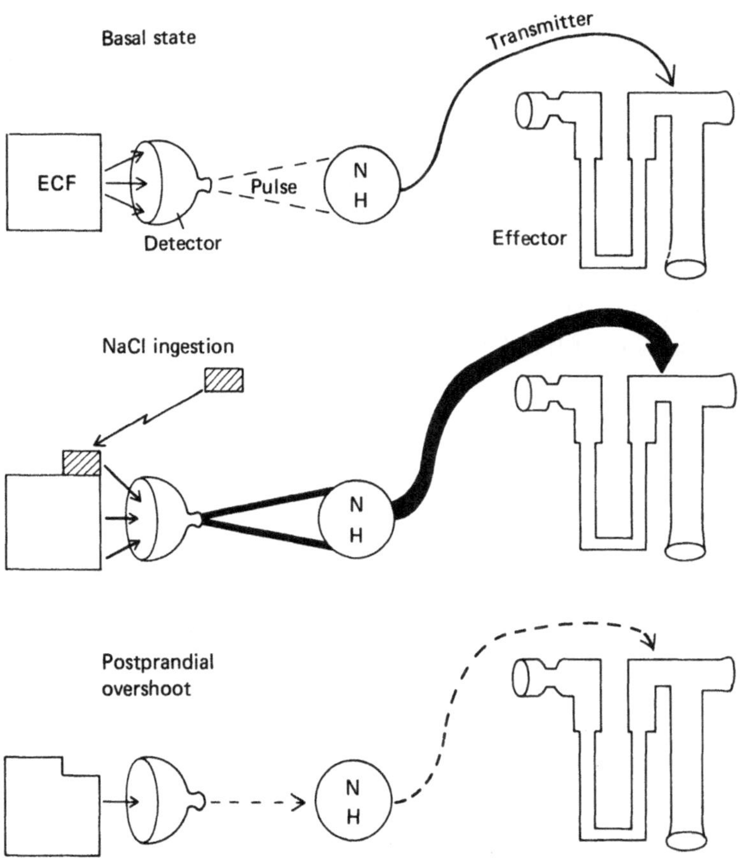

Fig. 5. Proposed model of the biologic control system for sodium. N. H. stands for putative natriuretic hormone.

assume for the present discussion is natriuretic hormone. In health, in the basal state, the level of the hormone in the circulation is low, the degree of inhibition of distal tubular sodium reabsorption is small, and urinary sodium excretion is minimal. This basal state would prevail some hours after the ingestion of a meal and perhaps would be most characteristic of the pattern observed during early morning.

The middle panel in Fig. 5 depicts the effects on the control system of the ingestion of sodium chloride. The entrance of the NaCl into the extracellular fluid leads to isosmotic expansion of the extracellular fluid as previously noted. The detector element then senses the expansion through a still-to-be-defined hemodynamic event induced by the expansion, and the activity of the detector is markedly increased over that which prevailed in the basal state. The result is that the pulses sent out to the organ producing the transmitter are increased; the thick black arrow in the figure depicts a marked increase in the rate of release of the transmitter substance. The transmitter, which again is assumed to act by inhibiting distal tubular sodium transport, will, after reaching the nephrons via the renal circulation, diminish net sodium reabsorption per nephron and thereby increase sodium excretion per nephron. The concentration of the inhibitor in the postglomerular blood should be identical for all nephrons (with the possible exception of the juxtamedullary units) and, if the number of receptor sites for the transmitter is proportional to SNGFR, and the affinity of the unoccupied sites is constant from nephron to nephron, the number of new transmitter molecules that will attach to the unoccupied receptors also should be proportional to SNGFR. Hence, the *percentage* change in distal tubular sodium reabsorption of the distal load of sodium would be identical in all nephrons and would be determined by (1) the concentration (or activity) of the transmitter element in the blood; (2) the affinity of the receptor sites for the inhibitor; and (3) the number of new receptor sites occupied. Despite the homogeneous change in the percentage of distal sodium reabsorption, as discussed previously, the actual number of sodium ions prevented from crossing the epithelial cells, and thus remaining in the tubular fluid to be excreted, will vary from one nephron to another in the same kidney depending on the distal load of sodium, and the latter will depend, in turn, on the value for SNGFR. The dispersion of values for sodium excretion rate per nephron, as shown in Fig. 2, thus will vary widely as does SNGFR. Nevertheless, the effect of the increased activity of the transmitter on the residual nephrons, regardless of their number, will be to increase total sodium excretion.

The bottom panel represents the system's status after the transmitter has exercised its effects on the nephrons. All the ingested sodium chloride has been excreted, but the possibility exists that an "overshoot" phenomenon might be involved. It seems likely that as the extracellular fluid volume is restored toward normal, the stimulus to the detector element will diminish pari passu. It also seems likely, however, that the system cannot operate with absolute precision and that the extracellular fluid volume will fluctuate about an "ideal" volume. Thus, despite the fact that the full amount of added sodium chloride has been excreted, the activity of the transmitter may persist at a level greater than basal for a finite period and result in a continuing, albeit diminished, natriuresis. The overshoot phase should be self-limited, and when additional sodium chloride is ingested, the extracellular fluid volume will first return to the basal level and then undergo expansion.

In essence, therefore, with a detector-oriented model, the natriuresis attendant on the addition of sodium chloride to the extracellular fluid will begin to abate as the extracellular fluid volume begins to diminish toward normal. Activation of the detector in this model plays a key role in determining the rate of release of the transmitter element. The model provides for the preservation of sodium homeostasis through the maintenance of external balance regardless of the number of nephrons or of the dispersion of single-nephron sodium excretion rates.

The Magnification Phenomenon

The question must be asked whether, in the progression from 2 million to 30,000 nephrons, the identical volume perturbation produces a progressively greater degree of activation of the detector element, thereby explaining the magnification phenomenon. Although this possibility cannot be ruled out, it seems to me extremely unlikely that each time a nephron is lost, a change will occur in the sensitivity of the detector element; for it should be noted that the magnification phenomenon is characteristic not only of sodium, but also of phosphate, magnesium, potassium, and probably a number of other solutes. The detector element for phosphate probably monitors a change in ionized calcium; that for potassium may monitor a change in transmembrane chemical or electrochemical potential gradient; and that for magnesium perhaps monitors a change in the concentration of ionized magnesium, and so forth. If the magnification phenomenon for even these few solutes were based on a stepwise and simultaneous increase in sensitivity of each element, one would have to invoke multiple separate mechanisms (one for each system) whereby each wave of nephron loss would "reset" the sensitivity of each detector mechanism.

The evidence for an increase in production of natriuretic factor in chronic renal disease already has been cited. What mediates this increase is unknown, but there is no consistent or compelling evidence to suggest that the change is due to a continuous expansion of extracellular fluid volume throughout the course of chronic renal disease. There are no data, however, concerning the rate of release of natriuretic factor in response to the addition of a given amount of sodium at each level of GFR throughout the entire course of chronic renal disease. Although such data will be quite difficult to obtain until a highly sensitive assay system is developed, they ultimately will be essential if the missing pieces of this puzzle are to be filled in. The possibility that the release rate of the transmitter element varies as an inverse function of GFR in response to the ingestion of a fixed amount of sodium thus cannot be dismissed until the requisite data are obtained. Another possible explanation for the magnification phenomenon is that there is an increase in end-organ sensitivity to the transmitter element and that this heightened response might be due either to an enhanced intrinsic sensitivity or responsivity of the nephron and/or to an increase in the number of receptors per unit of SNGFR or of tubular length. Indirect evidence supporting increased end-organ sensitivity was obtained in experiments in which a fixed amount of natriuretic factor was injected into the renal artery of normal and uremic rats. The estimated rate of sodium excretion *per nephron* increased substantially more in the uremic than in the normal animals [41].

In summary, the magnification phenomenon is essential for the preservation of sodium homeostasis in chronic renal disease and thus for the preservation of life in the presence of progressive nephron loss. Evidence suggests that the activity of the transmitter element, which inhibits sodium reabsorption by the distal tubule, may increase in response to a given load of sodium as GFR falls. Further, end-organ sensitivity might increase as chronic renal disease advances. This remarkable magnification phenomenon, the central element of the adaptation in sodium excretion in chronic renal disease, remains basically unexplained, although many aspects of the phenomenon should be readily amenable to experimental examination with modern techniques.

Conclusions

We have examined the processes involved in the maintenance of homeostasis of a single solute, sodium, in healthy individuals and in patients with chronic renal disease such as the one presented today. But homeostasis also is maintained with close precision for a host of other solutes, and for some of these, the homeostatic process adapts continuously as disease destroys greater than 90% of the original nephron population. If a biologic control system does oversee sodium homeostasis, we believe that biologic control systems probably exist for other solutes as well. At least some of these control systems, and perhaps all, could contain transmitter elements that modulate tubular transport of their specific solute. Some systems, such as the one for sodium, however, would require a transmitter that inhibits reabsorption; others would need a transmitter that stimulates secretion; and it is conceivable that still others might require a transmitter element that alters the balance between reabsorption and secretion. All the systems must be capable of overriding any interference produced by the action of other control systems. In general, the rates of acquisition of key solutes of body fluids vary both randomly and independently of one another in advancing renal disease as well as in the healthy state. It is obvious that an increase in sodium intake cannot lead to a persistent increase in phosphate or potassium excretion despite the fact that natriuretic factor has been shown to be phosphaturic and that natriuresis ordinarily increases potassium excretion; moreover, a decrease in sodium intake cannot lead to a reduction in phosphate excretion, potassium excretion, or the excretion of any other solute that is influenced by the reabsorption of sodium by tubular epithelial cells.

The unraveling of the nature of solute-specific biologic systems and the changes that take place in those systems in chronic renal disease, I believe, represent one of the most interesting and important biomedical challenges facing us in the coming decade. Indeed, I would submit that this area stands among the key unsolved mysteries of mammalian biology.

Questions and Answers

Dr. Barton Levine *(Assistant Professor of Medicine, Wadsworth VA Medical Center, UCLA School of Medicine, Los Angeles, California)*: In what tubular segment or segments is natriuretic hormone thought to have an effect?

Dr. Bricker: There are recollection micropuncture data that suggest a modest effect on the proximal tubule [42], but it would appear that the principal effect is on the cortical collecting tubule [35].

Dr. Leon G. Fine *(Director, Nephrology Division, Center for the Health Sciences, UCLA School of Medicine, Los Angeles)*: The data you showed regarding the effects of water immersion are interesting. However, before one can conclude that these observations reflect a change in the sensitivity of the end organ, one must know that the movement of fluid is the same with the patient on a low- or high-salt intake. You indicated that the measured blood volume was the same whether the patient was on a high- or low-salt diet. I would predict that if any part of the extracellular fluid composite was protected, it would be the blood volume. There is a good chance, however, that the total extracellular fluid volume or the interstitial volume would be significantly lower when the patient ingested a low-salt diet, and the differences you report could be explained by differences in the amount of fluid shifted. Unfortunately, in water immersion, neither the hematocrit nor a change in protein concentration can be used to reflect a change in extracellular volume.

Dr. Bricker: First, I did not intend to imply that the site of the increased responsivity in the adapted state is necessarily limited to the nephron. It could reside at any level, or multiple levels, of the control system. With respect to whether "deadaptation" was associated with extracellular fluid volume contraction, I agree that the equality of plasma volumes in the adapted and deadapted states is not in itself sufficiently strong evidence to rule out this possibility and that some index of central blood volume, cardiac index, or plethysmographic measurements of the legs would be helpful. Extracorporeal volume expansion in the adapted versus the unadapted state also would help to clarify this question, and such studies are being conducted by Dr. Michael Shapiro in our laboratories.

Dr. Gabriel M. Danovitch *(Director, Clinical Nephrology, Center for the Health Sciences, UCLA School of Medicine, Los Angeles)*: We recently reported a patient who manifested spontaneous changes in sodium excretion very similar to those seen in the two water immersion studies performed in the patient under discussion [43]. Our patient suffered the unusual combination of advanced polycystic renal disease and Crohn's disease. He had an ileostomy, from which he lost an appreciable amount of sodium-containing fluid daily. His diet contained 150 mEq of sodium per day, but he excreted only 5 or 6 mEq of sodium in his urine; the rest was lost in the ileal fluid. This unique set of circumstances had prevailed for approximately 10 years. Thus, as his renal failure advanced, he did not "need" to develop an adaptive natriuresis per nephron and, in fact, he remained "unadapted," excreting virtually no sodium in his urine. When he was subjected to marked extracellular fluid volume expansion, his urine contained little or no sodium. Thus he did not exhibit the magnification phenomenon. We interpreted this as an experiment of nature in which "deadaptation" occurred spontaneously. We believe the data are consistent with the results of the water immersion studies, in which a magnified natriuresis failed to occur in the absence of adaptation. Later in his course, however, after prolonged volume repletion, his sodium excretion increased.

Dr. Bricker: This fascinating experiment of nature bears directly on the key question of whether a preexisting adaptation is necessary for the magnification phenomenon to work for sodium. In the case of magnesium (Kirschenbaum MA, Liebross B, Bricker NS, unpublished observations) and probably potassium [44], adaptation does appear to be necessary for magnification to occur. In the case of phosphate, however, it does not [45].

Dr. Fine: One could conceive of a hormone-mediated natriuresis occurring without an increase in hormone concentration. If the number of nephrons decreased but an excess of hormone receptors still existed, more hormone-receptor complexes would be formed on those remaining nephrons, and a correspondingly greater natriuresis per nephron would ensue. But when you measure natriuretic hormone with existing bioassay techniques, the hormone concentration in serum is elevated; the question is why. Could this increase be related to "steady-state" blood volume? How adequate are the data on measured blood volume in uremic patients? If the hormone concentration is elevated simply because uremic patients have higher blood volumes than do nonuremic patients, then that elevation could simply reflect a different steady state and it might not play a role in governing the excretion of sodium.

Dr. Bricker: Your hormone-receptor theory, if validated, could help explain the magnification phenomenon. One might examine whether the isolated perfused cortical collecting tubule from normal versus uremic, and adapted uremic versus unadapted uremic, animals exhibits differences in sensitivity to the same amounts of natriuretic factor in vitro.

The question of whether blood volume or, more importantly, extracellular fluid volume is consistently elevated in uremia is beclouded somewhat by methodologic problems. Thus the existing methods, particularly those used for measuring extracellular fluid volume, are not sufficiently precise to allow for a definitive answer. Some years ago, Schultze studied normal dogs in which he measured inulin space and blood volume. He then made the dogs uremic, maintained the same salt intake, and repeated the space measurements; he found no changes [24]. More recently Dr. Michael Shapiro has found that inulin spaces are no greater in uremic than in normal rats and no greater in sodium-adapted than in sodium-unadapted uremic rats (unpublished observations). However, the conclusions drawn from these observations must be tentative because the error in inulin space measurements must be at least 5%.

Dr. Joel D. Kopple *(Professor of Medicine and Public Health, Wadsworth VA Medical Center, UCLA School of Medicine, Los Angeles)*: A shift of 700 ml of fluid into the upper half of the body during water immersion represents less than 3% of total body water. This is well below the accuracy of these measurements of extracellular space.

I have a question, Dr. Bricker. I find the welter of data strongly suggestive that there is a humoral factor. But I find problematic the length of time it takes to deadapt a uremic patient from the presumed effects of this hormone. With every other hormonal system I am aware of, the adaptive response is measured in terms of minutes or, at the most, hours; yet in this instance a patient can become profoundly volume depleted, including having marked reductions in blood volume, and still have inappropriate sodium excretion. Granted, it may be because not only is the circulating hormone increased but also because the receptors are increased. But don't you find it troublesome that it takes so many weeks to wean a patient from the natriuretic state?

Dr. Bricker: Yes. But there is at least one analogous situation, namely, the uremic patient with poorly suppressible hyperparathyroidism, in whom it may take a year or longer before the euparathyroid state is restored after successful renal transplantation. Also the salt-losing state does not seem to occur in uremic rats or dogs, possibly because the adaptation in laboratory animals generally evolves over a very much shorter period of time than in patients.

Dr. Jordan J. Cohen: Have you ever failed in an attempt to deadapt a patient? That is, do some uremic patients have unremitting salt wastage?

Dr. Bricker: Dr. Rever, would you like to respond to that?

Dr. Barbara L. Rever *(Assistant Professor of Medicine, Center for the Health Sciences, UCLA School of Medicine, Los Angeles)*: I have studied five patients and have encountered only one in whom we could not decrease the daily sodium intake below 15 mEq. Dr. Danovitch has studied five patients and was successful in all [20]. Thus deadaptation has been accomplished successfully in nine of ten patients.

Dr. Amnon Licht *(Assistant Professor of Medicine, Center for the Health Sciences, UCLA School of Medicine, Los Angeles)*: When deadaptation is attempted too quickly, volume depletion can develop, requiring saline infusion. However, with a slower rate of sodium "weaning," the same patient can be deadapted successfully. This was apparent in today's patient.

Dr. Kiyoshi Kurokawa *(Chief, Nephrology Division, Wadsworth VA Medical Center, UCLA School of Medicine, Los Angeles)*: In uncomplicated patients with chronic renal failure who ingest a stable sodium intake, have you found a good correlation between measured plasma volume or plasma renin activity on the one hand, and the level of sodium intake on the other?

Dr. Bricker: Renin values decrease during water immersion in uremic patients. However, I am not aware of a systematic set of data that would permit a clear answer to your question.

Dr. Kurokawa: If this sensor system is to be operative in the presence of chronic renal failure, say in a patient with a GFR of 10 ml/min and a sodium intake of 100 mEq/day, a small increase in sodium intake, of say 20 mEq/day, must result in an equivalent increase in sodium excretion, as would occur in normal individuals. Given that patients with reduced GFRs are thought to have high levels of natriuretic factor to start with, it is unclear how these patients can detect relatively small additional increments in volume and translate these increases into the appropriate change in sodium excretion. Because these patients have high levels of natriuretic factor to start with, it is hard for me to accept that the same small increase would produce the same increment in sodium excretion as it does in normal individuals.

Dr. Bricker: In preliminary studies, again by Dr. Michael Shapiro, natriuretic factor has been found in the urine of adapted uremic rats. It is highly likely that the animals used for the bioassay had high endogenous levels of natriuretic factor. The addition of 20 mEq/day of sodium, barring different rates of excretion, would produce the same increment in extracellular fluid volume in the patient as in the normal person; thus the increase in endogenous natriuretic factor should be equal.

Dr. Cohen: What, if any, influence might an altered diurnal pattern of sodium input and output have on sodium adaptation? After all, we don't ingest sodium continuously but rather in boluses with meals throughout the day. It is conceivable that the response of a normal individual and of a patient with marked renal insufficiency to the same increment in sodium intake could be identical when expressed as mEq/24 h but quite different when looked at in temporal profile over a typical day. Are there any data about the relative rates at which a given sodium increment, provided in bolus form, is excreted by a normal person versus a patient with chronic renal failure?

Dr. Bricker: There are both animal and human data, but there are contradictions. In one study, uremic dogs who received a 2.5-g sodium chloride load excreted approximately the same amount of sodium in 5 h as did the same dogs before they became uremic [24]. More recent studies from St. Louis showed a slower short-term rate of excretion in uremic dogs [46]. Finally, in studies currently being performed, Danovitch and Licht have found a consistent increase in excretion of natriuretic factor in *normal* individuals between midnight and 4:00 A.M.

Dr. Michael A. Kirschenbaum *(Assistant Professor of Medicine, Center for the Health Sciences, UCLA School of Medicine, Los Angeles)*: The elusiveness of the identification of the components of the volume regulation system is very disturbing. In many other biologic control systems, it has been a great deal easier to identify components. Yet in primate as well as subprimate studies seeking the elements of the detector limb, negative results have been obtained; these failures suggest that perhaps the detector, controller, and effector are located intrarenally. Maybe we are looking at a purely intrarenal event which, as Dr. Fine suggests, might overshoot substantially and which in most situations might not be very selective or sensitive.

Dr. Bricker: I can only reiterate the fact that the lower the GFR, the greater the change in tubular epithelial transport (at any given value for SNGFR) for a given change in intake of a single solute, and that the rates and direction of change for sodium, as well as for other substances, are solute specific and geared to the preservation of homeostasis. Also, the ability to "wean" a chronically uremic patient of dietary sodium with no consistent change in plasma sodium concentration, plasma volume, or GFR bespeaks a highly ordered control system.

Dr. Kurokawa: Dr. Fine has demonstrated that natriuretic factor modulates sodium transport in the cortical collecting tubule. It should be feasible, therefore, for one to compare the response of tubules obtained from animals with chronic renal failure with those obtained from normal controls. If one produces a dose-response curve using the same source of natriuretic factor in serial dilutions, shouldn't one be able to demonstrate differences in the sensitivity—i.e., a shift of the response curve to the right or left—as well as differences in the responsiveness—i.e., the magnitude—of tubular response?

Dr. Bricker: We are in the process of studying the natriuretic effect of urine fractions from adapted versus deadapted rats using adapted and deadapted rats for bioassay. The studies you suggest are important and I hope they will be done soon.

But let me make one other point with regard to your question. One can make dogs uremic by reducing nephron mass in serial steps; if salt in the diet is decreased in exact proportion to the decrease in GFR, such animals will become uremic and have no increase in natriuresis per nephron; moreover, the bioassay for natriuretic hormone will remain negative [34]. Your question could be answered by studying isolated perfused cortical collecting tubules from such nephrons and comparing the results to those obtained in nephrons from uremic animals with high levels of natriuretic factor.

Dr. Hector J. Rodriguez *(Assistant Clinical Professor of Medicine, UCLA School of Medicine, Los Angeles)*: You have included aldosterone in your scheme as a modulator of sodium excretion. Does available evidence permit one to exclude changes in sensitivity or responsiveness of the surviving nephrons to aldosterone levels?

Dr. Bricker: I think aldosterone plays a very important role in sodium homeostasis. But experimental observations suggest that if one maintains mineralocorticoid hormone levels in a uremic dog or patient at a fixed level, whether this be very low or very high, and if one modifies the sodium intake, sodium balance will be maintained [16,24].

Dr. Fine: Gruber et al. recently reported a circulating ouabain-like substance [40]. Do you think they have discovered the natriuretic hormone?

Dr. Bricker: Although samples have not been exchanged between laboratories—and in my view, there is an urgent need that this be done—they believe that their inhibitor can be measured using a radioimmunoassay for digoxin. I don't know whether their substance is natriuretic hormone, but as I noted earlier, natriuretic hormone could be an endogenous, digitalis glycoside-like compound. Many characteristics of the hormone resemble those of ouabain: the hormone is active only when added to the basolateral or blood surface, it increases intracellular sodium content, it blocks sodium efflux but doesn't affect sodium influx, it decreases oxidative phosphorylation, it has the right molecular weight, and there are other similarities.

Dr. Fine: Let's say then that Gruber et al. do have a circulating natriuretic substance. Does one stop there and say *the* natriuretic hormone has been discovered, or does one go on looking for another natriuretic hormone?

Dr. Bricker: I'd be happy with one!

References

1. Bank N, Aynedjian HS: Individual nephron function in experimental bilateral pyelonephritis, I. Glomerular filtration rate and proximal tubular sodium, potassium, and water reabsorption. J Lab Clin Med 68:713–727, 1966
2. Lubowitz H, Purkerson ML, Sugita M, Bricker NS: GFR per nephron and per kidney in the chronically diseased (pyelonephritic) kidney of the rat. Am J Physiol 217:853–857, 1969
3. Rocha A, Marcondes M, Malnic G: Micropuncture study in rats with experimental glomerulonephritis. Kidney Int 3:14–23, 1973
4. Lubowitz H, Mazumdar DC, Kawamura J, Crosson JT, Weisser F, Rolf D, Bricker NS: Experimental glomerulonephritis in the rat: Structural and functional observations. Kidney Int 5:356–364, 1974
5. Kramp RA, MacDowell M, Gottschalk CW, Oliver JR: A study by microdissection and micropuncture of the structure and the function of the kidneys and the nephrons of rats with chronic renal damage. Kidney Int 5:147–176, 1974
6. Schultze RG, Weisser F, Bricker NS: The influence of uremia on fractional sodium reabsorption by the proximal tubule of rats. Kidney Int 2:59–65, 1972
7. Hayslett JP, Kashgarian M, Epstein FH: Mechanism of the change in the excretion of sodium per nephron when renal mass is reduced. J Clin Invest 47:774–782, 1968
8. Allison MEM, Wilson CB, Gottschalk CW: Pathophysiology of experimental glomerulonephritis in rats. J Clin Invest 53:1402–1423, 1974

9. Blantz RC, Wilson CB: Acute effects of antiglomerular basement membrane antibody on the process of glomerular filtration in the rat. J Clin Invest 58:899–911, 1976
10. Blantz RC, Tucker BJ, Wilson CB: Acute effects of antiglomerular basement membrane antibody on the process of glomerular filtration in the rat. Influence of dose and complement depletion. J Clin Invest 61:910–921, 1978
11. Weber H, Lin K, Bricker NS: Effect of sodium intake on single nephron glomerular filtration rate and sodium reabsorption in experimental uremia. Kidney Int 8:14–20, 1975
12. Deen WM, Maddox DA, Robertson CR, Brenner BM: Dynamics of glomerular ultrafiltration in the rat. VII. Response to reduced renal mass. Am J Physiol 227:556–562, 1974
13. Bricker NS, Fine LG: The renal response to progressive nephron loss. In Brenner BM, Rector FC Jr (eds.): The Kidney, 2nd ed. Philadelphia, Saunders, 1981, pp. 1056–1096
14. Bricker NS, Fine LG, Kaplan MA, Epstein M, Bourgoignie JJ, Licht A: "Magnification phenomenon" in chronic renal disease. N Engl J Med 299:1287–1293, 1978
15. Bricker NS, Danovitch GM: Extracellular fluid volume regulation: On the evidence for a biologic control system. In Epstein M (ed.): The Kidney in Liver Disease. New York, Elsevier/North Holland (in press)
16. Slatopolsky E, Elkan IO, Weerts C, Bricker NS: Studies on the characteristics of the control system governing sodium excretion in uremic man. J Clin Invest 47:521–530, 1968
17. Epstein M: Cardiovascular and renal effects of head-out water immersion in man. Circ Res 39:619–628, 1976
18. Coleman AJ, Arias M, Carter NW, Rector FC, Seldin DW: The mechanism of salt wastage in chronic renal disease. J Clin Invest 45:1116–1125, 1966
19. Stanbury SW, Mahler RF: Salt wasting renal disease: Metabolic observations on a patient with "salt-losing nephritis." Q J Med 28:425–447, 1959
20. Danovitch GM, Bourgoignie JJ, Bricker NS: Reversibility of the "salt-losing" tendency of chronic renal failure. N Engl J Med 296:14–19, 1977
21. Bricker NS: Life beyond the earth's environment: The biology of living organisms in space. In Bricker NS, (ed.): Monograph for Space Science Board. Washington, D.C., National Academy of Sciences, 1979
22. Fitzhugh FW Jr, McWhorter RL Jr, Estes EH Jr, Warren JV, Merrill AJ: The effect of application of tourniquets to the legs on cardiac output and renal function in normal human subjects. J Clin Invest 32:1163–1170, 1953
23. Feldman D, Funder J, Edelman I: Subcellular mechanisms in the action of adrenal steroids. Am J Med 53:545–560, 1972
24. Schultze RG, Shapiro HS, Bricker NS: Studies on the control of sodium excretion in experimental uremia. J Clin Invest 48:869–877, 1969
25. Schrier RW, Regal EM: Influence of aldosterone on sodium, water and potassium metabolism in chronic renal disease. Kidney Int 1:156–168, 1972
26. Hormonal regulation of sodium excretion. In Lichardus B, Schrier RW, Ponec J, (eds.): Proceedings of the Satellite Symposium of the 28th I.V.P.S. Congress. Amsterdam, Elsevier/North Holland 1980
27. Bourgoignie JJ, Hwang KH, Espinel C, Klahr S, Bricker NS: A natriuretic

factor in serum of patients with chronic uremia. J Clin Invest 51:1514–1527, 1972
28. Bourgoignie JJ, Hwang KH, Ipakchi E, Bricker NS: The presence of a natriuretic factor in urine of patients with chronic uremia. The absence of the factor in nephrotic uremic patients. J Clin Invest 53:1559–1567, 1974
29. Brown PR, Koutsaimanis KG, de Wardener HE: Effect of urinary extracts from salt-loaded man on urinary sodium excretion by the rat. Kidney Int 2:1–5, 1972
30. Favre H, Hwang KH, Schmidt RW, Bricker NS, Bourgoignie JJ: An inhibitor of sodium transport in the urine of dogs with normal renal function. J Clin Invest 56:1302–1311, 1975
31. Epstein M, Bricker NS, Bourgoignie JJ: The presence of a natriuretic factor in urine of normal men undergoing water immersion. Kidney Int 13:152–158, 1978
32. Vanlanthan M, Louis F, Favre H: Importance relative du facteur natriuretique et de l'aldosterone dans le maintien du bilan sodique. J Urol Nephrol 85:569–573, 1979
33. Klahr S, Rodriguez HJ: Natriuretic hormone. Nephron 15:387–408, 1975
34. Schmidt RW, Bourgoignie JJ, Bricker NS: On the adaptation in sodium excretion in chronic uremia: The effects of "proportional reduction" of sodium intake. J Clin Invest 53:1736–1741, 1974
35. Fine LG, Bourgoignie JJ, Hwang KH, Bricker NS: On the influence of the natriuretic factor from patients with chronic uremia on the bioelectric properties and sodium transport of the isolated mammalian collecting tubule. J Clin Invest 58:590–597, 1976
36. Clarkson EM, Raw SM, de Wardener HE: Further observations on a low-molecular-weight natriuretic substance in urine of normal man. Kidney Int 16:710–721, 1979
37. Bricker NS, Licht A: Natriuretic hormone: Biologic effects and progress in identification and isolation. In Lichardus B, Schrier RW, Ponec J (eds.): Proceedings of Symposium on Hormonal Regulation of Sodium Excretion. Amsterdam, Elsevier/North Holland, 1980, pp. 399–408
38. Kaplan MA, Bourgoignie JJ, Rosecan J, Bricker NS: The effects of the natriuretic factor from patients with chronic uremia on the bioelectric properties and sodium transport of the isolated mammalian collecting tubule. J Clin Invest 58:590–597, 1976
39. Bricker NS, Licht A: Natriuretic hormone: Current status. In Massry SG, Glassock RJ (eds,): Textbook of Nephrology. New York, Elsevier/North Holland (in press)
40. Gruber KA, Whitaker JM, Buckalew VM Jr: Endogenous digitalis-like substance in plasma of volume-expanded dogs. Nature 287:743–745, 1980
41. Fine LG, Bourgoignie JJ, Weber H, Bricker NS: Enhanced end-organ responsiveness of the uremic kidney to the natriuretic factor. Kidney Int 10:364–372, 1976
42. Weber H, Bourgoignie JJ, Bricker NS: Effects of the natriuretic serum fraction of proximal tubular sodium reabsorption. Am J Physiol 226:419–425, 1974
43. Danovitch GM, Jacobson E, Licht A: Absence of renal sodium adaptation in chronic renal failure. Am J Nephrol 1:173–176, 1981

44. Fine LG, Yanagawa N, Schultze RG, Tuck M: Functional profile of the isolated uremic nephron. Potassium adaptation in the rabbit cortical collecting tubule. J Clin Invest 64:1033–1043, 1979
45. Slatopolsky E, Caglar S, Pennell JP, Taggart DD, Canterbury JM, Reiss E, Bricker NS: On the pathogenesis of hyperparathyroidism in chronic renal insufficiency in the dog. J Clin Invest 50:492–499, 1971
46. Altsheler P, Klahr S, Rosenbaum R, Slatopolsky E: Effects of inhibitors of prostaglandin synthesis on the renal excretion of sodium in normal dogs and dogs with decreased renal mass. Am J Physiol 235:F338–F344, 1978

Refractory Ascites in Cirrhosis

Principal Discussant
Norman G. Levinsky

Case Presentation

A 36-year-old man was admitted to the hospital for the eighth time because of confusion, lethargy, nausea, and vomiting of 3 weeks duration; he had been discharged from the hospital only 3.5 weeks earlier.

The patient is a known alcoholic with a daily intake of approximately one quart of wine and one-fifth of whiskey or vodka for at least 8 years. Four years ago, he was evaluated at another hospital for a seizure disorder thought to be due to alcohol withdrawal. Three years ago, he was admitted to the New England Medical Center for the first time for nausea, vomiting, abdominal pain, seizures, and fever. Examination at that time revealed normal blood pressure, asterixis, and an enlarged liver; he had no ascites, edema, or peripheral neuropathy. The weight was 75 kg. The hematocrit was 25%. Laboratory findings at that time were as follows: serum electrolytes, normal; blood urea nitrogen (BUN), 5 mg; serum creatinine, 1.2 mg; serum bilirubin, 2 mg; serum albumin, 4 g/100 ml; and alkaline phosphatase, 6.3 Bodansky U. Hemoglobin electrophoresis revealed sickle cell trait. Upper gastrointestinal series revealed "duodenitis" without a definite ulcer crater. An i.v. urogram was normal. He was treated with folic acid, thiamine, multivitamins, antacids, chlordiazepoxide, and phenytoin.

During the next 3 years, the patient was readmitted several times. A liver biopsy specimen obtained 2 years prior to the present hospitalization revealed hemosiderosis, mild to moderate cirrhosis, and mild alcoholic hepatitis. During one representative admission, initial laboratory findings were BUN, 45 mg; serum creatinine, 4.5 mg/100 ml; sodium, 136 mEq; potassium, 2.6 mEq; chloride, 85 mEq; and total carbon dioxide content, 36 mEq/liter. Diarrhea, thought to be related to lactulose therapy, resulted in a transient fall in the total carbon dioxide content to 12 mEq/liter. By the time of discharge, the serum creatinine had fallen to 0.8 mg/100 ml; the serum sodium was 138 mEq, potassium was 5 mEq, chloride was 105 mEq, and total carbon dioxide content was 20 mEq/liter.

Three months prior to the present hospitalization, the patient was admitted because of confusion. Weight was 63.9 kg; ascites and edema were noted. The bilirubin was 7.3 mg/100 ml. Serum electrolytes were sodium, 133 mEq; potassium, 2.4 mEq; chloride, 72 mEq/liter. Total carbon dioxide content was 43 mEq/liter. At the time of admission, the BUN was 88 mg, and the serum creatinine was 3.3 mg/100 ml; by the time of discharge, they were 31 and 2.3 mg/100 ml, respectively. The mental confusion, thought to be due to hepatic encephalopathy, disappeared completely before discharge. The patient was discharged on a regimen of spironolactone, folic acid, thiamine, and phenytoin.

Six weeks prior to the present admission, the patient was again hospitalized for mental confusion, nausea, vomiting, and weakness. Blood pressure was 90/70 mmHg, weight was 58.8 kg, and there was massive ascites. The patient was icteric; asterixis and a peripheral neuropathy were demonstrated. The serum concentration of sodium was 141 mEq, potassium was 2.6 mEq, chloride was 66 mEq, and the total carbon dioxide content was 53 mEq/liter. Arterial blood findings were pH, 7.6; arterial oxygen tension (Po_2), 51 mmHg; and arterial carbon dioxide tension (Pco_2), 53 mmHg. Random urinary values for electrolyte concentrations were sodium, 60 mEq; and chloride 0 mEq/liter; the patient was not receiving diuretics at this time. At the time of admission, the BUN was 60 mg, and the serum creatinine was 5 mg/100 ml; before discharge, the levels were 53 and 3.9 mg/100 ml, respectively. Upper gastrointestinal series was negative on two occasions. Renal echogram revealed the kidneys to be of normal size; there was no evidence of obstruction. The serum electrolytes and acid-base equilibrium returned toward normal. While the patient was being treated with nasogastric suction, however, the total carbon dioxide content rose to 49 mEq/liter and the arterial Pco_2 rose to 67 mmHg. Arginine hydrochloride (approximately 150 mEq, in 300 cc) was administered i.v. over a time period of approximately 4 to 6 h; during the infusion, serum potassium concentration rose from 5.3 to 7.3 mEq/liter despite the fact that no potassium was administered. The patient was discharged on a regimen of phenytoin, cimetidine, and multivitamins.

He was readmitted for the eighth time 3.5 weeks later. Physical examination disclosed the following findings: temperature, 36 °C; pulse, 70; respirations, 18/min; blood pressure, 82/60 mmHg supine and 72/58 mmHg standing; weight, 63 kg; abdominal girth, 98 cm; the liver edge was 5 cm below the right costal margin; there was massive ascites and no peripheral edema; the patient was mildly confused. Laboratory studies revealed the following data: hematocrit, 35%; white blood cell count, 5500/mm^2. Results of urinalysis revealed specific gravity, 1.012; pH, 7.5; and occasional white blood cells. Electrolyte concentrations in the serum were sodium, 130 mEq; potassium, 2.8 mEq; and chloride, 66 mEq/liter. Total carbon dioxide content was 49 mEq/liter. Arterial blood had a pH of 7.59, with a Po_2 of 53 mmHg and a Pco_2 of 47 mmHg. The BUN was 100 mg, serum creatinine was 5.8 mg, and albumin was

2.2 g/100 ml. Random samples for urinary electrolytes were sodium, 43 mEq; potassium, 42 mEq; and chloride, 0 mEq/liter. The serum enzyme values were alkaline phosphatase, 8.9 Bodansky U; glutamic oxaloacetic transaminase (SGOT), 24 U; serum glutamic pyruvic transaminase (SGPT), 11 U; lactate dehydrogenase (LDH), 103 U; and creatinine phosphokinase (CPK), 3 U. Chest x-ray revealed elevated hemidiaphragms; an electrocardiogram demonstrated normal rhythm at a rate of 70/min, and there were nonspecific ST-T wave changes. The patient was treated with a 500-mg sodium chloride diet, salt-poor albumin, arginine hydrochloride (approximately 300 mEq/day, for 3 days), potassium chloride, lactulose, cimetidine, and spironolactone (begun 1 week later). The serum concentrations of potassium and chloride rose (potassium, to 4.5 mEq; chloride, to 103 mEq), and the total carbon dioxide content fell to 20 mEq/liter.

Eleven days following admission, the patient was alert and oriented. Massive ascites persisted; abdominal girth was 96 cm, and weight was 63 kg.

On the 12th hospital day, a LeVeen peritoneal-jugular shunt was inserted because of the patient's severe ascites, impaired renal function, and reluctance to use vigorous diuretic therapy.

Preoperatively, the hematocrit was 32%, and the blood chemistry values were bilirubin, 2mg; serum albumin, 3.3 g; BUN, 64 mg; serum creatinine, 1.9 mg/100 ml; serum sodium, 133 mEq; serum potassium, 3.9 mEq; serum chloride, 103 mEq; and total carbon dioxide content, 20 mEq/liter.

For the first 7 days postoperatively, the patient received approximately 40 mg of furosemide and 50 mg of spironolactone daily, but thereafter no diuretics were given; while ingesting a 1-g sodium chloride diet, edema did not recur. Blood pressure was 105/80 mmHg, weight was 58.6 kg, and abdominal girth was 84 cm. The serum electrolyte concentrations were sodium, 135 mEq; potassium, 4.6 mEq; chloride, 103 mEq/liter. The total carbon dioxide content was 24 mEq/liter. The BUN was 19 mg, serum creatinine was 1.1 mg, and bilirubin was 1.2 mg/100 ml. The patient was discharged 17 days following surgery.

Discussion

Dr. Norman G. Levinsky *(Chairman, Department of Medicine, Boston University Medical Center, Boston, Massachusetts)*: Ascites and renal failure are the key nephrologic problems presented by this patient. I shall devote most of the discussion to these typical disorders of advanced cirrhosis and the new form of management undertaken in this case. The patient also developed a number of interesting fluid and electrolyte disturbances related to his individual clinical course, and I shall discuss some of these briefly.

We can discuss the patient's ascites and renal failure together, since they began at about the same time in his course and these problems probably are related pathophysiologically. The patient had a number of episodes of reversible azotemia during the first 3 years of his course here. I assume that these episodes were prerenal azotemia due to the volume depletion of vomiting. Each was associated with metabolic alkalosis and a history of vomiting; renal function became normal after treatment. Three months before this admission, the patient was first noted to have ascites, which increased in amount thereafter despite treatment with a low-salt diet and spironolactone. At the same time, moderately persistent azotemia was first noted; during three admissions thereafter, the serum creatinine concentration only fell to 2.3, 3.9, and 1.9 mg/100 ml after treatment. Although the patient was appropriately evaluated at one point for causes of azotemia not directly related to his cirrhosis, apparently no specific cause was found, such as ingestion of nephrotoxins, which should always be considered in alcoholic patients. The azotemia was not progressive and seems to represent moderate, chronic renal failure, intrinsic to his underlying liver disease.

The traditional view of the afferent mechanism for this man's condition can be summarized as follows (Fig. 1, *left*). Decreased albumin synthesis by the cirrhotic liver reduces oncotic pressure, while intrahepatic obstruction raises hydrostatic pressure in the hepatic and splanchnic circulation. These changes in pressure alter Starling's forces to favor transudation of plasma filtrate into the intraabdominal cavity. Resistance to blood flow through the liver also traps an increased vol-

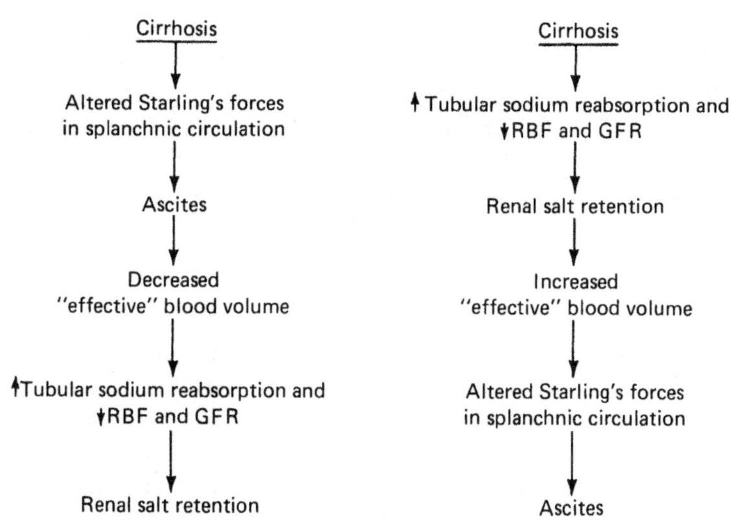

Fig. 1. Simplified schemata of the "underfilling" (*left*) and "overflow" (*right*) theories of the pathogenesis of the sodium retention in cirrhosis.

ume of blood in the splanchnic circulation. Both factors—trapping and transudation—diminish the central "effective" blood volume. Renal vasoconstriction, decreased renal blood flow, and sodium retention are secondary to the reduction of "effective" blood volume. Several conclusions relevant to this man's management follow from this formulation. Diuretics were used sparingly. Because these agents act on the kidney, their direct effect is to deplete the blood volume. Only if and when loss of fluid from the plasma leads to a change in Starling's forces in the hepatic/splanchnic circulation favoring uptake of edema fluid (reduction in capillary pressure and concentration of plasma proteins) will ascites diminish and the blood volume be restored to its initial, already inadequate, level. Thus, the well-recognized tendency for potent diuretics to precipitate hypotension and renal failure is seen to be an iatrogenic exacerbation of the fundamental pathophysiologic disorder, inadequate "effective" blood volume. These complications also occur after paracentesis and are explained, similarly, to be due to further contraction of the "effective" circulatory volume, when fluid shifts from the plasma to reform ascites. Based on this line of reasoning, some years ago attempts were made to maintain intravascular volume during diuresis by infusing ascites intravenously. Dramatic diureses were often obtained, even in patients otherwise resistant to diuretics, without inducing hypotension or renal failure [1]. As a practical matter, this form of treatment is necessarily short term.

In 1974 LeVeen and associates [2] described an ingenious peritoneovenous shunt suitable for chronic implantation by a minor surgical procedure under local anesthesia (Fig. 2). The key feature is a valve which opens at a pressure of 3–5 cm$H_2$0. This valve, implanted under the skin of the abdomen, connects an intraabdominal drain to a subcutaneous shunt, inserted in the jugular vein. Thus, when intraabdominal pressure exceeds venous pressure by 5 cmH_2O, ascites flows into the vein. If the rate of self-infusion is too rapid, venous pressure will rise a few centimeters and the valve will close, thereby preventing overloading of the central circulation. A number of papers have described the effects of this shunt [3,4] in cirrhotics. Ascites is rapidly reabsorbed, and losses of 10 kg in 10 days are reported in patients previously refractory to diuretics [5]. Ascites was relieved in more than 95% of patients in one large series [3], apparently indefinitely, although detailed follow-up observations have not yet been reported. The long-term effects on sodium retention by the kidney, need for diuretics, and ability of patients to tolerate increased sodium intake are as yet unclear, although the originators state that they have unpublished evidence that "avid reabsorption of sodium in patients with refractory ascites can be at least in part counteracted" [5]. Plasma aldosterone and renin fall to normal [4,5], but this observation should not be taken to imply a cause and effect relation to the accompanying natriuresis. At least two groups

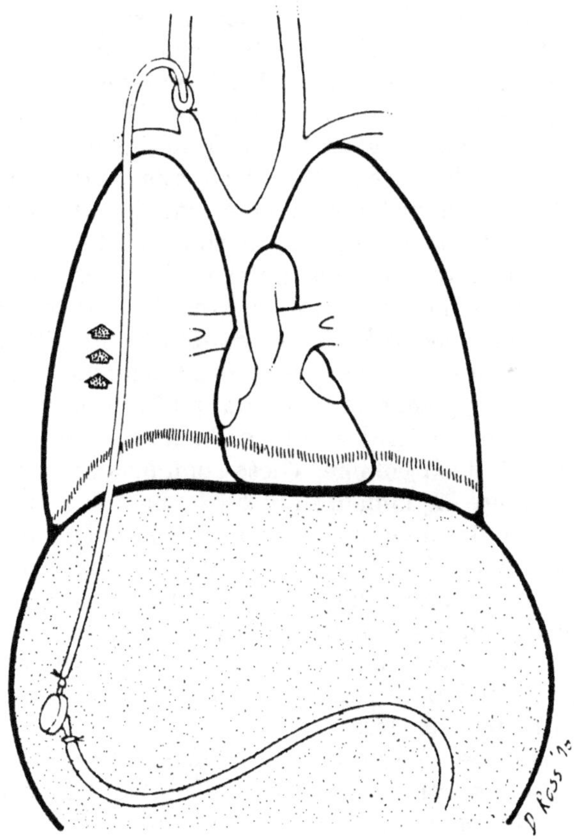

Fig. 2. LeVeen peritoneal-jugular shunt. Perforated silicone rubber tubing bathes in ascitic fluid compartment. Springlike valve is extraperitoneal and is connected to jugular vein by subcutaneous silicone rubber tube. (Reprinted with permission of JAMA [5].)

[6,7] have shown that volume expansion can lower plasma aldosterone and renin in cirrhotics with ascites, without inducing a natriuresis.

Although the point is not fully documented, it appears that relief of ascites is obtained without the adverse effects of hypovolemia, such as hypotension and deterioration of renal function. Indeed, the chronically reduced glomerular filtration rate (GFR) characteristic of patients with advanced cirrhosis actually improves. In 28 patients, plasma creatinine concentration decreased from 2.4 to 1.8 mg/100 ml 10 days after insertion of the shunt [5]. This improvement is presumably due to expanded central volume, since similar increases in GFR occur after infusion of ascites [1], and during bodily immersion [8], which shift blood volume centrally. The LeVeen shunt and paracentesis with reinfusion of ascites also lower intraabdominal pressure, a maneuver known to raise GFR acutely. The improvement of GFR after reduction in abdominal pressure, however, doesn't persist, and the favorable effect of immersion occurs without reduction in this pressure. Thus, decreased abdominal pressure is probably not the major mechanism for improved GFR after LeVeen shunting.

Most strikingly, it is reported that hepatorenal syndrome can be reversed by the LeVeen shunt. Four cases have been presented in detail [4,9], and LeVeen et al. [3] state that nine patients with the syndrome all improved. The relation between chronically reduced GFR in advanced cirrhosis and the hepatorenal syndrome is uncertain. Although the former is common, only a minority of patients develop the relentless progression of renal dysfunction to oliguria and clinically significant renal failure that characterizes the hepatorenal syndrome. It is not known what fraction of those who develop the hepatorenal syndrome are patients who previously had stable but reduced GFR for a prolonged period, and what fraction are individuals with wholly normal renal function who suddenly develop hepatorenal syndrome. The apparent ability of the LeVeen shunt to reverse these conditions for indefinite periods certainly suggests that both chronic reduction in GFR and hepatorenal syndrome may be volume-dependent phenomena. The familiar clinical observation that hepatorenal syndrome may be triggered by minor hypovolemia, such as after paracentesis or a small gastrointestinal hemorrhage, suggests a chronically inadequate "effective" circulation, from which irreversible renal failure can be generated by a small added volume deficit. Acute volume expansion has had limited, if any, benefit in patients with hepatorenal syndrome [10]. More than 10 years ago, one study [11], however, showed maintained renal hemodynamic and clinical benefit in a few patients treated by reinfusion of ascites for several days. The beneficial effects of the LeVeen shunt, the first practical method for chronic return of ascites to the central circulation, fit with these limited previous observations. The efferent mechanism of the effect is unknown. It has recently been suggested that renal failure in hepatorenal syndrome is due to the combination of increased vasoconstrictor (renin/angiotensin) and decreased vasodilator (prekallikrein/bradykinin) activity. As noted earlier, elevated plasma angiotensin in the hepatorenal syndrome is decreased after insertion of the LeVeen shunt. The effect of the shunt on plasma prekallikrein/bradykinin is as yet unknown.

Should the patient under discussion have been treated with a LeVeen shunt? He had massive ascites that had failed to respond to treatment with a low-salt diet and spironolactone in-hospital or at home. More potent agents had apparently been avoided for fear of adverse effects, especially deterioration of already diminished renal function. Thus, this man cannot be described as resistant to a full diuretic program, as were the patients treated with the shunt in published series [3]. The dangers of diuretic use are well known and include hypotension, electrolyte disturbances (such as hyponatremia, potassium depletion, and alkalosis), precipitation of hepatic coma, and hepatorenal syndrome. As discussed earlier, it is uncertain whether patients with chronic stable reduction of GFR, such as this man, are more prone to hepatorenal syndrome, but as a practical matter it is reasonable to be especially concerned about further deterioration of renal function in such patients. On the other hand, this patient's azotemia was moderate (BUN, 64 mg/100 ml; serum creatinine, 1.9 mg/100 ml) after initial in-hospital management. Although firm data are difficult to find, my own experience is that judicious, in-hospital use of potent diuretics causes minor, easily treatable complications, such as exacerbation of hyponatremia or azotemia, in about 5 to 10% of patients with cirrhosis and tense ascites. Severe complications, such as clinical hypotension, severe encephalopathy, serious deterioration of renal function, and hepatorenal syndrome, can be avoided in all but 1 to 2% of these patients by careful observation, slow diuresis not exceeding 1 kg of body-weight-loss/day, and intermittent rather than continuous use of the most potent agents such as furosemide. There is, of course, an old-fashioned but effective alternative treatment of tense ascites—paracentesis. When limited to removal of no more than 2 liters (sufficient, because of the hyperbolic relation between intraabdominal pressure and volume, to reduce pressure markedly), the risk of serious complications is low, perhaps 1% in my experience.

The complications of the LeVeen shunt have been reported, thus far, only by the originators [3], who note approximately 5% wound infections, 3% sepsis, 15% leakage of ascites, and 15% subcutaneous bleeding. Ten percent of the patients develop upper gastrointestinal hemorrhage, presumably due to increased pressure in varices as ascites is rapidly reabsorbed, a familiar complication of rapid expansion of blood volume in advanced cirrhosis. (Most of the patients had bled previously, and the orginators suggest that the shunt should not be used after recent variceal bleeding, unless a portosystemic shunt is performed first.) Thus, the frequency of complications from the shunt is comparable to that from careful use of diuretics, and probably exceeds that from limited use of paracentesis. Moreover, further complications from use of the shunt may appear after more prolonged and extensive observation.

The other part of the cost-benefit equation must be evaluated, however. Long experience indicates that relief of severe ascites by low-salt diets, diuretics, and paracentesis is limited and transient. Such relief, obtained by careful management in the hospital, is usually dissipated rapidly outside in the real world by erratic control of diet and casual adherence to diuretic programs. The LeVeen shunt apparently produces dramatic relief of ascites for an indefinite period in the majority of patients.

The question must be asked, however, why is relief of ascites important? Since the underlying hepatic dysfunction is not reversed, the greatly shortened life expectancy of patients with decompensated cirrhosis will presumably not improve. The potential benefits of decreased acites are relief of fullness and discomfort, improved appetite, and a greater sense of well-being. An improved self-image may contribute to greater willingness to follow therapeutic regimens, including abstinence from alcohol. Tense ascites may interfere with respiration, especially when the patient is recumbent. Abdominal skin and umbilical hernias may stretch excessively and break down. Uncomfortable peripheral and scrotal edema may be due, in part, to compression of the inferior vena cava by tense ascites. Patients are often remarkably asymptomatic, however, despite gross ascites. Hence, the conservative view has been to accept ascites, use cautious therapy to achieve the limited goal of relief of symptoms when necessary, and avoid the frequent complications of attempts to produce a patient who is free of ascites.

The dramatic relief of ascites for indefinite periods with the LeVeen shunt, however, is tempting to physicians, such as myself, who are frustrated by their inability to alter the underlying, lethal hepatic pathology. Moreover, the classical view that ascites is a consequence of diminished "effective" circulation suggests theoretical advantages for use of this procedure, since intravascular volume is thereby continuously restored to normal. Will this technique, for example, prevent the hepatorenal syndrome, since the initial reports cited above suggest it can treat this otherwise irreversible and lethal complication? The originators suggest that the incidence of hepatic encephalopathy is reduced, perhaps because improved renal function leads to a lower maintained level of blood urea, thereby decreasing ammonia formation from urea in the gut. They further report a markedly improved sense of well-being, which may not be entirely due to the psychologic benefit of a surgical procedure with a dramatic cosmetic effect. Wasting of muscles and facies has long been recognized as typical of cirrhotics with ascites—a big belly with thin face and limbs—and usually has been attributed to alcoholic malnutrition. The patient under discussion had lost 16 kg of dry body weight over 3 years. LeVeen and associates report rapid restoration of muscle and fat and loss of the cirrhotic facies within weeks after insertion of the shunt. Is there an effect beyond improvement of appetite? Is there a "cirrhotic cachexia" analogous to cardiac cachexia, attributable to diminished "effective" circulation, which can be overcome by chronic reinfusion of ascites to the central volume? These are all exciting possibilities suitable for careful study.

In terms of the management of individual patients today, I would be conservative. In patients who develop unequivocal hepatorenal syndrome, almost always irreversible and fatal with conventional treatment, a trial of the LeVeen shunt seems indicated. (It is important, of course, to rule out volume depletion due to excessive diuresis and acute tubular necrosis, both of which are frequent findings in patients with cirrhosis and are often confused with hepatorenal syndrome.) In patients who are symptomatic from tense ascites that cannot be managed with diuretic therapy, occasional paracentesis, and low-salt diets, a trial of the shunt may be in order. The patient under discussion had moderate, stable azotemia, but no evidence of hepatorenal syndrome. It is not clear whether he was symptomatic from ascites, but in any case, he had not been treated with potent diuretics or paracentesis. Hence, I probably would not have used the LeVeen shunt in this patient.

Whatever its ultimate place in the clinical treatment of ascites, careful study of the effects of the LeVeen shunt may make an important contribution to our understanding of the pathophysiology of this condition. Thus far, we have described the genesis of ascites according to the conventional view, in which renal sodium retention is secondary to underfilling of the "effective" circulation. Recently, this view has been challenged by clinical [12] and experimental [13] evidence in favor of an "overflow" mechanism (Fig. 1, *right*). According to this hypothesis, the sick liver releases or stimulates factors which directly cause renal vasoconstriction and excessive tubular sodium reabsorption. Excess salt and water ultimately "overflow" from the hepatic and splanchnic circulation, where abnormal Starling's forces favor transudation, to form ascites. The key difference between the two hypotheses is whether the "effective" circulation is underfilled or overfilled, a point with obvious consequences for the interpretation of a variety of clinical phenomena in cirrhotic patients with ascites. This is not the place for an extended discussion of the arguments for each view, but a few examples can be summarized. Numerous studies show that blood volume is usually increased in patients with cirrhosis and ascites. This fits directly with the "overflow" theory; the "underfilling" theory explains this observation by postulating that blood volume is increased because of increased vascular capacity in the dilated splanchnic vessels, but postulates that the (unmeasurable) "effective" circulation is inadequately filled. Some studies show that the rate of ascites formation does not increase after paracentesis, nor does plasma volume decrease [12] as would be expected according to the traditional, but not the "overflow," theory. Recently, Levy [13] has provided strong evidence for the "overflow" theory in cirrhotic dogs, in which he was able to study the evolution of ascites through all stages. He found that renal sodium retention preceded ascites by 10 days, that nonsplanchnic volume, measured directly, was increased, and that paracentesis did not cause reformation of ascites as long as dietary salt was restricted. Most pertinent to the present discussion is Levy's finding [14; Levy, personal communication, 1978] that mobilization of ascites with a LeVeen shunt does not eliminate renal sodium retention, although the natriuretic response to a diuretic is greatly enhanced. When placed on a high-salt diet, the cirrhotic dogs developed massive anasarca, although, strikingly, edema was now facial and pulmonary, since the LeVeen shunt prevented the formation of significant ascites. These data obviously fit easily in the "overflow" mechanism, but they are difficult to reconcile with the conventional view. Careful study of renal sodium-handling in patients with LeVeen shunts should contribute significantly to our understanding of the pathophysiology of ascites in man. The key point is whether patients treated with the shunt will regain the ability to excrete a normal dietary intake of sodium without diuretics. Although it has been reported that this was the outcome in one patient [4], data on this point are inadequate. Appropriate studies of the present patient would be very interesting.

Although this discussion has focused on the patient's principal clinical problem and its management, brief comments on several other problems of nephrologic interest are in order. The patient had hypokalemic alkalosis on several occasions, in each episode related to vomiting. Use of diuretics such as furosemide, a likely cause of this pattern in cirrhotics with ascites, was apparently not a factor here. Although mild hypokalemia, probably caused by poor dietary intake of potassium and secondary aldosteronism, is sometimes present in patients with cirrhosis and ascites, the alkalosis, the presence of the electrolyte abnormality on one occasion before ascites was present, and on another occasion during treatment with an aldosterone antagonist (assuming the patient was taking it as prescribed!), all point to vomiting as the principal cause of the hypokalemic alkalosis. At first glance, the high urinary potassium (42 mEq/liter on the last admission when serum potassium was 2.8 mEq/liter) may seem puzzling, since the usual teaching is that urinary potassium should be below 20 mEq/liter when hypokalemia is caused by extrarenal losses. Schwartz et al., however, have found that the pattern of urinary electrolytes during the *genesis* of hypokalemic alkalosis due to loss of gastric juice is different than that characteristic of *maintained* hypokalemic alkalosis [15]. If we assume that this patient was vomiting severely right up to the time of admission, the pattern of urinary electrolytes would be typical of that noted by Schwartz et al. during the genesis of experimental hypokalemic alkalosis by gastric aspiration. We can hypothesize that rapid loss of hydrochloric acid has elevated the patient's plasma bicarbonate above his renal tubular reabsorptive capacity, even though the latter is presumably elevated by volume contraction and possibly (to a lesser degree than once believed) by hypercapnia. Hence, significant bicarbonate escapes tubular reabsorption, as is evident from the alkaline urine (pH,

7.5). This bicarbonate acts, in effect, as an unreabsorbable anion, promoting delivery of sodium to the distal nephron and, especially in the presence of secondary aldosteronism, augmenting distal potassium secretion. The ability of bicarbonate, acting as an unreabsorbable anion, to force sodium excretion is especially striking in this patient who, despite cirrhotic mechanisms strongly favoring complete renal sodium retention, exhibited a urinary sodium concentration of 60 mEq/liter during one episode. At the same time, urinary chloride was 0 mEq/liter, correctly signaling the underlying state of sodium retentiveness. The formation stage of hypokalemic alkalosis due to vomiting is one of the few instances in which the clinical use of urinary sodium and potassium concentrations to separate renal from extrarenal losses of these ions may prove invalid.

The deleterious consequences of hypokalemic alkalosis in patients with cirrhosis are especially worth noting. This patient on several occasions entered with hepatic encephalopathy coincident with the electrolyte derangement. The encephalopathy cleared after a number of therapeutic maneuvers, important among them being treatment to reverse the hypokalemic alkalosis. It is well recognized that the distribution of ammonia between extracellular fluid and cells is determined, in part, by the hydrogen ion gradient between them. Experimental and clinical studies suggest that extracellular hypokalemic alkalosis probably does not cause cellular alkalosis. Indeed, the cells probably become more acid, especially if, as in the present patient, hypercapnia due to respiratory compensation supervenes. The absolute or relative acidification of the intracellular fluid, including that of the brain, will trap an increased fraction of the total body pool of ammonia inside cells. Experimental evidence suggests that this is one mechanism by which alkalosis may precipitate encephalopathy. The other postulated mechanism is renal. As is well known, potassium depletion stimulates ammonia production by the kidney, presumably in response to acidification of tubular cells. When ammonia production increases during metabolic acidosis, it is largely trapped by the acid urine. If, however, extracellular alkalosis accompanies potassium depletion, the urine will be relatively alkaline, as in this patient. In this event, less ammonia will be trapped in the urine, and more will diffuse into the peritubular blood. These phenomena have been demonstrated by renal venous catheterization in patients with cirrhosis. Moreover, as this patient demonstrates, the compensatory hypoventilation of metabolic alkalosis may cause significant hypoxia, which may contribute to the encephalopathy. (The estimated alveolar-arterial P_{O_2} gradient in this patient, however, was 35–40 mmHg on two occasions, indicating that his severe hypoxia was due to pulmonary disease as well as hypoventilation.) Thus, it is easy to see why hypokalemic alkalosis due to vomiting or diuretics may precipitate encephalopathy and justify treatment:

increased ammonia production by the kidney, increased movement of renal ammonia into blood rather than urine, increased movement of extracellular ammonia into brain cells, and hypoxia. Moreover, elevation of plasma urea, because of associated prerenal failure as occurred in this patient, may lead to increased intestinal ammonia production through enhanced urea breakdown by bacterial flora in the gut, as noted earlier.

Finally, a word should be included about the hyperkalemia precipitated on one occasion by attempts to treat the patient's severe alkalosis with arginine hydrochloride. After infusion of 150 mEq of this cationic amino acid, serum potassium concentration rose 2 mEq/liter, from 5.3 to 7.3 mEq/liter. The ability of all cationic amino acids to drive potassium out of muscle cells is well documented both *in vivo* and *in vitro* [16]. At the time he received the infusion, this patient was probably fully potassium-repleted, since his serum potassium concentration was 5.3 mEq/liter despite extracellular alkalosis. He still had reduced renal function, since even at discharge serum creatinine concentration had fallen only to 3.8 mg/100 ml. The combination of sudden release of potassium from tissues and limited renal excretory capacity accounts for the sharp rise in serum potassium. Similar increases were reported in several patients with advanced, chronic renal failure who were infused with comparable amounts of arginine [16].

Questions and Answers

Dr. John T. Harrington: We were reluctant to use potent diuretics in this individual because on several occasions in the past he had hepatorenal syndrome or, at least, renal insufficiency associated with hepatic insufficiency. We attributed this reduction in glomerular function in part to volume depletion, and we thought that perhaps a reduction in "effective" circulating volume was also responsible. On that basis, the LeVeen shunt was attempted after many hospitalizations [17]. In the past when I have heard you talk about treating patients admitted with cirrhosis, or at least hepatic decompensation, I seem to recall that you have discouraged the use of potent diuretics during that period. My question is, Are you drawing a distinction between the use of potent diuretics shortly after admission and a week or two later when the patient is stable?

Dr. Levinsky: Perhaps I should clarify my views on both points. First, with regard to the presence of hepatorenal syndrome, I can only reemphasize what I said earlier. I would not feel there was evidence that this patient had the hepatorenal syndrome. I would suggest that he had two types of renal failure at different points in his course. On many occasions, he was admitted with volume contraction due to vomiting and prerenal failure. Later in his course when the azotemia persisted after fluid repletion, I think he had chronic stable reduction in renal hemodynamics and glomerular filtration; this is seen in a significant fraction of patients with advanced cirrhosis who are not developing the hepatorenal syndrome. As I said earlier, I am not even sure that all those who develop the hepatorenal syndrome necessarily have a creatinine of, perhaps, 1.5 or 2.0 mg/100 ml for weeks or months and then deteriorate. In fact, my guess would be contrary: some start with relatively normal renal blood flow and then suddenly deteriorate. Thus, I think that distinctions should be drawn between the various forms of renal failure which are possible in the patient with cirrhosis and advanced ascites. Second, I would not wish to promulgate, in any way, the impression that I was advocating the use of potent diuretics in all cirrhotics with ascites. To clarify what I said, the physician may feel treatment is needed when ascites is very tense, skin is breaking down, breathing is labored, or the patient is grossly disfigured and uncomfortable. If he thinks relief of such symptoms is important in a particular patient, the doctor might perform a modest paracentesis or cautiously treat with potent diuretics, to see if the patient is responsive. I would not have used the shunt just yet in this patient because I think it is as safe to give a few doses of furosemide to see what kind of response you get, as it is to insert the shunt.

Dr. Harrington: You estimated earlier that the incidence of severe complications from intermittent use of potent diuretics is 1 to 2%. Is it possible that severe diuretic-induced complications are more likely in patients with preexisting renal insufficiency, than in patients with normal renal function?

Dr. Levinsky: It sounds reasonable but I don't know.

Dr. Jordan Cohen: Would you comment on the strategy of using intermittent albumin infusion coupled with diuretics as an alternative therapeutic approach to management of ascites when it is deemed to be necessary?

Dr. Levinsky: Like ascites reinfusion, albumin avoids blood volume depletion and increases the response to diuretics. Either may precipitate bleeding from varices or hepatic encephalopathy. If the hospital is appropriately equipped, I would favor ascites reinfusion because ascites is relieved directly. In practice, we rarely use either technique.

Dr. Cohen: That leads me to the next question. If one adopts the "overflow" hypothesis to account for the sodium retention, how would one explain the apparent diuresis that usually ensues after insertion of the shunt?

Dr. Levinsky: I think there is no problem as long as the sodium retention is not completely reversed. According to the "overflow" theory, cirrhosis directly stimulates sodium retention, which should not disappear unless the cirrhosis itself improves. The critical question is whether the patient is able to handle a normal sodium intake without any need for diuretics. If he is able to handle a wide range of sodium intakes, it would be evidence against the "overflow" hypothesis. But as long as you must give him any diuretics or reduce his salt intake, the findings would be perfectly compatible with the thesis that renal sodium retention is stimulated by a direct hepatic mechanism, which has not been reversed by the shunt.

Dr. Harrington: Actually, we don't know the sodium tolerance of the patient. He was given diuretics following the shunt prophylactically because of our lack of experience in handling such patients, and for the same reason, he was given a 1-g salt diet. He has not had a sodium challenge.

Dr. Jerome P. Kassirer: With regard to some of the issues you raised about metabolic alkalosis, perhaps there are some points worth making. First, I think your description of the difference in the composition of the urine between the nonsteady state and the steady state in patients with gastric alkalosis is quite accurate. We would have no quarrel with your physiologic analysis including the fact that a stimulus for sodium reabsorption is necessary in order to preserve bicarbonate reabsorption when a patient becomes hypochloremic and alkalotic, and that volume contraction is the factor that creates that stimulus. Certainly, when metabolic alkalosis is first developing or becoming more severe, that stimulus is lacking, and that is the reason for the sodium and alkali diuresis. This sequence was shown nicely in experiments with normal human subjects in which metabolic alkalosis was induced by selective depletion of hydrochloric acid [18]. The experience in patients with vomiting and nasogastric suction confirms this experimental observation because most of these patients have a fair amount of sodium and bicarbonate in their urine and the urine pH is typically high [19]. By contrast, the patient with metabolic alkalosis who is in a steady state has no sodium or alkali in the urine and, of course, the urine is acid. Second, metabolic alkalosis may be particularly deleterious for a patient with cirrhosis. The best evidence suggests that, of the many factors that have been invoked as responsible for hepatic encephalopathy, blood pH is one that seems to correlate fairly well with the level of awareness. Several studies show that a considerably larger fraction of patients with encephalopathy are alkalemic compared to those with normal central nervous system function [20]. Patients with cirrhosis may be uniquely at risk when they develop metabolic alkalosis because they often have a simultaneous mild respiratory alkalosis, the mechanism for which is not clear. Therefore, for any given elevation of bicarbonate concentration, cirrhotics tend to be more alkalemic than the noncirrhotic individual. The normal adaptive respiratory response to metabolic alkalosis is not well defined, but it appears that every increase in plasma bicarbonate of 1 mEq/liter is associated with an increase in arterial P_{CO_2} of approximately 0.6 to 0.9 mmHg. On two of the occasions that severe hyperbicarbonatemia occurred in this patient, the increment in arterial P_{CO_2} was only approximately 0.3 to 0.5 mmHg per mEq/liter increment in bicarbonate, suggesting that hyperventilation was contributing to alkalemia. Unfortunately, we don't know whether the patient was hypocapnic in the absence of metabolic alkalosis. Third, I have a final observation about your remark that patients with the LeVeen shunt seem to develop encephalopathy less frequently. One explanation that might account for this finding is that these patients are no longer being subjected to potent diuretics and, therefore, are not developing potassium depletion, volume contraction, and metabolic alkalosis, all factors that might predispose them to develop cerebral dysfunction.

Dr. David Bernard *(Renal Service, University Hospital, Boston)*: Could you comment specifically on the use of spironolactone? The British literature has placed tremendous emphasis on the value of inhibiting steroid effects. A couple of years ago, it was suggested that the dose of spironolactone be titrated against the sodium and potassium concentrations in the urine aiming for a ratio of one. You haven't discussed which diuretics you would recommend, but do you think spironolactone actually adds anything to diuretic therapy?

Dr. Levinsky: Yes, spironolactone is often used initially, and I think properly, because it is a relatively modest diuretic and, hence, is unlikely to cause some of the adverse effects of rapid volume contraction produced by the more potent agents such as furosemide. I think one should always start with a less potent agent. A second advantage is that it doesn't induce potassium depletion and alkalosis and, thus, some of the encephalopathic complications. Beyond that, I don't think it has any specific virtue. I noted earlier that two studies quite clearly separate reduction of plasma aldosterone from natriuresis in cirrhosis. I don't think there is any specific virtue in competing with aldosterone. Spironolactone is a good baseline diuretic which may mitigate the hypokalemia and alkalosis that occurs if you must use one of the more potent diuretics.

Dr. James Strom *(Renal Fellow, NEMC)*: You suggested doing paracentesis to remove 1 or 2 liters of fluid. Gabuzda has estimated that the formation of ascitic fluid occurs at approximately 800 cc/24h [21]. Given the same Starling's forces, wouldn't ascites simply reaccumulate in a few days thereby mitigating the treatment? In addition, isn't the risk of spontaneous peritonitis in the alcoholic—estimated at 10–15% by some authorities—worth consideration?

Dr. Levinsky: Yes, the latter is a very good point. I should have listed spontaneous peritonitis as a complication of ascites, although I think 10 to 15% is a generous estimate. With regard to your first point, you may have noticed that I made a contrary statement earlier: I pointed out that the Reynolds group did not find an increased rate of formation of ascites after paracentesis. The Reynolds group commented that the discrepancy could be attributed to sodium restriction in their patients, while Gabuzda's patients were not sodium restricted. If one accepts the "overflow" hypothesis, this is a critical point. According to the "overflow" hypothesis, the patient will not rapidly reform ascites on a low-salt diet, because ascites formation is secondary to renal salt retention.

Dr. Cohen: One of the striking occurrences in this patient was the hyperkalemia precipitated by the arginine infusion. I wonder whether you think arginine should be avoided as a treatment for metabolic alkalosis in favor of hydrochloric acid, which has been recommended by some.

Dr. Levinsky: There are other reasons to favor hydrochloric acid, but hyperkalemia is not a major problem if you are aware of it. I would administer the arginine slowly and check the serum potassium concentration after an hour or two.

Renal Fellow: Are there any instances of pulmonary edema following insertion of the shunt?

Dr. Levinsky: None has been reported, but I would add that most of the reports describe experiences occurring within the first 10 days after surgery. Most importantly, during that time the patients received diuretics, and dietary salt was restricted. The dogs who developed pulmonary edema, described earlier, were not receiving diuretics or a low-salt diet. According to the experimental results, extraabdominal edema might occur if patients with LeVeen shunts are taken off diuretics and placed on *ad lib* salt intake.

References

1. Eknoyan G, Martinez-Maldonado M, Yium JJ, Suki WN: Combined ascitic-fluid and furosemide infusion in the management of ascites. N Engl J Med 282:713–717, 1970
2. LeVeen HH, Christoudias G, Moon IP, Luft R, Falk G, Grosberg S: Peritoneovenous shunting for ascites. Ann Surg 180:580–590, 1974
3. LeVeen HH, Wapnick S, Grosberg S, Kinney MJ: Further experiences with peritoneovenous shunt for ascites. Ann Surg 184:574–579, 1976

4. Witte MH, Witte CL, Jacobs S, Kut R: Peritoneovenous (LeVeen) shunt. JAMA 239:31–33, 1978
5. Wapnick S, Grosberg S, Kinney MJ, LeVeen HH: LeVeen continuous peritoneal-jugular shunt. JAMA 237:131–133, 1977
6. Chonko AM, Bay WH, Stein JH, Ferris TF: The role of renin and aldosterone in the salt retention of edema. Am J Med 63:881–889, 1977
7. Epstein M, Levinson R, Sancho J, Haber E, Re R: Characterization of the renin-aldosterone system in decompensated cirrhosis. Circ Res 41:818–829, 1977
8. Epstein M, Pins DS, Schneider N, Levinson R: Determinants of deranged sodium and water homeostasis in decompensated cirrhosis. J Lab Clin Med 87:822–839, 1976
9. Fullen WD: Hepatorenal syndrome: Reversal by peritoneovenous shunt. Surgery 82:337–341, 1977
10. Conn HO: A rational approach to the hepatorenal syndrome. Gastroenterology 65:321–340, 1973
11. Tristani FE, Cohn JN: Systemic and renal hemodynamics in oliguric hepatic failure: Effect of volume expansion. J Clin Invest 46:1894–1906, 1967
12. Lieberman FL, Denison EK, Reynolds TB: The relationship of plasma volume, portal hypertension, ascites and renal sodium retention in cirrhosis: The overflow theory of ascites formation. Ann NY Acad Sci 170:202–206, 1970
13. Levy M: Sodium retention and ascites formation in dogs with experimental portal cirrhosis. Am J Physiol 233:F572–F585, 1977
14. Levy M, Wexler MJ: Urinary sodium retention and the "effective" plasma volume in dogs with experimental cirrhosis and ascites. Clin Res 25:706A, 1977
15. Schwartz WB, van Ypersele de Strihou C, Kassirer JP: Role of anions in metabolic alkalosis and potassium deficiency. N Engl J Med 279:630–639, 1968
16. Hertz P, Richardson JA: Arginine-induced hyperkalemia in renal failure patients. Arch Intern Med 130:778–780, 1972
17. Pladson TR, Parrish RM: Hepatorenal syndrome: Recovery after peritoneovenous shunt. Arch Intern Med 137:1248–1249, 1977
18. Kassirer JP, Schwartz WB: The response of normal man to selective depletion of hydrochloric acid: Factors in the genesis of persistent gastric alkalosis. Am J Med 40:10–26, 1966
19. Howe CT, LeQuesne LP: Pyloric stenosis: The metabolic effects. Br J Surg 51:923–932, 1964
20. Casey TH, Summerskill WHJ, Bickford RG, Rosevear JW: Body and serum potassium in liver disease. II. Relationship to arterial ammonia, blood pH, and hepatic coma. Gastroenterology 48:208–215, 1965
21. Gabuzda GH: Cirrhosis, ascites, and edema. Gastroenterology 58:546–553, 1970

Mechanisms of Urine Concentration

Principal Discussant
Robert W. Berliner

Preface

In this issue of "The Forum" we make a modest departure from our usual, case-oriented discussion. Because basic scientific principles form the backbone of all pathophysiologic reasoning, we present here a strictly physiologic discussion of the development of the countercurrent hypothesis of urine concentration and dilution. The way in which this theory developed exemplifies several recurrent themes in the history of science; valid hypotheses ignored for years, new observations forced into an outmoded theoretical framework, false pathways traversed because of erroneous experimental data, clinical acceptance of a new hypothesis, and lingering doubts that motivate additional studies forcing refinement of existing "truths."

Clinicians will have no difficulty recognizing the implications of the countercurrent hypothesis. Dilutional states, drug-induced concentrating disorders, and mechanisms of diuretic action are a few of the clinically relevant items that we comprehend better because of it, and we do a better job of treating the sick now that this mechanism is understood.

Discussion

Dr. Robert Berliner *(Dean, Yale University School of Medicine, New Haven, Connecticut)*: The mechanism for producing a urine more concentrated than other body fluids is one of the more spectacular adaptations of form to function, at least on the macroscopic scale, in vertebrate physiology. And it is remarkable that for many years the mainstream of renal physiology was totally able to disregard this relationship. Had renal physiologists been a little less parochial, perhaps they would not have missed the fact that studies in comparative anatomy, generally looked down upon then as now, pointed in the right direction almost half a century before the physiologists began to take note of their relevant findings.

In attempting to recount the story of how we arrived at our current understanding of the way in which the mechanism really works, I will try to follow the two paths that finally merged in the late 1950s and begin with the one that seemed to most of us working in renal physiology to be the only one before that time.

The development of renal physiology from the time of World War I to around 1960 can be associated largely with the names of a small number of outstanding investigators who set the style for the rest: A. R. Cushny, A. N. Richards, E. K. Marshall, Homer Smith, R. F. Pitts. The emphasis throughout most of this period was on the integration of glomerular filtration and the activity of the tubules to determine the rates of excretion of various substances. And throughout much of this period, the emphasis was on substances other than the strong electrolytes. This was a reflection, at least in part, of the fact that the methods for measuring most of the strong electrolytes—chloride being a major exception—were exceedingly laborious. In dealing with the major subjects of the studies of that period—inulin, glucose, paraaminophippurate, urea—it was relatively easy to neglect most of the anatomic features of the kidneys, and the nephron came to be regarded as simply a glomerulus, a proximal convoluted tubule, and a distal tubule, with the latter two joined together by an insignificant connecting segment, much as it is in the amphibian, the subject of the early micropuncture work in Richards's laboratory (Fig. 1). Although it was recognized that the effluent from the various nephrons eventually was gathered together in collecting tubules and collecting ducts, these structures usually were denigrated as having little or no significance. To quote Homer Smith's book of 1951, the major compendium on the kidney at the time: "The cytology of the collecting tubules does not suggest any specialized function other than service as conduits, and they are so treated by almost all writers." Smith did add that there was some evidence that might be interpreted as indicating that the collecting tubules had a reabsorptive function, particularly for water [1].

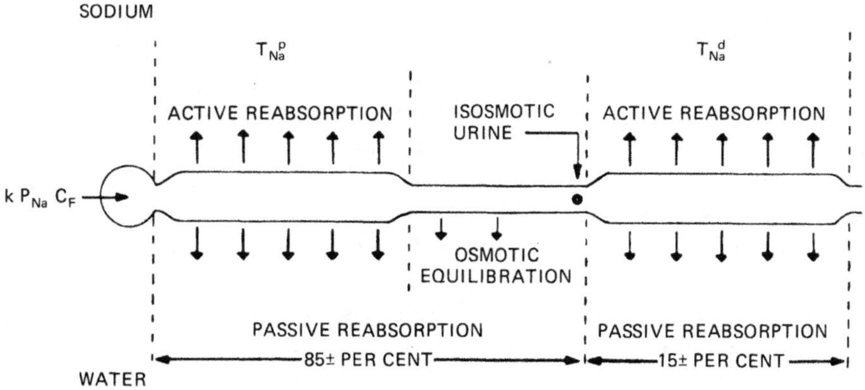

Fig. 1. "The rectilinear nephron as previously drawn by the writer [H. W. Smith] on several occasions with minor modifications." From Ref. 45.

The ability to form concentrated urine had long been of interest to clinicians because diminished capacity for urine concentration had been recognized as a relatively sensitive indicator of impaired renal function, and the determination of the urinary specific gravity was one of the easiest measurements one could make. For a long time, however, the subject was given little attention by renal physiologists. As attention turned in the late 1940s and 1950s to the regulation of salt and water excretion, stimulated particularly by the invention of the flame photometer, the formation of dilute and concentrated urines became a matter for explanation. The formation of dilute urine was easily explained by the removal of salt without water from the tubule lumen. The process required only a relatively low permeability to water in the epithelial lining of the tubule from the point of salt reabsorption until the urine left the kidney. Work with the antidiuretic hormone vasopressin had shown that it had the specific property of increasing the permeability of responsive epithelia to water. So there was no great difficulty in providing an explanation for the excretion of dilute urine in water diuresis and the increase of the urine concentration, at least to the point of isotonicity, when vasopressin was given or when an increase in the osmolality of body fluids was imposed so as to cause endogenous release of vasopressin.

The fact that osmolality rose to a value well above that of the blood was another matter, however, and it was considerably more difficult to explain. It was clear that the process involved removal of water rather than the addition of solute, because the concentration of the urine was relatively independent of the nature of the solute that it contained, and it would have been difficult to identify any solute that might have been added to produce the hypertonicity. The only solute whose excretion varied much with urine concentration was urea, and here the change was in the wrong direction, excretion falling as the urine concentration increased. For the same reason, i.e., the relative independence of solute excretion from the rate of water excretion, it was generally concluded that the removal of water was a final step in the elaboration of concentrated urine. In any case, we were forced to consider how water might be removed from the urine and transported against what appeared to be a large activity gradient—in other words, by a process of active transport. It was obvious that there was problems involved in the possibility of active water transport that did not apply to the transport of solutes; chief among these were the quantitative considerations. Isotonic fluids are about 55.2 molal with respect to water and less than 0.3 molal with respect to anything else; thus there are, in body fluids, nearly 200 water molecules for every particle of a solute. It would be difficult to imagine that water could be transported one molecule at a time by reversible combination with a carrier—it would require too high a concentration of the carrier molecules, or too high a rate of turnover, or both. So it seemed highly improbable that the process involved what we now would call primary active transport.

Attention was therefore directed to some process that might move water in bulk, the obvious one being something depending on osmosis. A model of such a process had been proposed by Frank and Mayer [2], and although little concern was raised whether this suggested mechanism was feasible, it was generally accepted that some such process could underlie the uphill movement of water. In essence, the Frank–Mayer model invoked the cyclic assembly and disassembly of a polymer within the transporting cell: the polymerization at one margin of the cell presumably decreased osmotic pressure and the depolymerization at the other surface increased osmolality, thus creating a gradient of osmotic pressure within the cell. Although the model was qualitatively sound, for a time not much attention was paid to its quantitative aspects. For example, the transporting cells would have had to contain an enormous quantity of the organic monomer involved in the process. It was not because of this consideration, however, that the illusion was dispelled that the model could serve the required function. Instead, Brodsky and his associates showed on thermodynamic grounds that the process could not generate a steep enough gradient over the short distance represented by the thickness of the cells that line the tubules [3].

The demise of the only hypothesis that had seemed to provide a plausible explanation for uphill water transport demanded new explorations to determine how the urine was made hypertonic to other body fluids. An entirely different approach to the problem already had been proposed by Wirz and his associates in Basel, but it had been almost totally disregarded. But rather than start in the middle of the story with the work of Wirz, Hargitay, and Kuhn [4], let me go back nearly another 50 years to the origins of their views in the work of the comparative anatomists that I mentioned earlier.

The study usually cited as first indicating that the medulla, and specifically the loop of Henle, had something to do with the formation of concentrated urine is that of Peter [5], who in 1909 described a correspondence between the length of the loop of Henle in various mammalian species and the specific gravity of the urine that these species produced. In fact there were even earlier studies pointing to the importance of the medulla that might have brought an alert physiologist close to our present views. Filehne and Biberfeld in 1902 had reported that the osmotic pressure of medullary tissue was higher than that of the cortex [6]. Hirokawa in 1908 reported similar findings [7] and wrote (I quote Carl Gottschalk's translation from the original German [8]:

> The urine present in the medulla has a much higher osmotic pressure than that of the convoluted tubules of the cortex; therefore the osmotic pressure of the urine increases considerably during its

> passage through the loops of Henle and collecting tubules. . . . The osmotic pressure of the medulla is extraordinarily variable; it is almost without exception higher than that of the cortex, and is higher the more concentrated the excreted urine.

I don't know whether these last two contributions had any influence at the time but, if they did, it had disappeared from the scene by 10 or so years later, and these findings remained more or less unheard of until confirmed much more recently by Wirz and others. Neither of these two papers are among the 2300 cited in Homer Smith's 1951 book [1].

The loop of Henle came back into consideration among students of urine concentration with a paper by Burgess, Harvey, and Marshall in 1933 [9]. In examining the effect of pitressin on representatives of each of the vertebrate classes, they found no effect on urine flow in either catfish or frog but did note a striking effect, often amounting to extended anuria, in the alligator; this effect was associated with what was apparently a very marked fall in glomerular filtration (no mention is made of possible dead-space errors). In the chicken and the dog, they found decreases in urine flow with relatively small changes in glomerular filtration. On the basis of these observations they concluded that antidiuretic hormone had its effect on the loop of Henle, which is the only renal structure present exclusively in birds and mammals, and that its effect was to stimulate water reabsorption. It is interesting that they said nothing about the production of a hypertonic urine, although their conclusions often have been interpreted that way. They did not, in fact, make any measurements of osmolality. Since it has more recently been shown that the frog does respond to vasopressin by producing a less dilute urine [10], the basis for their conclusions made a considerably greater impression than did the far more relevant one of Crane four years earlier that only birds and mammals produced hypertonic urine [11].

So for a few years it was believed that hypertonic urine was generated in the loop of Henle. This idea was dealt a fatal blow when Walker, Bott, Oliver, and MacDowell reported the first micropuncture studies in mammals. Three samples collected from rat distal tubules proved not to be hypertonic although the final urine was [12]. In fact, two of the three distal samples appeared to have significantly lower osmolalities than did the blood. At the time nobody knew how to interpret their finding although, of course, it later was recognized as particularly important.

The idea that the loop of Henle might be a countercurrent multiplier first came to the attention of renal physiologists in 1951 with publication of papers by Hargitay and Kuhn [13] and Wirz, Hargitay, and Kuhn [4]. An earlier paper in German by Kuhn and Ryffel published during World War II in the Swiss literature had gone relatively unnoticed [14].

Kuhn, a physical chemist, had developed the idea of the hairpin countercurrent multiplier as a way of carrying out processes of solute concentration. He recognized the hairpin shape of the loop of Henle and, knowing that the loop had been associated with the formation of concentrated urine, suggested that the loop behaved as a countercurrent multiplier. The hypothesis required that the medulla have an increasing osmotic pressure from its base to the tip of the papilla; Wirz, a physiologist, collaborated in an attempt to determine whether such a gradient of osmolality was in fact present [4]. By examining the frozen kidney in polarized light and watching the disappearance of ice crystals as the specimen was rewarmed, they measured the freezing point of the renal structures . Their results indicated that the predicted increase in osmolality was indeed present and that, furthermore, all the structures at the same depth in the renal medulla had the same freezing point (Fig. 2). It is now known that their method failed to detect the relatively small differences in osmolality between the ascending limb of Henle's loop and the other structures. Their findings confirmed those many years earlier of Filehne and Biberfeld [6] and of Hirokawa [7]. The concept

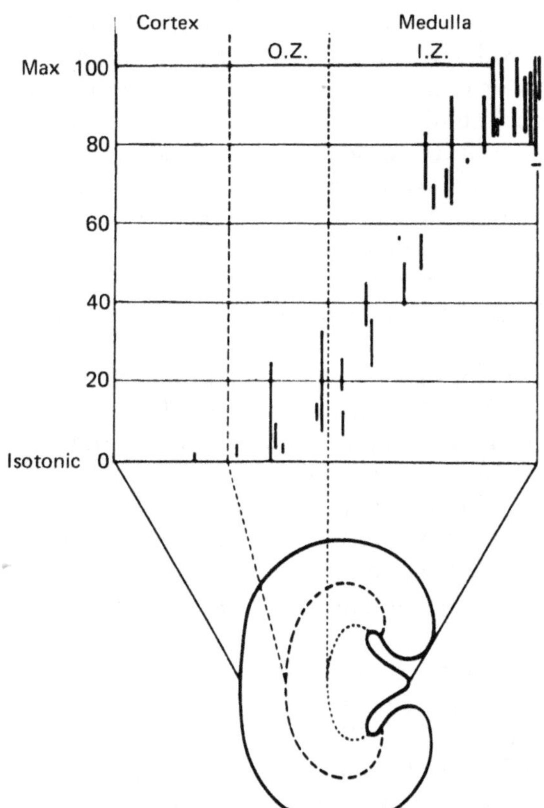

Fig. 2. Osmolality of fluids at various depths in the rat kidney. From Ref. 4.

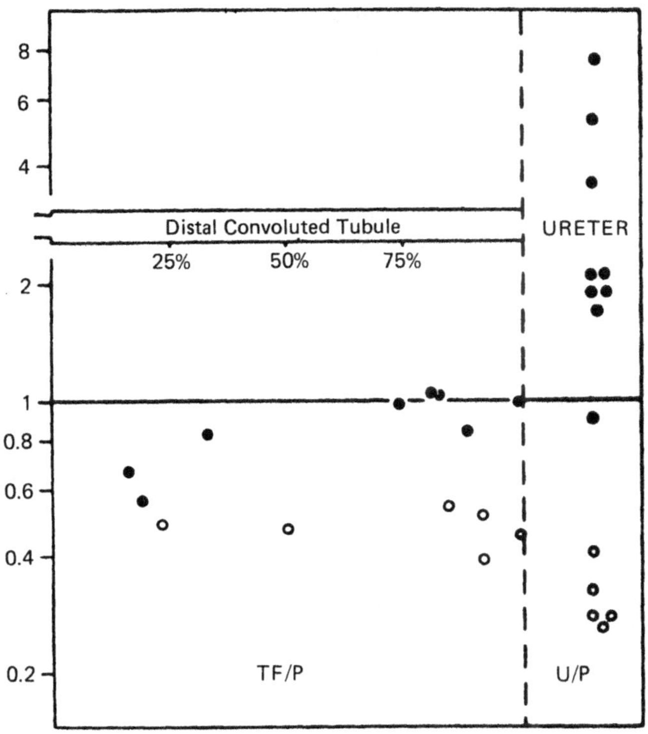

Fig. 3. Osmolality of fluid from distal tubule. From Ref. 17.

of an osmotic gradient was later confirmed by Ullrich and his associates from studies of the osmometric behavior of kidney slices and the finding of increasing concentrations of measured solutes at increasing depth within the medulla [15]. The latter findings of course have been confirmed by many investigators since.

In a series of continuing studies, Wirz made additional observations that were in conformity with the requirements of the countercurrent multiplier hypothesis. He found that blood obtained from superficial vessels at the tip of the hamster papilla had the same osmotic pressure as the urine [16]. He also confirmed the earlier findings of Walker and his associates [12] that the fluid in the early part of the distal tubule is dilute [17]. He found further that in water diuresis the urine remained dilute throughout the distal tubule whereas in animals producing concentrated urine, the fluid in later parts of the distal tubule approached, but did not exceed, isotonicity with the plasma (Fig. 3).

One might wonder why, with all these findings in conformity with the countercurrent multiplier hypothesis, acceptance of the model was delayed for such a long time. Aside from the expected resistance to a revolutionary way of thinking about a problem, we may get some idea of a more rational basis for the reluctance to accept the hypothesis if we look at the models that were used to illustrate it.

Figure 4 is from the paper of Hargitay and Kuhn [13]. The three channels in model *b*, the closest to the organization of the renal medulla, may be thought of as the analogs of, from top to bottom, the collecting duct, the descending limb of the loop, and the ascending limb. In this particular model, the driving force for the "single effect" is hydrostatic pressure applied to the central channel against the resistance of the constricted connection between the middle and lower channels, forcing water across the semipermeable membrane, SPM_{12}. This driving force produces an osmotic pressure that increases progressively from left to right in the central and lower channels. At the same time, a much smaller flow through the upper channel, leaving at the right end, is permitted to equilibrate across a semipermeable membrane, SPM_{R1}, and emerges with the same high osmotic pressure as the fluid in the multiplier itself. Although this model was driven by hydrostatic pressure, the authors recognized that the pressures in the kidney were not high enough to drive such a process in the kidney and pointed out that the same change in osmotic pressure could be accomplished by transporting solute across membrane SPM_{12} in the opposite direction,

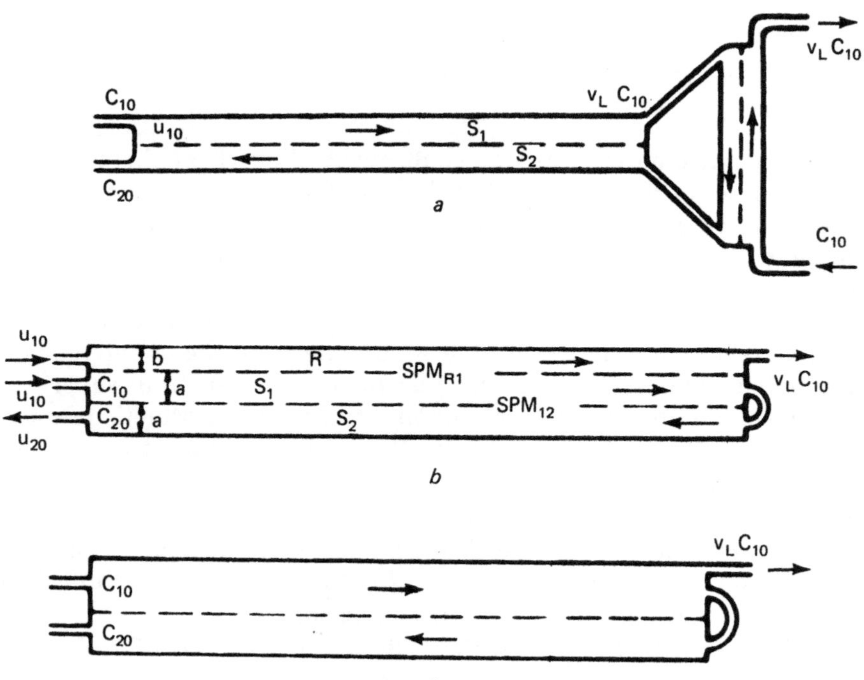

Fig. 4. Models of countercurrent multiplier. From Ref. 13.

assuming this membrane to be impermeable to water. The advantage of the hydrostatic pressure model was only that the authors were able to construct a mechanical working model. However, there are some problems in considering the model an analog of the renal medulla. First, it requires that the structures be contiguous to each other, at least for the hydrostatic pressure model. If we use the solute transport mode, we can allow separation of the two limbs of the loop if each transports solute in the right direction, but we cannot separate the collecting duct from one or the other limb because the model requires that the water lost from the collecting duct leave the system in the overflow from the ascending limb. Furthermore, if the water lost from the collecting duct is to enter the loop, the surface of the loop in contact with the collecting duct must have different properties than the remainder of the loop's surface, because the latter must be impermeable to water to prevent the movement of fluid along with the transported solute. Whether we assume water movement from the descending limb to the ascending limb, or solute movement in the reverse direction, the actual situation in the medulla, with the several structures separated by interstitial spaces, indicates that the loop cannot act on the surroundings because of the permeability characteristics that would be required. Thus, it became clear that Hargitay and Kuhn's model, which embodied the best theory of the time, was incomplete.

Davidson and I became interested in the problem of urine concentration as a result of our studies that showed that concentrated urine could be produced in the absence of antidiuretic hormone if the volume of fluid delivered to the concentrating site was sufficiently reduced by constricting the renal artery [18]. This observation led us to question the nature of the concentrating mechanism itself and the possible effects of vasopressin on it. Some features of the Wirz, Hargitay, and Kuhn model were attractive. It provided a function for the loop that corresponded to one that had been suspected for many years and offered an explanation for the adaptation that placed the loop and collecting ducts in isolation from the rest of the kidney. It made the abstraction of water the last step in the elaboration of concentrated urine as had been previously inferred. It explained the dilute character of urine emerging into the distal tubule. It accounted for the high solute concentration throughout the medulla as had then been abundantly demonstrated. And, perhaps most important, it envisioned the active process as salt transport, eliminating the need to invoke active transport of water. In trying to fit all these facts together and yet provide a more plausible function for the loop, Levinsky, Davidson, Eden, and I conceived the idea that the loop should be considered a pumping device delivering sodium salts to the interstitial space of the medulla rather than a countercurrent multiplier [19]. According to this hypothesis, the resulting increase in osmolality of the interstital space abstracts water from the collecting ducts, and the water from the collecting duct together with the salt pumped in by the loop leaves the medulla via the vasa recta rather than via the nephron. That much of the hypothesis fitted with all the observations. We further suggested that the loop was impermeable to water throughout its length and became progressively diluted as it pumped out sodium salts. This was not strictly in accord with Wirz's freezing point studies [4], but it was known that he had failed to detect the dilute character of urine in the thick ascending limb and distal tubule, and it seemed not unlikely that the method had failed to reveal the difference between the thin limbs and the rest of the medulla.

A good hypothesis is one that can be shown to be incorrect by a critical experiment. By that standard, our hypothesis was an excellent one because our paper was still in press when Gottschalk and Mylle proved it wrong by showing that fluid collected from the tip of the loop in the hamster papilla had the same high osmolality as did the urine in the collecting ducts and the blood in the vasa recta [8]. The latter was, of course, exactly as predicted by the countercurrent multiplier hypothesis. Had we been a little more imaginative, we would have recognized that our idea of the loop as a pump delivering sodium salts to the renal interstitium did not require abandonment of the countercurrent multiplier. The latter hypothesis required only that the descending limb be permeable to water, solute, or both and that the ascending limb be impermeable to water and be able to pump out salt. That was, of course, the way Gottschalk and Mylle interpreted their findings [8].

There never has been much question since then about the general outline of the mechanism. A few of the predictions that remained untested have since been determined to be accurate. Jamison, Bennett, and I found that the fluid in ascending limbs was more dilute than that in the descending limbs at the same level in the papilla (Fig. 5), the difference being fairly well accounted for by a difference in salt concentration [20]. If any question remained about whether the dilution was caused by loss of solute or by secretion of water (after all, one of the great virtues of the hypothesis was that it eliminated the need to think about active transport of water), Jamison showed that the dilution in the ascending limb was accompanied by a decrease in volume between descending and ascending limbs [21]. An examination of the medullary structures in the rat papilla showed that the permeability to osmotically induced water flow was about an order of magnitude greater in the descending limb than in the ascending limb and that the permeability was unaffected by vasopressin [22]. The permeability of the collecting duct, on the other hand, was responsive to vasopressin. Similar and much more precise studies of these structures isolated from the rabbit kidney have since been done by Kokko and his associates [23,24]. I will consider these later when we discuss yet another aspect of this problem.

One prediction from the hypothesis has never been convincingly demonstrated, namely, that the thin ascending limb has the capacity to extrude salt actively. No one has ever questioned the inference that the cells of the thick ascending limb would be able to transport salt actively. Indeed, it has been unequivocally shown by Burg [25] and by Kokko [26] that the isolated thick ascending limb does exactly that, although, contrary to what everyone had previously assumed, chloride rather than sodium is the actively transported ion. Although chloride's being the actively transported ion is important in other respects—particularly as it pertains to the action of diuretics—it is immaterial with respect to the concentrating mechanism. Because the thick ascending limb is limited to the outer medulla, there has not been any difficulty explaining the steep rise in salt concentration in that part of the medulla. The problem has been in accounting for the continuing rise in the inner medulla, which is clearly demonstrable, at least in hydropenic animals (Fig. 6), although the gradient is not as steep as in the outer medulla.

Given the relatively flat epithelium lining the thin limb, and a paucity of mitochondria in the lining cells, investigators always have questioned whether there was sufficient metabolic machinery to support active salt transport at the required rate. A few investigators have

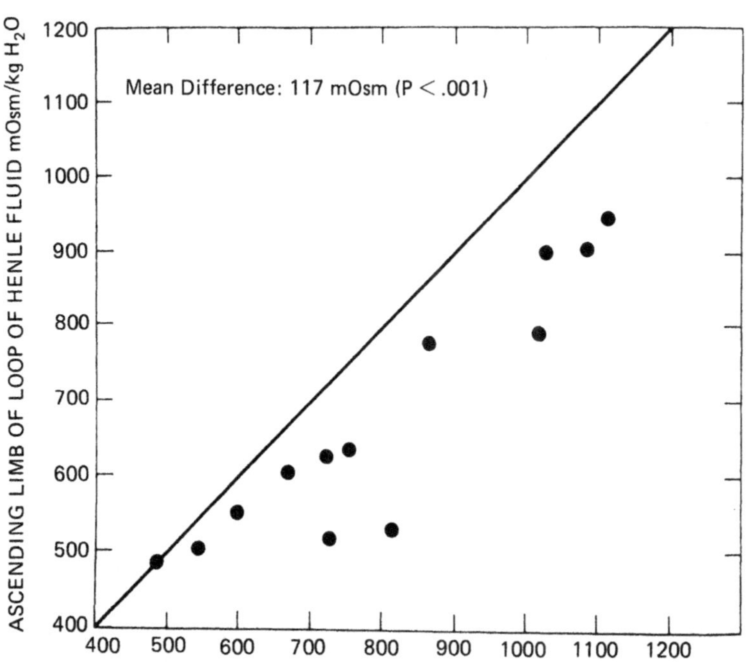

Fig. 5. Comparison of osmolalities of fluid from ascending limbs and adjacent descending limbs of the loop of Henle. From Ref. 20.

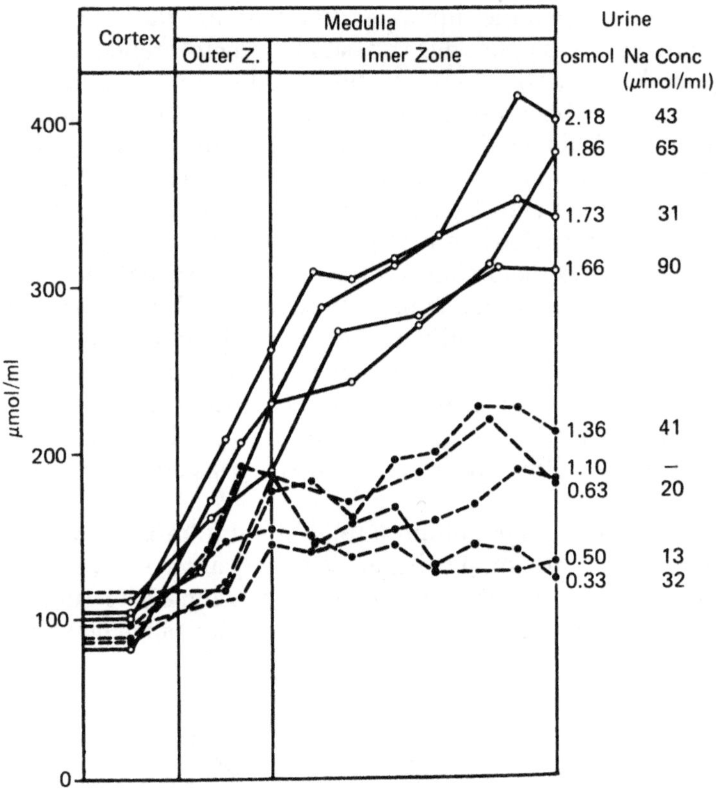

Fig. 6. Sodium concentration in tissue water of hydropenic (*open* circles) and hydrated (solid dots) dogs. From Ref. 15.

detected what might be interpreted as a very small amount of transport against a concentration gradient [27,28], but these findings have never been entirely convincing, and in other studies no evidence suggesting active transport of salt could be found [22,24,29]. Consequently there have been a number of attempts to account for the continued rise in salt concentration without invoking any active salt transport by the thin limbs. Several proposals have suggested that the collecting duct might be the site of the requisite salt transport [30,31], but it is difficult to see how transport of solute out of the urine in the collecting ducts could contribute to making the urine more concentrated. Other investigators have proposed that the only active transport of salt occurs in the outer medulla, but that the concentration could continue to rise in the inner medulla simply as a result of countercurrent exchange in the inner medulla [32,33]. These models were shown to be invalid when Stephenson demonstrated that, in a countercurrent system, no concentration greater than that of the inflow can be achieved *without an input of energy* [34]. I emphasize the phrase "without an input of energy" because Stephenson's proof generally was interpreted to mean without active transport of salt (i.e., in the ascending thin limb). There is, in fact, an alternative means of supplying free energy to effect transport out of the thin ascending limb. Stephenson did not have that alternative in mind when he published the proof; rather, 6 or 7 years later he [35] and Kokko and Rector [36] simultaneously and independently proposed that the source of additional free energy is the highly concentrated solution of urea in the collecting ducts which, in turn, is the source of a high concentration of urea in the interstitium of the medulla that surrounds the thin limbs of the loop of Henle.

This use of a solution of a second solute to produce a concentrating effect, not possible in a single solute system without a hydrostatic driving force or active solute transport, can be traced back to the 1942 paper of Kuhn and Ryffel [14]. Figure 7 shows their three-compartment model. It was in conncection with this model that Wirz said: "It is questionable that this paper was thoroughly studied by many who quoted it." Compartments A and B, each containing 0.1 M sucrose, are separated by a membrane (M_1) of copper ferrocyanide that is permeable to water but not to solute. Compartment C contains 0.1 M phenol and is separated from B by a rubber membrane (M_2) premeable to phenol but not to water or sucrose. Phenol diffuses into compartment B until B is 0.1 M with respect to phenol as well as sucrose or, in other words, until B has twice its original osmolality. Water then moves from A to B and raises the osmolality of A to equal that of B, but in A the solute is entirely sucrose at 0.2 M.

The proposals of Kokko-Rector and of Stephenson contain the same basic idea illustrated by this model. Compartment A corresponds to the descending thin limb, compartment B to the medullary interstitium, and C to the collecting duct. Sodium chloride is the solute in place of sucrose, and urea replaces phenol. If we now change the properties of membrane M_1 so that it corresponds to the epithelium of the ascending

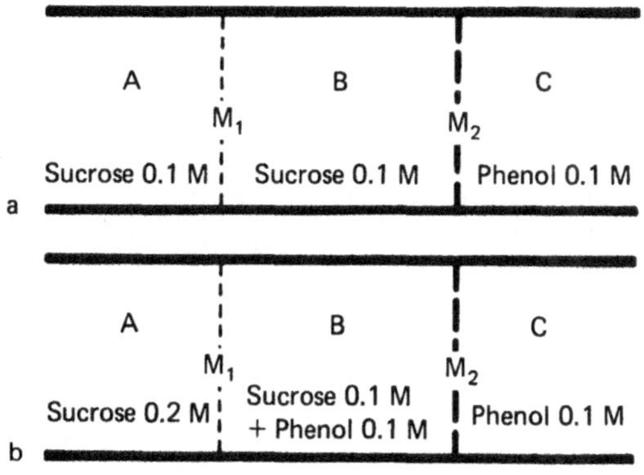

Fig. 7. Model of Kuhn and Ryffel [14]. See text.

thin limb, which is assumed to be permeable to salt but not to water, sodium chloride can diffuse *downhill* from A to B, diluting A below the concentration that has been reached when it leaves the descending limb. This increases further the osmolality of the interstitium and causes more water to be removed from the collecting ducts through membrane 2, M_2, here being considered permeable to water and urea but not salt.

These models, then, can explain the countercurrent multiplier function of the thin segment without requiring that the ascending thin limb transport salt by an active process. The free energy is supplied by a concentrated solution of urea. Urea is concentrated by the expenditure of metabolic energy in the cortex and outer medulla. In the cortex, salt and water are removed in the distal convoluted and collecting tubules, a process that leaves behind an isotonic solution containing mostly urea. In the outer medulla, urea in the collecting tubule is concentrated further by the movement of water into the medullary interstitium, which is made hypertonic by the active transport of salt by the thick ascending limb. It should be noted that Stephenson did not conclude that salt transport by some active process was absent in the thin ascending limb, but only that if salt transport did occur. it would be more efficient as a consequence of the less unfavorable (or possibly favorable) concentration gradient. In essence, the Kokko–Rector model is a special case of the Stephenson model.

The attractiveness of these models is obvious. Not only do they offer an attractive alternative to the hypothesis of an active transport mechanism in the thin segment of the loop (a mechanism that many thought was unlikely a priori), but they provide a critical role for urea, a role that explains some other old observations that often have been confirmed but never have been adequately accounted for. Gamble and his associates in 1934 studied the volume of urine excreted when various solutes were administered to rats on a low-protein diet and found that when pairs of solutes were administered, the volume in which these solutes were excreted was always the sum of the volumes in which each solute was excreted when given alone, except when urea was one of the solutes [37]. In the latter case, the volume in which the two solutes were excreted was lower than that when the nonurea solute was given alone, yielding what they called "an economy of water in renal function referable to urea." This finding has been confirmed several times [38,39]. Although some had tried to explain why urea might be excreted largely in water already required for the excretion of other solutes [19], there had not previously been an explanation of the observation that urea could reduce the volume in which other solutes were excreted.

The passive model of the operation of the thin segment of the loop of Henle imposes a number of requirements that are subject to experimental verification. The first of these relates to the permeability of the two limbs. If the system is to work, conditions must be such that a high concentration of urea in the interstitium produces a high concentration of sodium salts in the descending limb. And in the ascending limb, sodium chloride must be able to diffuse out into the interstitium (which is postulated to have a lower salt concentration) and in so doing render the fluid in the lumen more dilute than the surroundings. In other words, the descending limb must have a high permeability to water and a low permeability to both salt and urea, whereas the ascending limb must have a high permeability to salt, a lesser permeability to urea, and a low permeability to water. As I mentioned earlier, the permeability to water in the two limbs had been found generally to conform to these requirements [22]. The characteristics of the two thin limbs from the rabbit kidney were studied in detail by Kokko [23] and by Imai and Kokko [24] by perfusion in vitro. Their findings conform precisely to the model: they found the descending limb to be virtually impermeable to the relevant solutes and highly permeable to water, and the ascending limb to have the opposite characteristics.

Given that this model of a completely passive thin limb explains so many of the known observations, and given also that the permeability characteristics seem so well suited to this function, it would appear that the last piece of the puzzle has been fitted in and that we should be looking elsewhere for problems to work on. Almost, but not quite; a few bothersome facts remain that don't quite conform.

Or perhaps it is the sand rat *Psammomys obesus* that does not conform. At least it would be very difficult to explain the findings of de Rouffignac and his colleagues [40] on the basis of an unmodified version of the Kokko–Rector model. First of all, psammomys doesn't seem very dependent on urea for producing a highly concentrated urine. This animal, with the most highly developed thin segments of the loop of Henle of any animal so far encountered, seems able to produce a concentrated urine without much urea; osmolalities over 2000 mOsm have been obtained with urines containing only a little over 100 mM urea [40]. In most other animals, such a low concentration of urea would be associated with a marked lowering of the maximum concentration of the urine. Even more important is a number of observations suggesting that attainment of the high concentration of solute in the descending limb is largely attributable to salt entry rather than to water loss. Suggestive of the latter is the fact that the degree to which inulin is concentrated at the tip of the loop (a measure of water loss) is poorly related to the extent to which the osmolality is increased [40,41]. Perhaps even more difficult to fit with the passive mechanism is the relationship between the amount of sodium that reaches the tip of the loop and the amount of sodium that is filtered. On the average, in two separate studies, there was more sodium at the tip of the loop than ordinarily escapes reabsorption in the first half of a superficial proximal tubule and, in more samples than is likely to be attributable to experimental error, more sodium reached the tip of the loop than had been present in the glomerular filtrate of the punctured nephron [40,41]. Assuming these observations are correct, and I see little reason to doubt that they are, they seem to exclude the fully passive mode for the thin segments. But psammomys is unique in other respects, and perhaps it is an exception among mammals in transporting salt actively in the thin ascending limb.

Imai has extended in vitro perfusion studies of the isolated thin ascending limb to the rat and hamster [29]. The permeability properties were found to be similar to those previously found in the rabbit; again, he was able to detect nothing suggesting active transport. He had difficulty isolating adequate segments of descending limbs and found only that these segments had a high permeability to water. These studies suggest that the rat and the hamster are similar to the rabbit, but other studies in the rat do not completely support an entirely passive process. Perhaps most important is the concentration of urea in loop fluid relative to the concentration of urea in the medullary interstitium. The hypothesis of a passive process dependent on urea requires that the urea concentration outside the loop exceed that inside, at least to the extent that the salt concentration inside, exceeds that in the interstitium, since this difference is the driving force for the mechanism. Jamison and his associates have found that the concentration of urea at the bend of the loop is lower, but not much lower, than the concentration of urea in the collecting ducts, the latter setting an upper bound on the interstitial urea concentration [42]. They also found that the concentration of sodium in the loop fluid exceeds that in the vasa recta by a small margin [43]. The differences, althouth significant, are small enough to raise a question about whether they are sufficient to account for the passive reabsorption of enough salt. In addition, these differences set a low upper bound on the single effect for the countercurrent multiplier.

Bonventre and Lechene pointed out a somewhat different difficulty with the urea concentration in loop fluid; if the thin segment is to contribute any free water, the urea concentration in fluid at the bend of the loop in the completely passive model cannot exceed the concentration of urea in the interstitial space at the junction of inner and outer medulla [44]. In fact, since the thick ascending limb is virtually impermeable to urea, whatever urea is present at the junction of inner and outer medulla also will be delivered to the distal tubule, so that the concentration of urea at the inner medullary–outer medullary junction also will be found in the distal tubule and will limit the extent to which that fluid can be dilute. In other words, the urea concentration determines the extent to which that nephron generates free water and contributes to the entire concentrating process. It is doubtful that the urea concentration is low enough, at least in the rat, to conform to the requirements imposed by this analysis. Pennell, Lacy, and Jamison have found urea concentrations over 300 mM at the tip of the loop in Sprague-Dawley rats [42]. The urea concentration in the interstitium at the junction of inner and outer medulla is unlikely to be as high as this, and such a nephron, having a lower salt concentration than its environment at the inner medullary-outer medullary junction, will take up salt rather than contribute it to the medulla. The contents of the thin segment, not being more dilute than the surroundings, will not have contributed more solute than water to the inner medulla.

To circumvent the problem created by the relatively high urea concentrations, Bonventre and Lechene proposed elimination of one of the other assumptions of the Kokko-Rector model; they proposed that the thin descending limb does not have the same osmolality as its surroundings at the junction of inner and outer medulla. What is required for the thin limb to contribute excess solute to the inner medulla is that the fluid leaving the inner medulla be more dilute than that entering. This state can be achieved by making the ascending limb contents more dilute or the descending limb contents more concentrated than their environment, and Bonventre and Lechene suggest that the latter is the case. I must confess that I am less than enthusiastic about this proposal. It makes critical the rate at which descending limb fluid attains the same osmolality as its surroundings so that, for example, the figure with which their model is illustrated would permit the inner two-thirds of the inner medulla to make no contribution to the concentrating process [44]. I also have reservations about hypotheses that can't be subjected to experimental test and, at least at this time, there is no way to ascertain whether the postulated hypertonicity of the descending limb at the inner medullary-outer medullary junction actually is present.

This is the point at which one customarily draws things together and reaches some conclusion, but I'm afraid that for now we will have to leave things hanging. Attractive as the passive model of the thin segment is, there are some apparently hard facts that leave it in doubt. We can hope that in time the contradictions will be resolved.

Questions and Answers

Dr. Jordan J. Cohen: On at least a couple of occasions during your historic review, you pointed to observations that were published in the literature but virtually ignored. You intimated that had those reports been more widely read, our thinking about urinary concentration might have evolved quite differently. We are now living at a time when Current Contents, Medlars, Citation Indexes, and the like make access even to obscure literature very easy. In your judgment, could such a thing happen now? Are there important observations in the literature that we have ignored for 20 years?

Dr. Berliner: There are two reasons why things get ignored. One, nobody reads them, and two, they read them but don't believe them or it doesn't seem to fit into their way of thinking, so they disregard them. And I think in this case it is more the latter that we were dealing with rather than the former. It is probably true that until Wirz, Hargitay, and Kuhn published their paper, nobody in the medical field had read a paper of Kuhn and Ryffel that was published, not only in German during the war, but also in a physical chemistry journal. That is very likely to be missed by biologists. But, other than that I don't think it was that nobody read the papers. I just think they read them and said, "What am I going to do with that?" and threw them away.

Dr. Joseph Bonventre *(Renal Unit, Massachusetts General Hospital, Boston, Massachusetts)*: I would like to answer your criticisms regarding our model of the renal concentration process. Our model does account for concentration throughout the inner medulla. This is demonstrated in the numerical illustration of the model that we present in our paper [44]. The collecting ducts play an important role in interstitial concentration in the deeper portions of the inner medulla. The sodium chloride that comes out of the loop of Henle in the upper portion of the medulla results in withdrawal of water from the collecting ducts. You have shown that the reflection coefficient of the collecting duct in the inner medulla is greater for sodium chloride than it is for urea [22]. Since the fluid in the collecting duct is high in urea and low in sodium chloride, while the interstitial fluid has a greater portion of its total solute content made up of sodium chloride, equilibration of effective osmotic pressure across the collecting duct epithelium will result in a higher ideal osmotic pressure in the collecting duct than in the surrounding interstitium. This difference in ideal osmotic pressure accounts for the necessary net solute addition to the inner portions of the inner medullary interstitium.

Dr. Berliner: You can provide urea, but you can't provide any salt then, and it is the salt concentration that I am concerned about. You are quite right. You can get more urea; obviously, that is quite true. And I know that the mass balance equations work. But then the mass balance equations work out in Kokko and Recor's model, and that model doesn't work for exactly the reason that you pointed out: the urea concentration is too high. So, mass balance is not a sufficient condition for establishing that a model will work.

Dr. Bonventre: The profile in the inner medulla for sodium chloride is certainly much flatter than it is for urea. Our model does provide for salt concentration throughout the inner medulla. As we have demonstrated, active reabsorption of nonurea solute in the collecting duct in the inner medulla together with the net nonurea solute reabsorption from the loops of Henle can readily account for a sodium chloride gradient throughout the inner medulla. Finally, I would agree that mass balance is a necessary but not sufficient condition for establishing that a model will work. The model is testable, however, and attempts are being made to compare solute concentrations in the various compartments of the medulla near the outer medullary–inner medullary junction using techniques of electron microprobe analysis.

Dr. Berliner: Obviously it is much steeper in the outer medulla. When the animal is producing a dilute urine, almost all the increase in salt concentration is in the outer medulla. When it is producing a concentrated urine, the concentration of salt goes up much more steeply in the outer medulla, but it does continue to rise in the inner medulla and that is what I am concerned about. Urea doesn't worry me. It is true that if we have urea on the same scale it is much steeper in the inner medulla and relatively not steep at all in the outer medulla.

Dr. Cohen: Dr. Berliner, you noted the striking correlation between form and function for this particular aspect of renal physiology and how the thin ascending limb just doesn't have the requisite form to carry out a heavy active transport function. The present theory rests heavily on differential permeabilities of the descending thin limb versus the ascending thin limb. Are there morphologic correlates that would argue one way or the other about such permeability differences?

Dr. Berliner: Let me put it this way. Whether they are correlates of that particular difference I don't know, but there are differences. It was always said that one couldn't tell the difference between ascending and descending thin limbs, but in more modern work with electron microscopy there are clear differences. Permeability is pretty difficult to see. I don't think anybody has ever detected what it is that changes in making a membrane permeable or impermeable. That is a characteristic of the plasma membranes, and the plasma membranes are pretty thin; they don't appear to have very much in the way of structure. So even if one can't see any morphologic differences between them, the physiologic observations are quite clear; there is no doubt that there is a big difference in the permeability characterisitics.

Dr. Cohen: What about at the level of embryology? Is there any embryologic reason for thinking that the hairpin turn should demarcate two different sets of anlagen?

Dr. Berliner: Not that I am aware of, but I can't say that I really would know if there were. As a matter of fact, the change occurs almost certainly just a very little bit before the turn. So it's in the descending limb rather than at the tip of the loop. But you would have to ask an embryologist, which I am not.

Dr. Frank Epstein *(Director, Renal Division, Beth Israel Hospital, Boston, Massachusetts)*: One of the most striking pathologic situations in which this system seems to be disturbed is potassium deficiency. The disturbance is all the more striking since diluting ability is very often preserved and glomerular filtration rate is very often normal. To my knowledge, no one has pinpointed the precise locus of the disturbance but, as the grand master and super thinker of concentrating mechanisms, where would you look if you had to direct an eager investigator?

Dr. Berliner: I would look for somebody else! I think you would have to look at the effects of vasopressin on the membranes under those circumstances because I suspect it's not in the concentrating mechanism itself, but in the permeabilities that expose this mechanism.

Dr. Jerome P. Kassirer: If there is little urea in the highly concentrated urine of sand rat, what solute accounts for the high osmolality? Is it salt?

Dr. Berliner: Yes, it's salt. They live on so-called halophile plants, plants that grow in highly salty soils and are loaded with sodium chloride. They don't have much protein intake to require that they get rid of urea. They do have an enormous intake of sodium chloride, and they probably have a very high potassium intake also. As far as I know, all the studies on them have been done in Paris. When Rex Jamison tried to find out whether he could find the same thing as de Rouffignac did, he very wisely chose to go there instead of having them send him the rats.

Dr. Kassirer: There appears to be a large evolutionary gap in renal structure between animals that do not have countercurrent mechanisms and those that do. Does this remarkable evolutionary jump require some special explanation?

Dr. Berliner: No. Actually, I have always been struck by the fact that it doesn't. All it requires is an overgrowth of that particular part of the nephron. If you just take that connecting segment that is present in the amphibian and attach a hook to it and pull it down, it's all done. If you keep the descending part with characteristics somewhat like those in the proximal tubule and the ascending part with characteristics resembling those in the distal tubule, you have a look of Henle that behaves just the way you want it to. So, although it is a striking morphologic difference, it's not really an entirely new structure but one that could easily be adapted from what was there before.

References

1. Smith HW: The Kidney. Oxford Univ. Press, New York, 1951, p. 10
2. Frank J, Mayer JE: An osmotic diffusion pump. Arch Biochem 14:297–313, 1947
3. Brodsky WA, Rehm WS, Dennis WH, Miller DG: Thermodynamic analysis

of the intracellular osmotic gradient hypothesis of active water transport, Science 121:302–303, 1955
4. Wirz H, Hargitay B, Kuhn W: Lokalisation des konzentrierungsprozesses in der niere durch direkte kryoskopie. Helv Physiol Acta 9:196–207, 1951
5. Peter K: Untersuchungen uber bau und entwicklung der niere, Jena, Fischer, 1909
6. Filehne W, Biberfeld H: Beitrage zue diurese. Arch Ges Physiol 91:569–573, 1902
7. Hirokawa W: Ueber den osmotischen druck des nierenparanchyms, Hofmeisters Beitr Physiol Pathol 11:458–478, 1908
8. Gottschalk CW, Mylle M: Micropuncture study of the mammalian urinary concentrating mechanism: Evidence for the countercurrent hypothesis. Am J Physiol 196:927–936, 1959
9. Burgess WW, Harvey AM, Marshall EK Jr: The site of the antidiuretic action of pituitary extract. J Pharmacol Exp Ther 49:237–249, 1933
10. Sawyer WH: Increased renal reabsorption of osmotically free water by the toad (Bufo marinus) on response to neurohypophysial hormones. Am J Physiol 189:564–568, 1957
11. Crane MM: Observations on the function of the frog's kidney. Am J Physiol 81:232, 1927
12. Walker AM, Bott PA, Oliver J, MacDowell MD: The collection and analysis of fluid from single nephrons of the mammalian kidney. Am J Physiol 134:580–595, 1941
13. Hargitay B, Kuhn W: Das multiplikationsprinzip als grundlage der harnkonzentrierung in der niere. Z Elektrochem 55:539–558, 1951
14. Kuhn W, Ryffel K: Herstellung konzentrierter losungen aus verdunnten durch blosse membranwirkung. Ein modellversuch zur funktion der niere. Z Physiol Chem 276:145–147, 1942
15. Ullrich KJ, Drenckhahn FO, Jarausch KH: Untersuchungen zum problem der harnkonzentrierung und verdunnung. Ueber das osmotische verhalten von nierenzellen und die begleitende elektrolytanhaufung im nierendewebe bei verschiedenen diuresezunstanden. Arch Ges Physiol 261:62–77, 1955
16. Wirz H: Der osmotische druck des blutes in der nierenpapille. Helv Physiol Acta 11:20–29, 1953
17. Wirz H: Der osmotische druck in den corticalen tubuli der rattenniere. Helv Physiol Pharmacol Acta 14:353–362, 1956
18. Berliner RW, Davidson DG: Production of hypertonic urine in the absence of pituitary antidiuretic hormone. J Clin Invest 36:1416–1427, 1957
19. Berliner RW, Levinsky NG, Davidson DG, Eden M: Dilution and concentration of the urine and the action of antidiuretic hormone. Am J Med 24:730–733, 1958
20. Jamison RL, Bennett CM, Berliner RW: Countercurrent multiplication by the thin loops of Henle. Am J Physiol 212:357–366, 1967
21. Jamison RL: Micropuncture study of segments of thin loop of Henle in the rat. Am J Physiol 215:236–242, 1968
22. Morgan T, Berliner RW: Permeability of the loop of Henle, vasa recta, and collecting duct to water, urea, and sodium. Am J Physiol 215:108–115, 1968
23. Kokko JP: Sodium chloride and water transport in the descending limb of Henle. J Clin Invest 49:1838–1846, 1970

24. Imai M, Kokko JP: Sodium chloride, urea, and water transport in the thin ascending limb of Henle: Generation of osmotic gradients by passive diffusion of solutes. J Clin Invest 53:393–402, 1974
25. Burg MB, Green N: Function of the thick ascending limb of Henle's loop. Am J Physiol 224:659–668, 1973
26. Rocha AS, Kokko JP: Sodium chloride and water transport in the medullary thick ascending limb of Henle. J Clin Invest 52:612–623, 1973
27. Morgan T: Permeability of the thin limbs of the loop of Henle. Proc 5th Intl Congr Nephrol 2:105–111, 1972
28. Marsh DJ, Azen SP: Mechanism of NaCl reabsorption by hamster thin ascending limbs of Henle's loop. Am J Physiol 228:71–79, 1975
29. Imai M: Function of the thin ascending limb of Henle of rats and hamsters perfused in vitro. Am J Physiol 232:F201–F209, 1977
30. Marsh DJ: Hypo-osmotic re-absorption due to active salt transport in perfused collecting ducts of the rat renal medulla. Nature 210:1179–1180, 1966
31. Hilger HH, Klumper JD, Ullrich KJ: Wasserruckresorption und ionentransport durch die sammelrohrzellen der saugetiernier. Pfluegers Arch 267:218–237, 1958
32. Pinter GG, Shohet JL: Origin of sodium concentration profile in the renal medulla. Nature 200:955–958, 1963
33. Marumo F, Yoshikawa Y, Koshikawa S: A study on the concentration mechanism of the renal medulla by mathematical model. Jpn Circ J 31:1309–1317, 1967
34. Stephenson JL: Concentration in renal counterflow systems. Biophys J 6:539–551, 1966
35. Stephenson JL: Concentration of urine in a central core model of the renal counterflow system. Kidney Int 2:85–94, 1972
36. Kokko JP, Rector FC Jr: Countercurrent multiplication system without active transport in inner medulla. Kidney Int 2:214–223, 1972
37. Gamble JL, McKhann CF, Butler AM, Tuthill E: An economy of water in renal function referable to urea. Am J Physiol 109:139–154, 1934
38. Crawford JD, Doyle AP, Probst JH: Service of urea in renal water conservation. Am J Physiol 196:545–548, 1959
39. Levinsky NG, Berliner RW: The role of urea in the urine concentrating mechanism. J Clin Invest 38:741–748, 1959
40. De Rouffignac C, Morel F: Micropuncture study of water, electrolytes, and urea movements along the loops of Henle in Psammomys. J Clin Invest 48:474–486, 1969
41. Jamison RL, Roinel N, De Rouffignac C: Urinary concentrating mechanism in the desert rodent Psammomys obesus. Am J Physiol 236:F448–F453, 1979
42. Pennell JP, Lacy FB, Jamison RL: An in vivo study of the concentrating process in the decending limb of Henle's loop. *Kidney Int* 5:337–347, 1974
43. Johnston PA, Battilana CA, Lacy FB, Jamison RL: Evidence for a concentration gradient favoring outward movement of sodium from the thin loop of Henle. J Clin Invest 59:234–240, 1977
44. Bonventre JV, Lechene C: Renal medullary concentrating process: An integrative hypothesis. Am J Physiol 239:F578–F588, 1980
45. Smith HW: The fate of sodium and water in the renal tubules. Bull NY Acad Med 35:293–316, 1959

Neurogenic Diabetes Insipidus

Principal Discussant
Alexander Leaf

Case Presentation

A 15-year-old girl was admitted to the New England Medical Center Hospital (NEMCH) for investigation of the hypothalamic-pituitary axis. Four years earlier, an eosinophilic granuloma was discovered in the left mandible and was treated with excision and irradiation (1000 rads). Two years earlier she developed polyuria, and a diagnosis of diabetes insipidus was made at another hospital. She was treated with synthetic lysine vasopressin nasal spray (Diapid) several times a day and noted some symptomatic improvement. Eighteen months before admission, her menstrual periods, which had been normal for the previous 14 months, ceased and she complained of cold intolerance, constipation, and weight gain. She claimed to have grown 0.5 in. over the year prior to admission. She had occasional mild headaches when she did not take her medication but noted no visual disturbances. Family history was unrevealing. Her mother was 61 in. tall.

Physical examination revealed the following findings: blood pressure, 110/70; heart rate, 60/min; weight, 51.5 kg; height, 62 in.; skin was pale and dry; optic fundi were normal; formal testing for visual fields revealed no defects; there was a pale, white lesion on the inner aspect of the right-lower jaw; the thyroid gland was not palpable; breast development was stage III to IV; rectal examination was normal; neurologic examination was normal.

Laboratory findings revealed the following data: hematocrit, 39%; white blood cell count, 6700 with a normal differential; erythrocyte sedimentation rate, 10 mm/h; urine sediment, unremarkable; blood urea nitrogen (BUN), 12 mg; serum creatinine, 1 mg; serum calcium, 10.8 mg; serum phosphorus, 3.6 mg/100 ml; serum electrolytes were normal; the chest radiogram was normal; both bone scan and gallium scan revealed an area of increased uptake over the right mandible.

Various tests of hypothalamic-pituitary function revealed the following: an elevated resting prolactin level; a low T3 and T41 with an inappropriately low level of thyroid-stimulating hormone (TSH); an inappropriately low level of luteinizing hormone (LH) for a patient with amenorrhea; a decreased growth hormone response to insulin infusion;

and a normal cortrosyn stimulation test. Both TSH and LH responded normally to infusion of the appropriate releasing hormones. Data from a water deprivation test are shown in Table 1.

The lesion in the right mandible was biopsied and again revealed an eosinophilic granuloma. A second course of radiation (800 rads) was delivered to the right mandible on an outpatient basis. She was treated with L-thyroxine (150 μg/day), estrogen, and lysine vasopressin nasal spray.

One year later, lysine vasopressin was discontinued in preparation for the institution of dDAVP (1-desamino-8-D arginine vasopressin) therapy. Urine volume rose promptly to over 10 liters/day, but fell dramatically to less than 1 liter/day in response to dDAVP (15 μg, twice daily, intranasally). A repeat biopsy of the right mandible revealed recurrent eosinophilic granuloma. Cerebral computerized tomographic (CT) scan showed a questionable shift of the third ventricle and deformity of the basal cisterns. Pneumoencephalogram revealed a slight flattening of the infundibular recess of the third ventricle and asymmetry of the optic chiasm, but these findings were judged to be probably normal. Visual field examination was again normal. Repeat insulin tolerance test and an arginine infusion test revealed normal growth hormone responses. The right mandibular lesion was surgically excised; no fur-

Table 1. Water deprivation test.

	Weight (*kg*)	Posm	Uosm	Urine Volume (*ml*)
Day 1		Vasopressin discontinued		
10:00 P.M.	51.5	283	200	–
		—NPO—		
Day 2				
8:00 A.M.	50.9	291	154	530
9:00 A.M.	–	–	–	420
10:00 A.M.	50.1	–	53	280
11:00 A.M.	–	–	57	280
12:00 noon	49.3	309	67	500
	—Pitressin tannate in oil, 5U— at 12:00 noon			
1:30 P.M.			–	400
2:00 P.M.			–	38
4:00 P.M.			747	30
5:00 P.M.			802	17
6:00 P.M.			823	10
Day 3				
8:00 A.M.	51.5	–	1169	–

Note: Posm, plasma osmolality; Uosm, urine osmolality; NPO, nothing by mouth (after 10:00 P.M.).

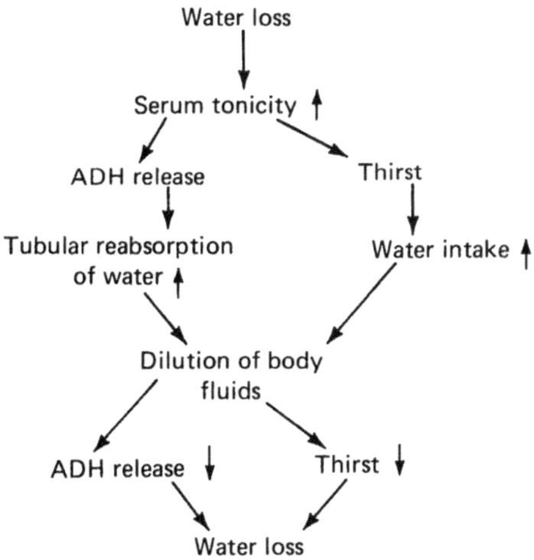

Fig. 1. The thirst-ADH-renal axis that functions to preserve the normal osmolality of body fluids—a double-negative feedback control system.

ther radiation was given. The patient has been evaluated biannually and continues to do well 2 years later. The dose of dDAVP has been reduced to 15 μg in the morning and 10 μg in the evening. She is asymptomatic and plans to pursue a career in nursing.

Discussion

Dr. Alexander Leaf *(Professor of Medicine and Ridley Watts Professor of Preventive Medicine, Harvard Medical School; Physician, Massachusetts General Hospital, Boston, Massachusetts)**: Neurogenic diabetes insipidus is a clinically rare but physiologically important disturbance of water balance. Its pathophysiology is as clearly understood as is any aspect of renal physiology and endocrine homeostasis. It results from a failure of antidiuretic hormone (ADH) secretion in response to the physiologic stimulus of water deficiency. This is the condition that our patient has and for which she exhibits all the classical and essential diagnostic criteria.

Since the classic studies of Verney [1] in the mid-1940s, it has been evident that the neurohypophysis plays a fundamental role in the economy of body fluids and in the regulation of the tonicity of the body fluids. This it does in combination with the thirst mechanism as established a decade later by Andersson [2]. The resulting "double-negative" feedback system which sustains our serum sodium concentrations constant between some 136 and 143 mEg/liter and the corresponding serum osmolality between 275 and 290 mOsm/kg H_2O is shown in Fig. 1. Cell membranes are generally so permeable to water that a single tonicity—chemical potential of water—exists throughout all body fluid

*At the time of this forum, Dr. Leaf was Jackson Professor of Clinical Medicine, Harvard Medical School; Chief, Medical Services, Massachusetts General Hospital

compartments. Thus this neurohypophysis-thirst-renal axis accounts for the constancy of serum sodium concentration and of osmolality of intracellular as well as extracellular fluids. It is so effective that the range of values that we accept as normal probably represents largely analytic rather than biologic variation.

With loss of neurohypophyseal function the situation changes as shown in Fig. 2. Thus, even when the ADH limb of the "double-negative" regulatory feedback is lost, the thirst mechanism still preserves a serum sodium and osmolality within the normal range but at the expense of pronounced polydipsia and polyuria. It is true that statistically the serum sodium concentration or osmolality of an untreated patient with diabetes insipidus may be slightly higher than the mean normal value, but the range of the latter prevents such small increases from having any diagnostic significance. Thus Barlow and de Wardener [3] found the plasma osmolality of patients suffering from diabetes insipidus to average 295 ± 15 mOsm/kgH_2O (SD), whereas that for normal subjects averaged 280 ± 6 mOsm/kgH_2O (SD). Since this statistically significant difference is associated with considerable overlap this determination if of little help diagnostically in the individual patient.

When unconsciousness or lack of water occurs, however, the patient with diabetes insipidus will continue to lose water with resulting weight loss and increase in serum osmolality. Dehydration of a serious degree can occur rapidly in such circumstances. This sequence is depicted nicely in the provacative diagnostic tests shown for our patient in Table 1. When fluids were withheld after 10 P.M., the bladder contained a large volume of urine the following morning. The hourly urine flow remained high, its concentration fell to minimal levels, the patient lost weight, and her serum osmolality increased from a normal level of 283 to 309 mOsm/kgH_2O. The values show good internal consistency since the patient lost 2.2 kg during the 14 h of water restriction and had a negative fluid balance by urine losses alone of 2.01 kg; her serum osmolality increased thereby to 309 mOsm/kgH_2O whereas the theoretical expected final osmolality would be some 305 mOsm/kgH_2O, assuming

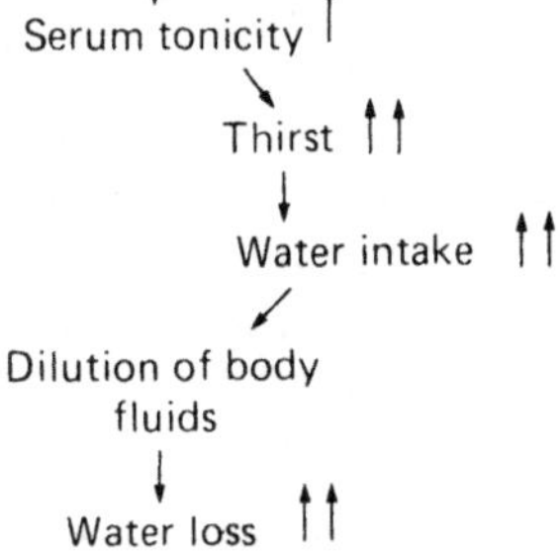

Fig. 2. Schemata of neurogenic diabetes insipidus. In neurogenic diabetes insipidus, the control of the osmolality of body fluids depends solely upon the operation of the thirst mechanism because the ADH-renal feedback control is lost. Serum tonicity can be maintained within normal limits but only at the expense of polyuria and polydipsia.

an initial total body water content of 60% of body weight. Her urine concentration fell to values close to maximal dilution capacity despite the increasing dehydration. Thus, her kidneys failed to show any ability to conserve body water in the face of increasing dehydration. It remained only to demonstrate that her renal tubules could conserve water when exposed to ADH: in fact, when pitressin tannate in oil was administered, her urine volume fell rapidly and urine osmolality rose to high levels. Her tubules could respond to ADH and her diabetes insipidus, therefore, was neurogenic due to insufficiency of ADH secretion.

In summary, the patient demonstrated the two physiologic features which are the *sine qua non* for the diagnosis of neurogenic diabetes insipidus: (1) she failed to concentrate her urine despite serum osmolality rising to abnormally high levels; (2) her kidneys responded to exogenous vasopressin by elaborating a concentrated urine. Without both features, one cannot make a diagnosis of neurogenic diabetes insipidus since polyuria with a dilute urine, which is unresponsive to vasopressin, occurs in a variety of disorders including nephrogenic diabetes insipidus, chronic renal disease, kaliopenic nephropathy, and hypercalcemia.

Nephrogenic diabetes insipidus is congenital, makes its appearance shortly after birth, occurs predominantly in males, and appears to result from genetic deficiency of adenylate cyclase responsive to ADH in the renal tubules. The other three conditions usually show stigmata of the disease or disturbance causing them and should not be difficult to diagnose.

Other provocative tests have been utilized in the diagnosis of diabetes insipidus. Infusion of hypertonic saline to elevate serum osmolality and thus to provide the stimulus for ADH release has been used, as has pharmacologic stimulation of ADH release with nicotine. The simple overnight dehydration test, however, as applied to this patient is by far the most satisfactory diagnostic test. Nonetheless, one must be aware that in the youngster with presumptive diabetes insipidus dangerous levels of negative water balance may develop rapidly; thus, urine volumes and weight must be followed carefully to avoid serious consequences of dehydration. Similar precaution must be exercised in testing the obtunded or mentally confused adult.

A more troublesome differential diagnosis occasionally exists in relation to primary polydipsia. This disorder is generally a manifestation of a functional mental illness, usually called compulsive water drinking or psychogenic polydipsia. The diagnostic difficulty arises from the fact that prolonged very high fluid intake itself impairs renal concentrating ability. Figure 3 shows the serum and urine osmolalities of normal subjects, patients with diabetes insipidus, and two patients with psychogenic polydipsia [4]. After 8 h of fluid restriction, the normal subjects had serum osmolalities within the usual range and were excreting a

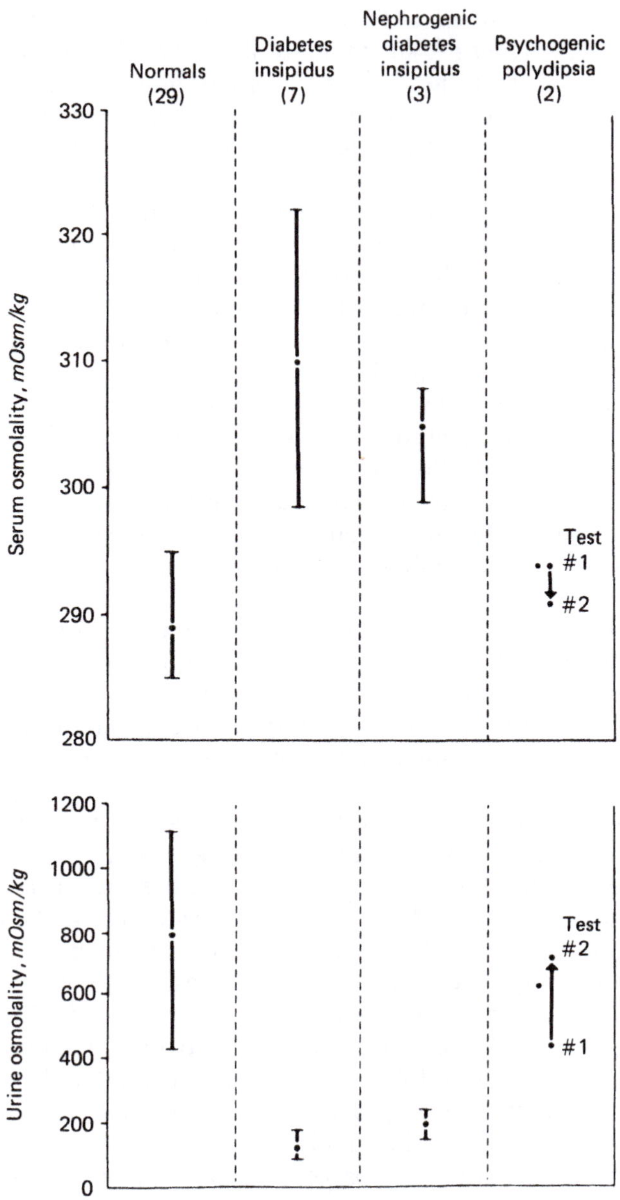

Fig. 3. Mean and range of serum and urine olmolalities after 8-h dehydration. Data taken from Ref. 4 by permission of *Journal of Clinical Endocrinology and Metabolism.*

concentrated urine. The patients with diabetes insipidus, both neurogenic and nephrogenic, developed high serum osmolalities while their urine tonicity persisted very dilute. The patients with psychogenic polydipsia had serum osmolalities that were normal and urine concentrations that were low, but overlapped the lower limits of the normals. When neurohypophyseal insufficiency is not complete, overlap may occur between psychogenic polydipsia and incomplete diabetes insipidus. It is useful, however, to remember a point made by Barlow and de Wardener, namely, that patients with neurogenic diabetes insipidus concentrate their urine better with exogenous ADH than following dehydration; whereas normal subjects or those with psychogenic polydipsia elaborate a more concentrated urine following water restriction than in response to exogenous ADH, irrespective of the absolute levels of the urine concentration attained [3].

At the level of the kidney, the major action of the neurohypophyseal hormone has been characterized. Specifically, ADH increases the permeability of the luminal plasma membranes of the cortical collecting ducts of water and of the medullary collecting ducts to water and urea. It may also enhance salt reabsorption in the thick ascending limb of Henle's loop, which generates the hypertonic medullary interstitium and makes possible the elaboration of a concentrated urine.

Diabetes insipidus is itself a benign condition so long as adequate water, or replacement therapy, or both is available. However, because loss of neurohypophyseal function may have different etiologies, not all of which are benign, it is important to learn if possible the cause in each case. Randall has suggested an etiologic classification of diabetes insipidus with two major categories, primary and secondary [5]. Primary diabetes insipidus includes familial and idiopathic cases. Idiopathic cases constitute the major group in any such classification, comprising 45% of Blotner's series [6], but perhaps exceeded today by head injuries, iatrogenic or accidental. Idiopathic diabetes insipidus may become manifest at any age and may affect either sex. It is unusual for the idiopathic type to appear early in infancy, as does nephrogenic diabetes insipidus, although it may develop in childhood. Familial diabetes insipidus, on the other hand, is very uncommon and constitutes less than 1% of cases. It may become manifest in infancy and may affect either sex. The condition has been described in seven generations of one family [7].

In the group with secondary diabetes insipidus, head trauma—accidental or neorusurgical—and neoplasms—primary or metastatic—constitute the major causes. In older series, primary intracranial tumors constituted nearly one-third of all cases. The currently increasing incidence of automobile injuries, surgical pituitary stalk sections, and other neurosurgical procedures in the neighborhood of the neurohypophyseal system has affected the frequency of secondary diabetes insipidus.

Of the metastatic tumors, breast cancer and lung cancer seem to have special predilection for the hypothalamus. Other etiologic factors contribute only small numbers to any series. However, sarcoidosis, birth injuries, eosinophilic granuloma—as our patient has—and a variety of local infections appear on any listing of extensive causes of diabetes insipidus.

Even with disease or tumor within the hypothalamus, diabetes insipidus is unusual. With loss or destruction of the posterior pituitary gland, diabetes insipidus may be short lived or nonexistent because the active hormone, which is synthesized in the supraoptic nuclei and to a lesser degree in the paraventricular nuclei, is transmitted down the supraopticohypophyseal tract and stored for release in the posterior pituitary. The hormone can be released from the higher levels of the tract when lower portions are damaged or destroyed, thus preventing manifest diabetes insipidus.

This capability of higher levels within the hypothalamus to subsume the secretion of ADH when lower portions of the supraopticohypophyseal tract have been damaged was described by Fischer, et al. [8] in experimental diabetes insipidus and probably accounts for the variable clinical course. I have seen complete diabetes insipidus following head trauma, which after maintaining a flagrant course for 3 years subsided, with replacement therapy no longer needed and with return of concentrating ability. On the other hand, I have seen diabetes insipidus start at 1 P.M. on a Saturday afternoon, cease abruptly 2 weeks later, and never return!

Given the evidence from biopsies of the mandible, we can presume that eosinophilic granuloma is the cause of diabetes insipidus in the patient under discussion today. Eosinophilic granuloma is frequently multifocal, often involves the mandible, and may affect both the bones and viscera. In the brain, the hypothalamus is most commonly affected but sometimes the cerebellum and cortex are involved. A lesion in the hypothalamus in our patient would account not only for the diabetes insipidus but also for the other endocrine changes elicited by the provocative tests of hypothalamic-pituitary function.

Thus, the elevated resting prolactin level is consistent with loss of the hypothalamic prolactin inhibitory factor (PIF). The low peripheral thyroid hormone levels and low level of the pituitary thyroid-stimulating hormone (TSH) are consistent with decreased or absent hypothalamic thyrotropin-releasing hormone (TRH). The normal response of TSH to infusion of TRH confirms the hypothalamus as the site of the primary deficiency. The low level of LH and its normal response to infusion of luteinotrophin-releasing hormone (LRH) has the same interpretation as does the diminished growth hormone response to hypoglycemic stress, which points to a deficiency of hypothalamic growth hormone-releasing factor (GHR). All of these tests indicate a lesion of the hypothalamus. The normal cortrosyn stimulation test of the adrenal cortex is reassuring evidence that glucocorticoid function is adequate. Although adrenal insufficiency may result from eosinophilic granuloma, we had strong evidence of normal adrenal cortical function in this patient from the observation that she could elaborate large volumes of very dilute urine. This capability is lost with adrenal or anterior pituitary failure even in the presence of neurogenic diabetes insipidus, though the mechanism of the lost ability to excrete a copious dilute urine with loss of both ADH and adrenal cortical secretions is still not well understood.

Although the function of this exercise is to discuss the disturbance in water metabolism, a word should be said regarding the patient's underlying problem, multifocal eosinophilic granuloma—a very confusing clinical entity or entities! Multifocal eosinophilic granuloma often makes its first appearance as a bony lesion of the mandible, mastoid, or skull. But when diabetes insipidus is the first manifestation, it is caused by granulomas within the hypothalamus, as in our patient, and not by pressure from the adjacent bony tumors. Other soft tissue organs, such as the liver, spleen, lymph nodes, and skin, may also be involved. Evidence for cerebral and cerebellar dysfunction may also be present. Anterior pituitary failure rarely develops in the course of this enigmatic disease, but whether this complication is the result of loss of hypothalamic trophic factors or direct destruction of the anterior pituitary by granuloma has not been settled by either hormone assays or postmortem studies to my knowledge.

Treatment of eosinophilic granuloma by surgical excision or radiation of local solitary bone lesions is usually successful. In multifocal eosinophilic granuloma beneficial results have been reported with chemotherapy including vinblastine, prednisone, mercaptopurine, or methotrexate singly or in various combinations. Once the diabetes insipidus is established, however, it does not respond to treatment of the underlying eosinophilic granuloma.

Finally, a word should be said regarding the therapy of diabetes insipidus. The condition has no known deleterious effect on health so long as its cause is benign and so long as water is available, the subject is conscious, and the thirst center is functioning. Thus, the indications for replacement therapy may not be pressing. The marked polyuria and polydipsia with complete lack of ADH activity usually is disturbing and socially distressing during the day and may interfere with sleep at night. For reasons of convenience and comfort replacement therapy is usually justified.

Fortunately, several modes of therapy are available. A variety of ADH sprays and powders for intranasal insufflation, as well as ADH for injection, have been the standard replacement therapy. Lysine vasopressin spray provides control of polyuria for relatively short periods of 2–6 h, insufficient for an undisturbed night's sleep. Moistening a pledget of cotton, however, with this solution of hormone and inserting it into a nostril at bed time is used by some to obtain an undisturbed night. Pitressin tannate in oil (5 U/ml) is potent and effective for 24–72 h. It requires a deep subcutaneous or intramuscular injection by a fairly large gauge needle because of the viscosity of the oil vehicle. This material causes sterile abscesses in some subjects. Care must be taken to allow return of polyuria and polydipsia between injections in order to avoid cumulative water retention and severe hyponatremia. The main drawbacks of pitressin tannate are, however, the discomforts and inconvenience attended upon any preparation that must be administered parenterally. Aqueous vasopressin (20 pressor units/ml), when it is available, plays virtually no role in the management of chronic diabetes insipidus. It does allow a readily controllable method of treating the comatose patient with head trauma and polyuria when the pitressin is diluted and administered intravenously. Since aqueous pitressin is degraded very rapidly its action ceases within minutes after the infusion is stopped. This property makes it worthless in the management of chronic diabetes insipidus. One young patient of mine had a sister who was a nurse. The sister injected the patient subcutaneously with 1 ml of aqueous hormone preparation four times daily—a total of 80 pressor units! With each injection the patient experienced general abdominal and uterine cramps, perioral blanching, and 30–60 min of decreased urine output. Later we found that 2 units of pitressin administered as the long-acting pitressin tannate in oil controlled her symptoms for over 24 h.

In the mid-1960s, structure-activity investigations were performed in Czechoslovakia with a variety of synthetic analogs of vasopressin [9]. From these studies emerged a substitution of D- for L-arginine at position 8 which resulted in a peptide, DAVP, with diminished vasopressor activity. Deamination of the hemicystein at position 1 gave rise to a second peptide, dAVP, with enhanced antidiuretic-to-pressor activity and prolonged duration of action. Combining both changes in one molecule, i.e., deamination at position 1 and substitution of D- for L-arginine in position 8 results in a peptide, dDAVP, with high antidiuretic-to-pressor potency (approximately 2000:1) and a prolonged duration of action (6–24 h), as compared with the natural hormone AVP (AD:P = 1; duration of action 2–4 h) [10,11]. This compound, dDAVP, is available for administration intranasally, and the experience to date indicates it to be a safe and effective means of control. Generally, administration twice daily in doses as low as 5–20 μg suffices in many patients. Local nasal irritation and systemic reactions are rare. An occasional patient may complain of headaches, and that is about all the side reactions that have been noted. The medication is readily self-administered intranasally by a plastic catheter (Rhinyle; A. B. Ferring Company, Malmo, Sweden).

Although intranasal dDAVP is the treatment of choice for diabetes insipidus, it is well to remember that alternatives to hormone replacement may be helpful at times. Since, with a very dilute urine of fixed osmolality, the urine volume is determined by the solute load requiring excretion, a reduction chiefly of salt and protein in the diet will reduce the major urinary solutes and thus the volume of urine necessary to accommodate their excretion. A diuretic such as chlorothiazide administered chronically will maintain a state of mild sodium depletion which impairs "free water" excretion by the kidneys and thus reduces urine volume from distressing levels of 6–10 liters daily to volumes of 2–4 liters. Chlorpropamide seems to potentiate the action of even small amounts of circulating antidiuretic hormone and may thereby enhance antidiuresis when neurohypophyseal failure is not complete. Severe hypoglycemia may be a complicating aspect of this therapy and is especially harmful in the young patient. Thus dDAVP in intranasal administration seems today the safest and most effective form of therapy for this distressing condition.

Questions and Answers

Dr. Seymour Reichlin *(Chief, Endocrinology Division, NEMC)*: We assessed the location of the lesion in this patient to be precisely where you did. It is really the only site where a small lesion can destroy antidiuretic function and some, but not all, anterior pituitary functions without producing other gross physiologic abnormalities [12]. A very small lesion is responsible it seems.

Dr. Jordan J. Cohen: Dr. Reichlin, considering the propensity of lesions such as this to recur and to grow, is it surprising to you that the patient has not shown more evidence of difficulty over a rather long period of time? Is it safe to follow a patient in this fashion?

Dr. Reichlin: It has been difficult to decide how to manage this patient. The possibility of an expanding granulomatous mass in the hypothalamus that might produce progressive damage has concerned us because some cases have been reported in which rapid expansion of an eosinophilic granuloma has caused death. On the other hand, we feel we can monitor the lesion by the use of the CT scan and by careful clinical evaluation. We have been concerned about exposing the hypothalamus to a tumoricidal dose of radiation and thus endangering the patient's residual hypothalamic function. We have been on the horns of a dilemma, i.e., to produce further damage versus protect her from tumor growth. We have elected to follow a conservative approach of watchful waiting. The lesion has not progressed for 5 years, and as Dr. Leaf mentioned, these lesions have a rather variable course, sometimes remitting spontaneously.

Dr. Leaf: I certainly support your decision. We have seen comparable lesions appear in a bone and disappear spontaneously. The deaths that have been reported from this condition generally occur when the viscera are involved, and this patient shows no evidence of such involvement. The condition can remain stable for many years, and for this reason I think it is wise to be conservative. Do you wish to comment, Dr. Reichlin, on the relationship of diabetes insipidus secondary to eosinophilic granuloma and other hormonal disturbances?

Dr. Reichlin: Dr. Goodman reviewed this literature recently after we encountered a patient with direct pituitary destruction due to the eosinophilic granuloma. Perhaps he could comment.

Dr. Richard H. Goodman *(Fellow in Endocrinology, NEMC)*: We were not able to find any cases in which there was involvement of the anterior pituitary by eosinophilic granuloma, but the posterior pituitary was sometimes involved. It is interesting that in this patient, as in some others previously described, growth hormone responses increased after a period of vasopressin therapy for the diabetes insipidus. Treatment with either thyroxin or estrogen or both may also have improved the growth hormone response in the patient described today.

Dr. Reichlin: Although growth hormone is released following vasopressin administration, innumerable studies show that vasopressin is not a GHR. Normal growth hormone secretory dynamics can be demonstrated in rats with the Brattleboro strain of congenital diabetes indipidus. Studies have shown that these animals have cyclical growth hormone secretion. It is possible that improvement of the general physical condition of the patient improves growth hormone secretion in a fairly nonspecific way.

Dr. Mark E. Molitch *(Endocrinology Division, NEMC)*: We have seen several instances of transient diabetes insipidus after pituitary surgery in which the condition persisted for several months or longer. The pathophysiology of the diabetes insipidus and the slow recovery of antidiuretic function have never been clear to me. Can you clarify it?

Dr. Leaf: I can refer you to the excellent study by Fischer et al. [8]. They produced stereotactic lesions in cats and found that the animals went through several phases. Immediately after surgery there was a very intense antidiuresis, then a phase in which polyuria occurred and was followed by mild antidiuresis, and finally permanent diabetes insipidus developed if the lesion was produced in the right location. They attributed the intial antidiuresis to release of stored hormone and the subsequent polyuria and mild anitdiuresis to a period of decreased hormone availability. The final permanent diabetes insipidus resulted if a lesion had been produced that prevented further hormone secretion. They found that even if they transsected the supraopticohypophyseal tract low down, the mamillary bodies in the hypothalamus could actually take over the hormone secretion; thus, the posterior pituitary could be destroyed and yet permanent diabetes insipidus not develop. I think the slow recovery that sometimes occurs is due to the subsiding of the response to the trauma in the higher portions of the tract. This restoration allows the hormone to be released at higher levels, closer to the supraoptic nuclei where it is formed. That is my interpretation of the physiologic events when recovery is delayed as long as a year.

Dr. Cohen: There is convincing evidence that volume "receptors" and other nonosmolar factors also control ADH release. Do the osmolar and nonosmolar mechanisms operate through the same neurons or are there different pathways involved? Also, do nonosmolar factors affect hormone synthesis or just hormone release?

Dr. Reichlin: The supraoptic neuron is played upon by a variety of impulses. The opiates should be mentioned because recent evidence indicates that endorphins activate the supraoptic neurons directly. This mechanism apparently accounts for morphine-induced antidiuresis. These very same neurons are responsive to acetylcholine, which mediates the right auricular and volume controls. They are also responsive to norepinephrine and to both sodium shifts and osmotic changes. Angiotensin II also appears to act directly on supraoptic neurons. This provides a mechanism through which decreased blood volume could signal ADH release. The osmoreceptor area contains integrating cells, the membranes of which process a great deal of neurotransmitter information from all parts of the body: blood chemistry, volume receptors, and probably psychologic data as well. They are impressively versatile neurons.

Dr. Cohen: I was trying to determine whether all cells in this area serve this integrating function or whether separate cells have different roles, which in the aggregate give rise to the observed, integrated behavior.

Dr. Reichlin: It has not been possible to answer the question with confidence because the best data are obtained by placing an electrode into the neuron itself. Hayward [13] found that a certain proportion of such cells will discharge repetitively when hypertonic saline is injected into the carotid artery.

Dr. Nicolaos E. Madias *(Renal Service, NEMC)*: Could you comment on recent observations that show a linkage between ADH and prostaglandins; namely, that ADH stimulates the production of prostaglandins, and that prostaglandins antagonize the hydroosmotic effect of ADH [14–17]. A study in the Brattleboro rat shows that the excretion of prostaglandin E_2 is very low and that it increases significantly after injection of ADH [14]. Do you envision a role for this system in the diagnosis and treatment of diabetes insipidus?

Dr. Lear: I think this area needs more exploration. You described the state of the art as well as I know it in your comments: ADH seems to effect the synthesis of prostaglandins by releasing arachidonic acid and evoking synthesis. There are many potential for interplay that must have some physiologic and clinical significance, but they need to be developed.

Dr. Jerome P. Kassirer: We've seen in recent years an explosion in the number of drugs that have notable effects on water balance. Some, in particular chlorpropamide, appear to have some important therapeutic properties. What are the current thoughts on the mechanism of action of chlorpropamide?

Dr. Leaf: I haven't studied chlorpropamide myself. Two studies have described differing physiologic mechanisms at work. One study in the toad bladder demonstrated evidence that chlorpropamide potentiates the effects of small amounts of ADH on the permeability to water [18]. Another study argued that the drug caused the release of ADH from the neurohypophysis [19]. The presence of ADH seems to be necessary for chlorpropamide to work. If there is still some residual function, that effect may be of therapeutic value. I think today with other modes of therapy available it is probably advisable not to use chlorpropamide, particularly in children because of the risk of hypoglycemia.

Dr. William E. Cobb *(Endocrinology Division, NEMC)*: Several patients have been described in the literature with diabetes insipidus and absolute diminished thirst. Some have had essential hypernatremia, high sodium levels, and no response to osmotic stimuli. It has been suggested that chlorpropamide is probably the drug of choice for treating this group of patients. It has also been suggested that perhaps chlorpropamide has an effect on the thirst center. Do you know of any data that would support this hypothesis?

Dr. Leaf: I don't. I think that this entity does not result from a single etiology. I think that it is possible to have a lesion in the hypothalamus that destroys the neurons responsible for thirst and also those responsible for osmoregulation. Although these neurons are apparently separable, both centers are located close together in the lateral preoptic and supraoptic areas of the anterior hypothalamus, respectively. I have no experience with possible effects of chlorpropamide on thirst or its use in these vary rare cases.

Dr. Kassirer: Dr. Cobb, would you elaborate a bit on your studies of therapy with a synthetic analog of vasopressin?

Dr. Cobb: As Dr. Leaf mentioned before, dDVAP has a longer duration of action and a much higher antidiuretic-to-pressor potency than the parent compound, AVP. We studied intranasal dDAVP in 29 patients with chronic and two patients with acute—i.e., postoperative—diabetes insipidus [20]. Twenty-eight patients with chronic neurogenic diabetes insipidus, who have now been followed for up to 35 months, achieved excellent control of symptoms at a dose of 2.5–15.0 μg, once every 8 to 24 h. One patient, initially well controlled on 10 μg, twice daily, developed partial resistance to dDAVP and presently requires a dose of 15–20 μg, four times daily. Headache occurred in the "resistant" patient at high doses (over 20 μg) and in one additional patient at a dose of 10 μg. In each of two patients who developed acute diabetes insipidus after transfrontal removal of a craniopharyngioma, 5 μg intranasal dDVAP every 14 to 18 h was effective. We have not used dDAVP to treat acute diabetes insipidus after transsphenoidal hypophysectomy because of surgically induced contusion and swelling of nasal mucous membranes.

In patients with chronic diabetes insipidus, dDAVP resulted in a degree of control superior to that of chlorpropamide or lysine vasopressin nasal spray and as good as that obtained with vasopressin tannate in oil. The frequent occurrence of side effects with chlorpropamide—hypoglycemia, reactions similar to those seen with Antabuse—and vasopressin tannate in oil—sterile abscesses, abdominal pain—especially in children, was in marked contrast to the low frequency and minor nature of side effects with dDAVP. We feel that intranasal dDAVP is the preferred treatment of chronic diabetes insipidus in both children and adults, and of acute postoperative diabetes insipidus following transfrontal surgery. Hopefully, the cost of the drug will fall in the near future and thus make it possible to exploit its advantages widely.

References

1. Verney EG: The absorption and excretion of water: the antiuretic hormone. Lancet 2:739–744, 781–783, 1946
2. Andersson B: Polydipsia, antidiuresis and milk ejection caused by hypothalamic stimulation, In Heller H (ed.): The Neurohypophysis, London, Butterworth, 1957
3. Barlow ED, de Wardener HE: Compulsive water drinking. QJ Med 28:235, 1959
4. Price JDE, Lauener RW: Serum and urine osmolalities in the differential diagnosis of polyuric states. J Clin Endocrinol Metab 26:143–148, 1966
5. Randall RV, Clark EC, Bahn RC: Classification of the causes of diabetes insipidus. Proc Mayo Clin 34:299, 1959
6. Blotner H: Primary or idiopathic diabetes insipidus: a system disease. Metabolism 7:191, 1958
7. Blotner H: The inheritance of diabetes insipidus. Am J Med Sci 204:261, 1942
8. Fischer C, Ingram WR, Ranson SW: Diabetes Insipidus and the Neurohormonal Control of Water Balance. Ann Arbor, Edwards Brothers, 1938

9. Zaoral M. Kole J, Sorm F: Amino acids and peptides. LXXI. Synthesis of 1-deamino-8-D-aminobutyrine vasopressin, 1-deamino-8-D-lysine vasopressin and 1-deamino-8-D-arginine vasopressin. Coll Czech Chem Commun 32:1250–1257, 1967
10. Sawyer WH, Acosta M, Balaspiri L, Judd J, Manning M: Structural changes in the arginine vasopressin molecule that enhance antidiuretic and specificity. Endocrinology 94:1106–1115, 1974
11. Sawyer WH, Acosta M, Manning M: Structural changes in arginine vasopressin molecule that prolong its antidiuretic action. Endocrinology 95:140–149, 1974
12. Reichlin S: Regulation of the endocrine hypothalamus. Med Clin North Am 62:235–250, 1978
13. Hayward JN: Functional and morphological aspects of hypothalamic neurons. Physiol Rev 57:574–658, 1977
14. Walker LA, Whorton AR, Smigel M, France R, Frolich JC: Antidiuretic hormone increases renal prostaglandin synthesis in vivo. Am J Physiol 235:F180–F185, 1978 or Am J Physiol (Renal Fluid Electrolyte Physiol.) 4:F180–F185, 1978
15. Anderson RJ, Berl T, McDonald KM, Schrier RW: Evidence for an in vivo antagonism between vasopressin and prostaglandin in the mammalian kidney. J Clin Invest 56:420–426, 1975
16. Urakabe S, Takamitsu Y, Shirai D, Yuasa S, Kimura G, Orita Y, Abe H: Effect of different prostaglandins on the permeability of the toad urinary bladder. Comp Biochem Physiol 52:1–4, 1975
17. Zusman RM, Keiser HR, Handler JS: Vasopressin—stimulated prostaglandin E biosynthesis in the toad urinary baldder: effect on water flow. J Clin Invest 60:1339–1347, 1977
18. Lozada ES, Gouanx J, Franki N, Appel GB, Hays RM: Studies on the mode of action of sulfonylureas and phenylacetamides in enhancing the effect of vasopressin. J Clin Endocrinol Metab 34:704–712, 1972
19. Moses AM, Numann P, Miller M: Mechanism of chlorpropamide induced antidiuresis in man: evidence for release of ADH and enhancement of peripheral action. Metabolism 22:59–66, 1973
20. Cobb WE, Spare S, Reichlin S: Neurogenic diabetes insipidus: management with dDAVP (1-desamino-8-D arginine vasopressin) Ann Intern Med 88:183–188, 1978

Hyperkalemia and Hyporeninemic Hypoaldosteronism

Principal Discussant
Ralph A. DeFronzo

Case Presentation

This 68-year-old black male has had sickle cell disease since childhood and has suffered the typical sickle cell crises that are characterized primarily by bone pain. The patient's longevity is probably attributable to a high percentage of fetal hemoglobin—65% hemoglobin SS by electrophoresis. From age 25, he underwent blood transfusion at approximately 6-month intervals, maintaining a hematocrit of approximately 30%. Sickle cell crises, managed with analgesics and hydration, occurred one to two times per year from age 25 to his most recent admission. From ages 28 to 30, the patient developed leg ulcers and acute cholecystitis for which he underwent sympathectomy and a cholecystectomy, respectively. At age 30, he developed tophaceous gout, which was managed with probenecid. Laboratory findings at that time included a serum uric acid of 10.8 mg/dl and a serum urea nitrogen of 16 mg/dl. A marked defect in urinary concentration—U_{max} = 320 mOsm/kg—was observed following a 12-h overnight dehydration test. At age 40, the patient developed angina pectoris as well as congestive heart failure and peripheral edema; his blood pressure was 170/100 mmHg, and cardiomegaly was evident on chest x-ray. The patient was started on a regimen of digitalis and diuretics.

At age 63, the patient was hospitalized with a myocardial infarction and congestive heart failure. Hypertension with a blood pressure of 200/100 mmHg and cardiomegaly again were present. Hyperkalemia was documented for the first time with a serum potassium concentration of 5.7 mEq/liter. Other laboratory findings were as follows: serum sodium, 141 mEq/liter; serum chloride, 104 mEq/liter; serum bicarbonate, 24 mEq/liter; serum creatinine, 1.4 mg/dl; serum urea nitrogen, 26 mm/dl; serum uric acid, 11.2 mg/dl. Results of urinalysis revealed 10–12 white blood cells (WBC) per high-power field (HPF); 5–10 red blood cells (RBC) per HPF; and proteinuria (3+). Urine culture was negative. Over the next 3 years, the patient was hospitalized on numerous occassions for congestive heart failure, chest pain, leg ulcers, and gout; he was treated with digoxin, furosemide, α-methyldopa, colchicine, and occasionally indomethacin. During this time, the serum potassium concentration never fell below 6 mEq/liter and ranged as high as 7.8 mEq/liter. Because of the persistently high serum potassium concentration, the patient was admitted to the clinical research center for further diagnostic evaluation.

On admission, the physical examination revealed the following: blood pressure, 200/100 mmHg; pulse, 84/min and regular; respirations, 16/min; temperature, 37° C. The skin showed old ulcer disease and stasis dermatitis; the optic fundi had moderate arteriolar narrowing and arteriovenous nicking without hemorrhages or exudates; the neck veins were distended 6 cm above the clavicle at 45°. Moist rales were heard one-third of the way up both lung fields posteriorly; the point of maximal impulse was diffuse in the 6th to 7th intercostal interspaces and 15 cm to the left of the midsternal line; S3 and S4 gallops were present; a grade III/VI systolic ejection murmur was heard at the base and radiated to the lower left sternal border. Abdominal examination revealed no organomegaly or tenderness. Rectal examination was normal and the prostate was enlarged (1+). Examination of the extremities revealed markedly diminished peripheral pulses, tophi over both elbows, and deforming arthritis of the hands and big toes, which had been affected previously with gout. Neurologic examination was unremarkable except for absent reflexes in the lower extremities and decreased sensation below the knees.

Laboratory findings included the following: hematocrit, 28%; WBC, 6800 with a normal differential; reticulocyte count, 1.2%; serum potassium, 7.2 mEq/liter, with a simultaneous plasma potassium of 6.8 Eq/liter; serum sodium, 140 mEq/liter; serum chloride, 109 mEq/liter; serum bicarbonate, 19 mEq/liter; serum urea nitrogen, 39 m/dl; serum creatinine, 2 mg/dl; serum uric acid, 11.8 mg/dl; serum calcium, 9 mg/dl; serum phosphate, 4.7 mg/dl; blood pH, 7.33; carbon dioxide tension, 31 mmHg; a simultaneous urine pH obtained under oil, 5.1; 24-h urine protein excretion, 2.4 g; 24-h uric acid excretion, 500 mg; creatinine clearance, 35 ml/min. Results of urinalysis revealed 2–5 WBC/HPF; 5–10 RBC/HPF. A urine culture was negative. Liver function studies were normal and glucose concentration while fasting was 105 mg/dl. A chest radiogram revealed marked cardiomegaly with redistribution of blood flow to the upper lobes. An electrocardiogram revealed evidence of an old anterior myocardial infarction and nonspecific ST-T wave changes.

Additional studies were performed to define the mechanism of the hyperkalemia and these findings will be discussed.

Discussion

Dr. Ralph A. DeFronzo *(Associate Professor of Medicine, Yale University School of Medicine, New Haven, Connecticut)*: This 68-year-old black man is the oldest known living patient with sickle cell disease. Today I plan to discuss only one of his renal and electrolyte problems—hyperkalemia. A full understanding of the etiology and management of this patient's severe hyperkalemia requires a brief review of the normal renal handling of potassium.

Renal Potassium Handling

Recent studies indicate that the majority of the potassium excreted in the urine is derived from secretion in the distal tubule and collecting duct [1–3]. Although approximately 600 to 700 mEq of potassium are filtered daily by the glomerulus, most potassium is reabsorbed proximally and only approximately 10% remains by the early distal tubule. This fraction remains fixed despite a variety of maneuvers that are known either to increase or decrease the rate of urinary potassium excretion. Approximately 60% of the filtered potassium load is reabsorbed by the accessible portion of the proximal convoluted tubule, and an additional 25% to 30% has been reabsorbed by the time the fluid reaches the first accessible segment of the distal tubule. Although some potassium may be added to the tubular fluid by the ascending loop of Henle [3], the mid-to-late distal convoluted tubule is the first major site of potassium secretion [1–3]. Cells of the cortical collecting duct are morphologically similar to those of the distal tubule; it is not surprising therefore that this segment of the collecting duct is also capable of net potassium secretion [3,4]. Although the contribution of the medullary collecting duct to final potassium excretion remains uncertain, several recent studies have indicated an important role of this nephron segment in renal potassium excretion [5–7].

Figure 1 illustrates a model depicting distal tubular potassium secretion using data gathered from micropuncture, microperfusion, and other techniques [3,8]. This model contains several salient features: (1) The luminal membrane is electronegative by approximately 50 mV as compared with the pericapillary membrane. (2) An active pump located in the pericapillary membrane transfers potassium into the cell against a large concentration gradient. Once within the cell, the potassum either back diffuses into the capillary blood or enters the tubular lumen, but the electrical gradient, which is lumen negative, favors the net secretion of potassium into the tubular fluid. (3) The transport of potassium by the active pump is coupled in some loose fashion to sodium transport, and the activity of the pump appears to be influenced by the enzyme sodium-potassium ATPase. (4) The pump system is dependent on the presence of aldosterone and in the absence of this hormone the ability to secrete potassium is markedly impaired. (5) The activity of the pump is exquisitely sensitive to small changes in the potassium concentration in the pericapillary blood: hyperkalemia provides a potent stimulus to enhanced potassium uptake by the distal

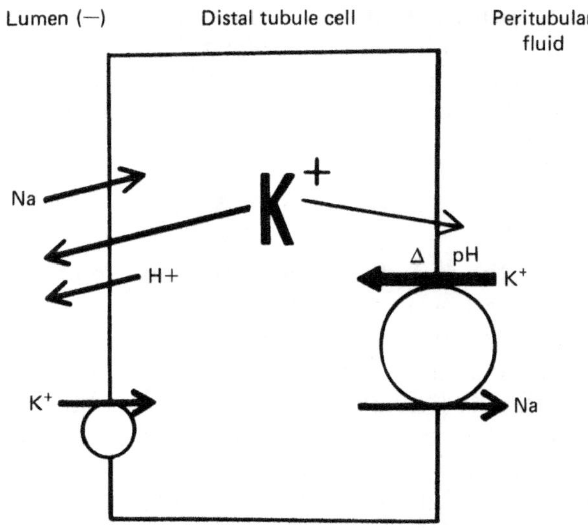

Fig. 1. Schematic representation of potassium secretion by the distal tubule.

tubular cell. Once inside the cell, potassium passively diffuses down the electrochemical gradient into the tubular fluid. (6) An increase in sodium delivery alone and an increase in urine flow independent of sodium delivery stimulate potassium excretion [9]. (7) The activity of the pump is strongly influenced by changes in acid-base status: acute acidosis inhibits, and acute alkalosis stimulates, potassium secretion. (8) A potassium reabsorptive mechanism also must exist in the distal tubule because urinary potassium excretion can approach zero under conditions of severe dietary potassium restriction despite delivery of 5–10% of the filtered load to the early distal tubule.

The pathophysiology of the clinical disorders complicated by impaired potassium secretion, and consequently, hyperkalemia follows directly from this model of renal potassium handling. Thus, decreased renal excretion of potassium and the potential for hyperkalemia can result from inadequate sodium delivery to the distal nephron; decreased urine flow; a defect in the renin-angiotensin-aldosterone axis; a primary tubular secretory defect; inhibition of the potassium pump; or the presence of renal disease, which directly affects the integrity of the potassium secretory cells located in the distal nephron.

Differential Diagnosis of Sustained Hyperkalemia

The search for the cause of hyperkalemia can be approached in a logical sequence. Table 1 lists nine general cuases of increased serum potassium levels. Before initiating an extensive investigation, factitious causes should be excluded. In the patient presented today, laboratory error was excluded by repeated plasma determinations. "Pseudohyperkalemia" was excluded by the observation that simultaneous determinations of potassium concentration in serum and plasma agreed within 0.2 mEq/liter and by the normal white blood cell and platelet counts. Acute acidemia is a well-known cause of true hyperkalemia [10]. Two mechanisms are involved: first, acute acidemia inhibits renal potassium secretion [3]; second, as acidosis develops, hydrogen ions move into cells and this shift is associated with an efflux of potassium from cells. Since hyperkalemia was present in this patient when the blood pH and plasma bicarbonate concentration were normal, the disturbance in potassium homeostasis cannot be related to an acid-base disorder.

Table 1. Etiology of hyperkalemia.

I. Factitious
   1. Laboratory error
   2. "Pseudohyperkalemia"—in vitro hemolysis, thrombocytosis, leukocytosis
II. Acidemia (acute)
III. Increased input
   1. Exogenous: diet, salt substitutes, low-sodium diet, medications
   2. Endogenous; hemolysis, GI bleeding, catabolic states, crush injury
IV. Inadequate distal delivery of sodium and decreased distal tubular flow
V. Renal failure
   1. Acute
   2. Chronic: GFR $<$ 15–20 ml/min
VI. Impaired renin-aldosterone axis
   1. Addison's disease
   2. Enzyme deficiency
   3. Primary hypoaldosteronism
   4. Primary hyporeninism
   5. Angiotensin deficiency or insensitivity
   6. Other (prostaglandin deficiency)
VII. Primary renal tubular potassium secretory defect
   1. Systemic lupus erythematosus
   2. Sickle cell disease
   3. Post-renal transplantation
   4. Amyloidosis
   5. Congenital (children with short stature)
   6. Familial
VIII. Inhibition of tubular secretion
   1. Spironolactone
   2. Triamterene
   3. Amiloride
   4. Digitalis
IX. Abnormal potassium distribution
   1. Insulin deficiency
   2. Aldosterone deficiency

Increased input of potassium, from either exogenous or endogenous sources, can also result in hyperkalemia, but the rise in plasma potassium concentration is usually transient unless an underlying defect in renal potassium excretion is present as well [11]. During sustained intravenous potassium chloride infusion, the plasma potassium concentration can rise into the 5.0–5.4 mEq/liter range initially, but it returns to normal within 24–36 h because of enhanced renal potassium excretion and increased cellular influx of potassium [12,13]. Thus, the persistence of hyperkalemia even in the face of an increased potassium load should suggest an underlying defect in the potassium homeostatic system. In the patient under discussion, no obvious cause of excess potassium input was discernible and, of course, hyperkalemia was sustained for long periods of time.

Diminished sodium delivery to the distal sites of potassium is commonly cited as a cause of hyperkalemia. However, this explanation is not sufficient unless urinary sodium excretion markedly falls to levels below 10–20 mEq/day; sodium delivery to the distal tubule, the major site of potassium secretion, is rarely rate-limiting, even when dietary sodium intake is markedly reduced [3]. Furthermore, recent studies suggest that flow, rather than sodium delivery, may be the primary determinant of potassium secretion [9]. In the patient we are discussing, neither decreased sodium excretion nor decreased urine flow were present and thus cannot account for the development of hyperkalemia.

The patient did have moderate chronic renal insufficiency secondary to a combination of "sickle cell" kidney disease, nephrosclerosis, gouty nephropathy, and as we will see later, mesangiocapillary glomerulonephritis. However, it is uncommon for a patient with chronic renal failure to have hyperkalemia unless the glomerular filtration rate is less than 10–15 ml/min. Such patients are protected from hyperkalemia by a remarkable adaptive increase in potassium secretion by the remaining renal tubular cells [13–15], enhanced gastrointestinal potassium secretion [16], and increased movement of potassium into tissues [17,18].

None of the previously discussed abnormalities can explain the patient's hyperkalemia; one must consider therefore the possibility of either a defect in the renin-angiotensin-aldosterone axis or a primary tubular potassium secretory defect. In previously published studies from our laboratory, we demonstrated impaired potassium excretion in patients with sickle cell disease who had normal aldosterone secretion [19]. Thus, on a priori grounds, a primary defect in renal tubular potassium secretion seemed the most likely cause of hyperkalemia in this patient. We studied six patients with sickle cell disease who ranged in age from 19 to 37 years; all were normokalemic and had normal inulin and paraaminohippurate clearances. In these individuals, the increase in urinary potassium excretion following the intravenous administration of potassium chloride, furosemide, and sodium sulfate was markedly impaired. This impairment occurred despite normal basal aldosterone levels and a normal plasma aldosterone response to volume contraction, ambulation, ACTH, and angiotensin II [19]. Impaired potassium secretion in the presence of an intact renin-aldosterone axis is evidence of a renal tubular defect in potassium secretion. The inability to augment potassium excretion after intravenous sodium sulfate administration is particularly characteristic of a renal tubular secretory defect. Delivery of the impermeant sulfate anion, which significantly increases the negativity within the lumen, markedly increases potassium secretion in normal individuals, and this stimulatory effect, although somewhat blunted, persists in the absence of aldosterone [20,21]. Despite these findings, clinically significant hyperkalemia is an exceptional occurrence in patients with sickle cell disease [22]. On the basis of histologic changes in the papilla and medulla [5–7], however, one might anticipate that hyperkalemia would occur if such patients lived long enough for the renal lesion to progress.

To examine whether a tubular defect in potassium secretion was present in this patient, he was given an intravenous infusion of sodium sulfate (1.8 mmol/kg over 2 h). The increase in urinary potassium excretion was determined over the subsequent 6 h (Fig. 2A). Baseline urinary potassium excretion was 55 μEq/min and increased to a maximum of only 73 μEq/min as compared with a greater than twofold increase in control patients. The response to furosemide was also markedly blunted (Fig. 2B). This agent increases urinary potassium excretion by augmenting aldosterone secretion, by increasing both distal sodium delivery and tubular fluid flow. The latter two factors are not dependent on an increase in aldosterone. The blunted response to both sodium sulfate and furosemide in in this patient indicates a primary renal tubular potassium secretory defect similar to that found in six patients with sickle cell disease described previously [19].

But the patient we are considering here presents an even more complicated picture, because a defect in the renin-aldosterone axis also was found. In this individual, the aldosterone response to angiotensin II was blunted, and no increase in plasma aldosterone occurred following ACTH administration (Table 2). Following volume contraction with furosemide and ingestion of a low-sodium diet, the plasma aldosterone response approximated that of normal controls (Table 3), but the plasma potassium concentration at this time was 6.5 mEq/liter. Since hyperkalemia is the most potent stimulus to aldosterone secretion on a chronic basis [11], when this patient's plasma aldosterone response is veiwed in light of the prevailing plasma potassium concentration, aldosterone secretion is deficient. The defect in aldosterone secretion became more obvious when the subject was ambulated for 2 h following volume depletion. In contrast to the control subjects in whom the plasma aldosterone concentration rose from 26 to 66 ng/ml, no increase was observed in this patient. With regard to plasma renin activity, both the baseline as well as the stimulated values were markedly diminished as compared with those of age-matched controls (Table 3). Thus, the patient we are discussing here might be considered to have "hyporeninemic hypoaldosteronism" [23]. It should be pointed out, however, that

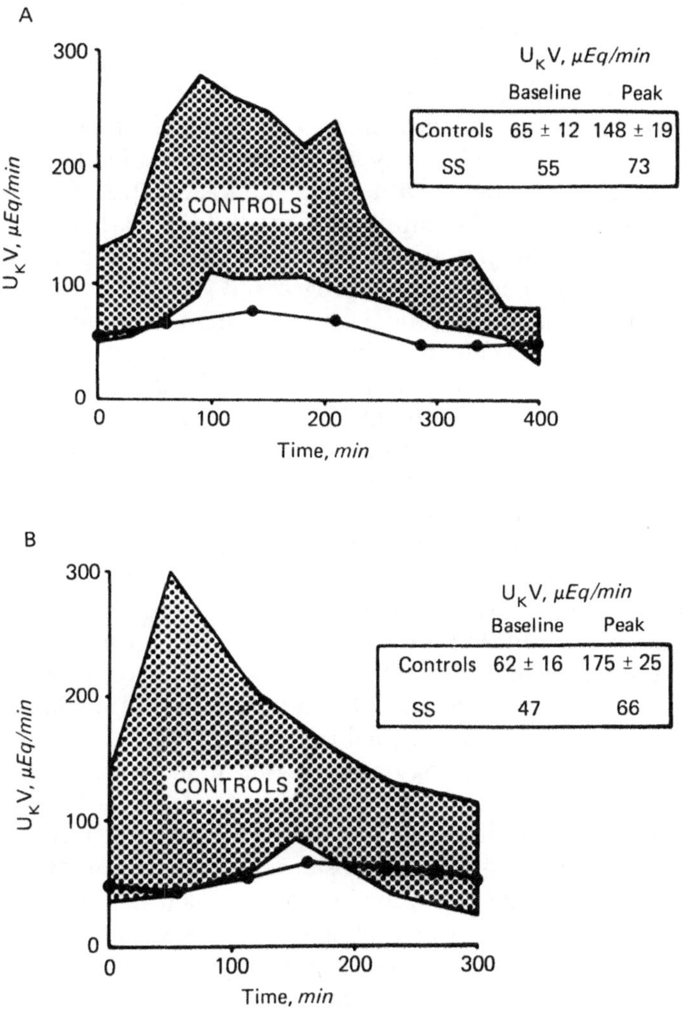

Fig. 2. **A** The increase in urinary potassium excretion (U_KV) following sodium sulfate infusion in the patient discussed here (SS) and control subjects. **B** The increase in U_KV following furosemide (80 mg orally) in the patient (SS) and controls. The *stippled* area represents the range of potassium excretion in the control group. Baseline and maximum peak rates of U_KV are shown in the inserts.

Table 2. Plasma aldosterone concentration following angiotensin II and ACTH infusion in the patient with sickle cell disease discussed here (SS) and in controls.

	Preinfusion (ng/dl)	Postinfusion (ng/dl)
Angiotensin II infusion		
Controls	7± 3	22± 3
SS	8	13
ACTH infusion		
Controls	8± 2	19± 2
SS	14	13

Note: control values represent the mean ± SEM.

the plasma aldosterone response to both angiotensin II and ACTH, substances known to stimulate aldosterone secretion [24,25], was impaired. Most importantly, persistent hyperkalemia, which normally provides a potent stimulus to aldosterone secretion [11], also *failed* to enhance its secretion. These observations suggest that, even though hyporeninemia was present, defects at the level of aldosterone biosynthesis, aldosterone release, or both may have contributed to the hypoaldosteronism in this patient.

Before returning to the question of defective aldosterone secretion, I would like to review the literature on the syndrome of "hyporeninemic hypoaldosteronism."

Review of Hyporeninemic Hypoaldosteronism

To date, 81 cases of this syndrome have been reported in the English literature [26–61]. The clinical findings are quite typical (Table 4). The mean age is 65 ± 7 years, with a range from 32 to 82 years. This observation may be important, as both renin and aldosterone secretion are known to diminish with advancing age. Approximately 75% of the

Table 3. Plasma aldosterone concentration (ng/dl) and plasma renin activity (ng of angiotensin generated/ml/h) following volume contraction and ambulation in the patient with sickle cell disease (SS) discussed here and in controls.

	Plasma Aldosterone		Plasma Renin Activity	
	Controls	SS	Controls	SS
Baseline	13 ± 2	15	0.6 ± 0.2	0.3
Volume contraction	26 ± 4	26	5.0 ± 1.0	0.6
Volume contraction + ambulation	66 ± 13	26	11.0 ± 2.0	1.1

Note: control values represent the mean ± SEM.

Table 4. Clinical and laboratory characteristics in 81 patients with the syndrome of "hyporeninemic hypoaldosteronism."

I. Mean age, 65 years; range, 32–82 years
II. Findings at presentation:
  1. Asymptomatic hyperkalemia (75%)
  2. Muscle weakness } (25%)
  3. Cardiac arrhythmia } (25%)
  4. Hyperchloremic acidosis (≃ 50%)
  5. Salt wasting (unusual)
III. Normal glucocorticoid function
IV. Mild to moderate renal insufficiency, 57/81 (70%)
V. Diabetes mellitus, 40/81 (49%)
VI. Low or low-normal baseline plasma aldosterone levels; all patients had a subnormal increase following volume contraction, 81/81 (100%)
VII. Normal baseline and/or stimulated plasma renin levels, 13/74 (18%)
VIII. Normal aldosterone response to angiotensin II infusion, 4/27 (15%)
IX. Normal aldosterone response to ACTH administration, 7/34 (21%)

Source: Data from Refs. 26–61.

patients are asymptomatic, and hyperkalemia is discovered on routine laboratory screening or during studies for an unassociated illness. The remainder of the patients come to medical attention because of symptoms referable to the hyperkalemia, such as muscle weakness or cardiac arrhythmias. Hyperchloremic metabolic acidosis is found in about 50% of the patients. Salt wasting is distinctly uncommon; most patients have a partial defect in aldosterone secretion, but their plasma aldosterone levels, although reduced, are sufficient to maintain normal sodium balance unless the dietary sodium intake is markedly restricted. Even though sodium balance is normal, however, the low circulating aldosterone levels are insufficient to prevent hyperkalemia. Baseline cortisol levels as well as the cortisol response to ACTH have been reported as normal in all patients.

Two underlying disorders, chronic renal failure and diabetes mellitus, are present in such high frequency in this syndrome as to preclude a chance association. Chronic renal failure was present in 57 of the 81 patients. The types of renal disease are listed in Table 5; diabetic glomerulosclerosis leads the list and is followed by a variety of renal diseases including interstitial nephritis, hypertensive nephropathy, presumed gouty nephropathy, nephrolithiasis, analgesic nephropathy, and some others. The syndrome also has been described in patients with glomerulonephritis. Diabetes mellitus was present in 40 of the 81 patients. We will return to a possible link between diabetes and hypoaldosteronism later.

I noted with interest that the patient we are discussing here had hyperuricemia with clinical gout as well as chronic hypertension. But he had neither a family history nor clinical or laboratory evidence of diabetes mellitus. The fasting glucose concentration was not elevated and an intravenous glucose tolerance test was minimally abnormal, but the latter finding could easily be explained by a combination of age and renal insufficiency, both of which are associated with decreased glucose tolerance.

In the 81 reported patients, baseline plasma aldosterone concentrations were low or low-normal; after volume contraction, a subnormal increase occurred in all 81 (Table 4). None of the patients demonstrated an absolute increase close to that expected for normal subjects. Two studies examined the effect of normalization of the serum potassium concentration (by a sodium-potassium exchange resin) on plasma aldosterone secretions [51,59]. In all 11 patients studied, plasma aldosterone levels fell significantly following reduction of the plasma potassium concentration. These results emphasize the importance of relating the plasma aldosterone level to the plasma potassium concentration. Thus, although some patients may have low-normal or even occasionally normal basal plasma aldosterone levels, these plasma concentrations must be considered abnormal in the presence of increased plasma potassium levels.

Reinterpretation of the Syndrome

Although this syndrome has been called "hyporeninemic hypoaldosteronism," several lines of evidence suggest that the primary defect responsible for the hyperkalemia in many patients resides in the adrenal gland and is not related to hyporeninemia (Table 4). First, baseline

Table 5. The causes of renal disease in 57 patients with the syndrome of "hyporeninemic hypoaldosteronism."

Diabetes mellitus	25
Interstitial nephritis[a]	7
Hypertension	7
Gout[b]	6
Glomerulonephritis	3
Nephrolithiasis	2
Analgesic nephropathy	1
Urinary tract obstruction	1
Mixed cryoglobulinemia	1
Unknown	4

[a]Type unspecified.
[b]Gouty nephropathy not documented histologically.
Source: Data from Refs. 26–61.

renin levels, stimulated renin levels, or both were normal in 13 of the 74 patients in whom it was measured. Thus, in at least a substantial minority of the cases, hypoaldosteronism cannot be explained on the basis of hyporeninemia. Second, the response to intravenous angiotensin II infusion was normal in only four of 27 patients. Since angiotensin II directly stimulates aldosterone release by the zona glomerulosa [24,25,62], the response should be normal if the adrenal gland is intact. Likewise, the aldosterone response to ACTH, another agent that directly stimulates the adrenal production of aldosterone, was normal in only seven of 34 patients. Although one could argue that more prolonged adrenal stimulation—i.e., several days as opposed to a few hours—with angiotensin II and ACTH is needed to elicit a normal aldosterone response because prolonged hyporeninemia had led to disuse atrophy of the zona glomerulosa, I would counter the argument by pointing out that nephrectomized patients have normal basal aldosterone levels that increase normally following provacative stimuli even though these patients have no demonstrable circulating renin [63–65].

These observations strongly suggest that the syndrome of "hyporeninemic hypoaldosteronism" is of mixed cause. In some patients the hypoaldosteronism is indeed secondary to hyporeninemia. In others, however, the primary defect probably resides in the adrenal gland. In the absence of sufficient circulating aldosterone, renal potassium excretion is impaired; the resulting hyperkalemia in turn suppresses renin secretion [66–68]. If this causal link is correct, prolonged normalization of the plasma potassium concentration would be expected to correct the hyporeninemia, whereas aldosterone levels would remain suppressed. Unfortunately, this important study has yet to be performed.

A third possibility is that two primary defects exist: one in the adrenal gland, leading to hypoaldosteronism, and another in the kidney, causing hyporeninemia. Resolving this issue would require a prolonged study in which the adrenal gland is stimulated for 7 to 10 days with angiotensin II, ACTH, or both. If plasma aldosterone levels did not increase despite prolonged daily administration of these agents, one could conclude that a primary adrenal defect in aldosterone secretion exists, since chronic adrenal stimulation with ACTH, angiotensin, and hyperkalemia failed to elicit an aldosterone response. Unfortunately such a study has not been done.

The hormonal and renal defects that could possibly result in hyperkalemia are summarized in Fig. 3 and include a primary renal defect leading to decreased renin secretion; a primary adrenal defect in aldosterone biosynthesis, release, or both; and a primary renal tubular potassium secretory defect. This figure also provides a possible explanation of why hyperkalemia and hypoaldosteronism are so common in diabetic patients. I should now like to turn to this problem.

Special Characteristics of the Diabetic

As discussed earlier, approximately one-half of the cases of "hyporeninemic hypoaldosteronism" have occurred in patients with diabetes. We know that insulin stimulates potassium uptake by a variety of tissues including muscle and liver [69-73]. In addition, we previously have shown that even basal insulin levels play an important regulatory role in potassium homeostasis: inhibition of basal insulin secretion by as little as 50% results in both a predictable rise in plasma potassium concentration and a decreased tolerance to exogenous potassium [12]. If insulin is also responsible for potassium uptake by the adrenal gland,

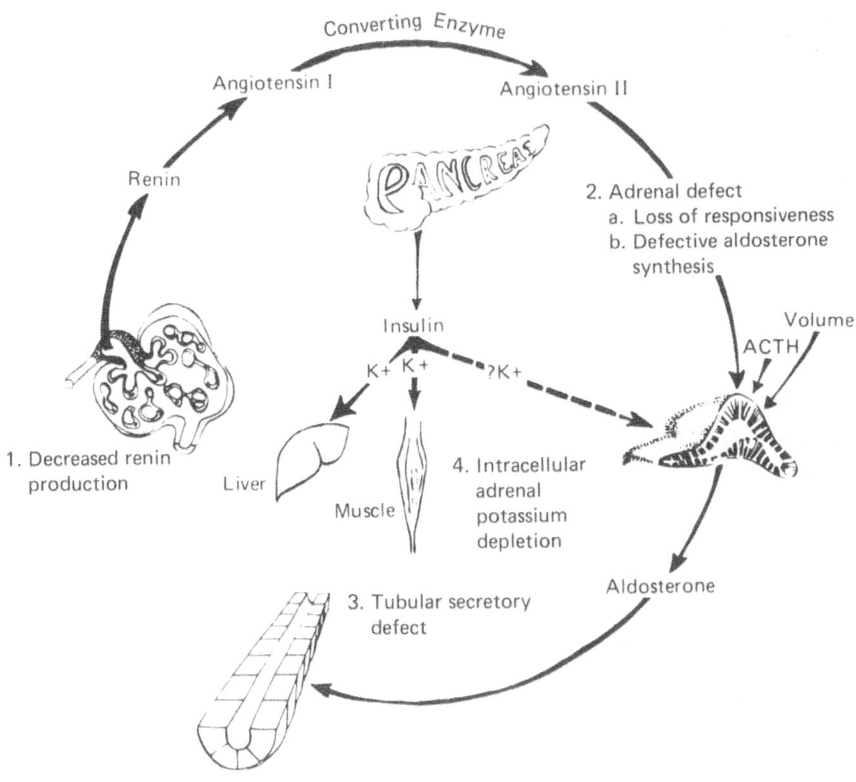

Fig. 3. Schematic representation of potential hormonal and renal defects resulting in hyperkalemia. Hyperkalemia might result as a consequence of the following: (1) decreased renin production; (2) decreased aldosterone production despite normal renin secretion (adrenal defect); (3) a renal tubular secretory defect; (4) insulin deficiency leading to failure of cellular potassium uptake, possibly involving cells of adrenal zona glomerulosa, and thereby contributing to hypoaldosteronism. (Reprinted with permission of *Arch Intern Med* 137:842–843, 1977.)

Table 6. Plasma aldosterone and renin responses to tilting in 59 normokalemic diabetic patients.

Aldosterone	N	↓	N	↓
Renin	N	N	↓	↓
Number	31	5	13	10
Percentage	53%	8%	22%	17%

Note: N, normal; ↓, decreased.
Source: Data summarized from Ref. 75.

then a state of intracellular potassium depletion may exist in diabetic patients (Fig. 3). Previous studies have shown that the ability of ACTH and angiotensin II to stimulate aldosterone secretion by cultured zona glomerulosa cells is impaired in the presence of low potassium concentrations [24,62]. These observations are consistent with the known stimulatory effect of potassium on the aldosterone biosynthetic pathway, which involves the conversions of cholesterol to deoxycorticosterone and corticosterone to aldosterone [25,74]. Indeed, two recent reports have documented the presence of acquired enzymatic defects in aldosterone biosynthesis in diabetic patients [40,51]. These defects involve deficiencies of both the 18-hydroxylase and 18-dehydrogenase reactions. Whether the enzymatic defects are secondary to cellular potassium depletion or some other aspect of the diabetic state remains to be determined. Because of discrepant results regarding whether diabetics have a primary defect in renin or in aldosterone secretion, deChatel et al, studied 59 normokalemic diabetics in an attempt to characterize further the nature of the defect in the renin-aldosterone axis [75] (Table 6). In 31 of 59 patients, the renin and aldosterone responses to tilting were normal. In the other 28 patients, however, a variety of defects was observed: five had diminished aldosterone responses with a normal renin response, 13 had impaired renin release with a normal aldosterone response, and ten demonstrated impaired release of both renin and aldosterone. These results clearly demonstrate that multiple defects in the renin-aldosterone axis can occur in diabetic patients and that the hyperkalemia probably results from a spectrum of disorders.

In addition to a primary adrenal defect in aldosterone production, which leads to diminished renal potassium excretion, and insulin deficiency, which results in decreased potassium movement into cells, hyperkalemia in the diabetic can result from a variety of other factors (Table 7). Perez et al, [52,55] and Christlieb et al, [61] have demonstrated a high frequency of renal insufficiency in their hyperkalemic patients who have hypoaldosteronism, but neither group has determined which aspect of the renal disease—decreased glomerular filtration rate, interstitial disease with subsequent tubular dysfunction, or juxtaglomerular scarring with resultant hyporeninism—if any, is the most important factor contributing to the development of the hyperkalemia. As discussed earlier, diminished renal function rarely leads to impaired renal potassium excretion unless the glomerular filtration rate is very low (< 10–15 ml/min). The glomerular filtration rates of most of the reported diabetic patients with hyperkalemia and hypoaldosteronism have exceeded 20 ml/min; reduced renal function therefore is not a convincing explanation for the hyperkalemia. Furthermore, deChatel failed to find any correlation between the defect in the renin-angiotensin-aldosterone axis and decreased glomerular filtration rate [75].

In addition to the well-known glomerular changes, interstitial scarring and tubular atrophy are prominent features of diabetic nephropathy [76,77]. Because of accelerated vascular disease, ischemic tubular injury and papillary necrosis occur with increased frequency in the diabetic population [78]. What role the development of these tubulointerstitial lesions might play in impaired potassium excretion is unclear. However, correction of hyperkalemia in diabetic patients often requires very large doses of mineralocorticoids, and reduced tubular responsiveness thus becomes suspect. We recently examined the ability of four normokalemic patients with longstanding diabetes to excrete an intravenous potassium chloride load. Despite a normal or only slightly decreased glomerular filtration rate and an intact renin-aldosterone axis, the increase in urinary potassium excretion was significantly impaired in these individuals as compared with that in control subjects. These preliminary results, combined with the inability to augment renal potassium secretion with physiologic doses of mineralocorticoids, raise the possibility that some diabetic patients might have a primary defect in tubular potassium secretion. Finally, Schindler and Sommers have postulated that in the diabetic patient, selective damage to the juxtaglomerular apparatus by the angiopathic process might lead to a state of hyporeninemia [79]. Of course, this hypothesis does not explain the lack of adrenal responsiveness to chronic hyperkalemia, angiotensin II, and ACTH in many diabetics.

Table 7. Possible mechanisms contributing to hyperkalemia in patients with diabetes mellitus.

I. Primary adrenal defect in aldosterone production
II. Insulin lack resulting in decreased hepatic and muscle potassium uptake
III. Renal disease
  1. Decreased glomerular filtration rate
  2. Interstitial damage leading to a tubular secretory defect
  3. Juxtaglomerular damage leading to hyporeninemia
IV. Inactive ("big") renin
V. Decreased catecholamines
VI. Elevated blood volume leading to suppressed renin
VII. Decreased prostaglandin synthesis

Recently Day et al. [80] and deLeiva et al. [51] suggested another explanation for the high prevalence of hyperkalemia in diabetic patients. These authors identified an association between high concentrations of the inactive renin precursor "big renin" and reduced levels of plasma renin activity in diabetic patients (Table 7). This finding raises the possibility that the hyporeninemia might result from the impaired conversion of prorenin, or "big renin," to active renin.

Decreased circulating levels of catecholamines and automatic neuropathy also have been postulated as causes of hyporeninemia in diabetic patients (Table 7). Sympathetic nerve terminals have been demonstrated in the juxtaglomerular apparatus [81], and epinephrine has been shown to stimulate renal secretion [82]. Because autonomic neuropathy is common in diabetes, and because patients with longstanding diabetes have decreased circulating levels of catecholamines [83], decreased sympathetic activity has been postulated as a cause of the hyporeninemia. Support for this hypothesis comes from a recent report by Tuck et al., who found a decreased plasma renin response to isoproterenol in five hyperkalemic diabetics who had "hyporeninemic hypoaldosteronism" as well as autonomic or peripheral neuropathy or both [84]. However, plasma and/or urinary catecholamines were normal in all six previously studied patients with "hyporeninemic hypoaldosteronism" [34,35,43,44], and no relation between decreased plasma epinephrine levels and defects in the renin-aldosterone axis was detected in 59 diabetic patients [75]. It seems possible nevertheless, that, at least in some diabetics, decreased sympathetic nervous system activity, low circulating plasma epinephrine levels, or both might contribute to hyporeninemia. How frequently this mechanism is responsible, however, remains to be determined.

Other Possible Explanations for Renin Suppression

Oh et al. postulated that extracellular fluid volume expansion secondary to sodium retention is responsible for a state of physiologic renin suppression in the "hyporeninemic hypoaldosteronism" syndrome [46]. However, none of the patients reported showed a normal aldosterone response to volume contraction that had been induced with diuretics, a low-sodium diet, or both. A two- to three-fold increase in plasma aldosterone levels was observed in many patients, but the absolute values were always well below those reported in healthy controls with an equivalent degree of volume contraction. Oh et al. reported patients whose plasma renin activity rose into the normal range following volume contraction for 3 to 6 weeks, but whose plasma aldosterone levels, although significantly increased, remained below normal. The disproportionate increase in plasma renin as compared to plasma aldosterone levels in this study is another observation that points to a primary adrenal defect in aldosterone secretion.

Finally, decreased circulating concentrations of prostaglandins have been suggested as a cause of "hyporeninemic hypoaldosteronism." Prostaglandin E_2 is known to stimulate renin release [85]; the administration of prostaglandin synthesis inhibitors impairs renin release [86,87]. Some prostaglandins, E_1 and E_2, also stimulate aldosterone and corticosterone synthesis in vitro [88]. Recently, hyperkalemia was observed in association with hyporeninemia and hypoaldosteronism in a 28-year-old woman treated with indomethacin [89]. Both the hyperkalemia and the impairment of the renin-aldosterone axis were corrected after withdrawal of indomethacin; both recurred when treatment with indomethacin was resumed. Two subsequent studies have demonstrated diminished urinary prostaglandin E levels in patients with the "hyporeninemia hypoaldosteronism" syndrome [58,90], but this observation has been refuted by other reports [91,92]. Although the possible association between prostaglandin deficiency and "hyporeninemic hypoaldosteronism" is interesting, further studies are needed to clarify these conflicting observations.

Management of Hyperkalemia

Once the diagnosis of hypoaldosteronism has been established, several different therapeutic regimens can be employed to lower the plasma potassium concentration. The physician should keep in mind, however, that the majority of patients suffering from this syndrome are elderly and have associated medical complications such as diabetes mellitus, atherosclerotic cardiovascular disease, chronic renal failure, and hypertension. Caution should be taken therefore to ensure that the side effects of therapy do not outweigh the benefits of correcting the hyperkalemia. Mineralocorticoid replacement, usually given as fludrocortisone acetate, is the mainstay of therapy (Table 8). Studies of 51 patients treated with a mineralocorticoid report a reduction of the plasma potassium concentration in 43, but large doses of the steroid, often as high as 0.4–1.0 mg daily, were frequently required to reduce the plasma level to normal [26–61]. As indicated above, this observation suggests that the renal tubular cell is resistant to the action of mineralocorticoids, at least with respect to their effect on potassium secretion. Sensitive to the sodium-retentive effects of fludrocortisone appeared to be less affected, because marked sodium retention with edema, exacerbation of hypertension, and congestive heart failure were common consequences. In many patients, the administration of a loop diuretic was required to prevent or treat these complications.

The patient presented today underwent a trial of deoxycorticoste-

Table 8. Possible modalities of therapy in patients with hyperkalemia and hypoaldosteronism.

- I. Mineralocorticoids: 43/51 (84%) responded
  1. Large doses often required
  2. Urinary potassium excretion does not always increase despite normalization of plasma potassium levels
- II. Diuretics
- III. Sodium bicarbonate
- IV. Sodium polystyrene sulfonate
- V. No therapy
- VI. Avoid drugs that predispose to hyperkalemia
  1. Spironolactone
  2. Triamterene
  3. Amiloride
  4. Heparin
  5. Indomethacin
  6. Propranolol?
- VII. Avoid volume contraction

Note: Data from Refs. 26–61.

rone acetate (DOCA), 10 mg twice a day, under metabolic balance conditions; the results of treatment are shown in Fig. 4. The dotted lines represent the dietary sodium and potassium intake. During the 3 days prior to DOCA administration, the plasma potassium concentration was 6.3 mEq/liter, and the potassium excretion in both the urine and stool approximated the dietary potassium intake. Following DOCA administration, the plasma potassium concentration fell to 5.2 mEq/liter, but this improvement was associated with a weight gain and a worsening of hypertension. Because of the plasma potassium response to DOCA, the patient was started on fludrocortisone acetate; at a dose of 0.4 mg/day the potassium concentration ranged from 4.9 to 5.2 mEq/liter. However, treatment was again associated with marked sodium retention and a 7-kg weight gain that was difficult to control even with large doses of furosemide. Finally, fludrocortisone was discontinued because the patient developed congestive heart failure. An interesting aspect of this patient's initial response to DOCA was that his plasma potassium concentration fell without a significant increase in net potassium excretion. Urinary potassium excretion did increase slightly on DOCA, but this small increase could not account for the progressive decline in the plasma potassium concentration. More importantly, the net potassium balance did not change; this finding suggests that the mineralocorticoid primarily increased the movement of potassium from the extracellular compartment.

Four previous reports also document correction of hyperkalemia by mineralocorticoid therapy in patients with "hyporeninemic hypoaldosteronism" without a concomitant increase in urinary potassium excretion [32,33,54,58]. This observation is consistent with the known effect of aldosterone on extrarenal potassium homeostasis [93,94]. These reports and the response of the patient under discussion underscore the existence of tubular unresponsiveness, which has not previously been emphasized in this syndrome. Whether this tubular defect in potassium secretion is related to the underlying renal disease in most of these patients or to some other as yet unrecognized factor remains to be determined.

If the hyperkalemia fails to respond to fludrocortisone acetate or if excessive sodium retention is encountered, a trial of potassium-wasting diuretics is warranted. In many patients, particularly those with a primary tubular potassium secretory defect, thiazide diuretics are effective [95]. Sodium bicarbonate may improve potassium excretion and correct the hyperkalemia in some patients. In this setting, the kaliuresis is probably caused by many factors including increased luminal negativity of the distal tubule. The presence in the lumen of the poorly reabsorbable

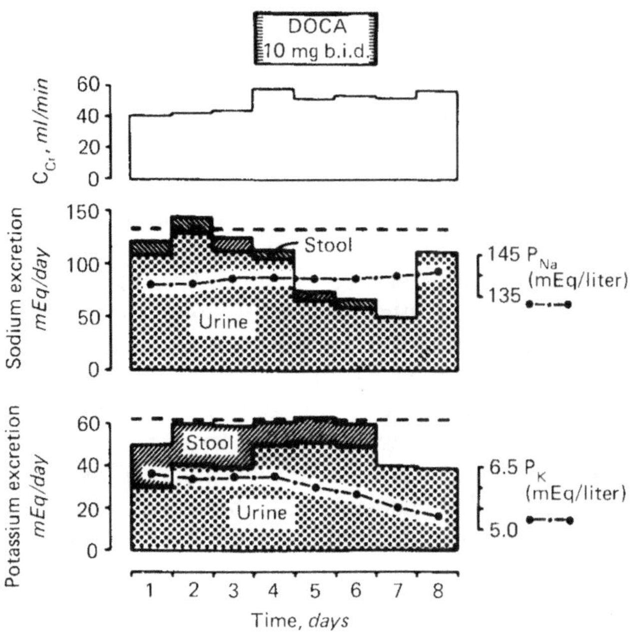

Fig. 4. The effect of deoxycorticosterone acetate (DOCA) on potassium and sodium balance. Following DOCA administration (10 mg b.i.d.), the plasma potassium concentration fell from 6.3 to 5.2 mEq/liter with a minimal increase in urinary potassium excretion and no change in net potassium balance. Despite the lack of effect of DOCA on urinary potassium excretion, urinary sodium excretion fell significantly. Dotted lines represent the dietary intakes of sodium and potassium.

bicarbonate anion, increased delivery of sodium to the distal tubule, and a direct stimulatory effect of alkalosis on distal potassium secretion all combine to produce the kaliuresis. The increase in blood pH and bicarbonate concentration also helps shift potassium into cells. If these measures fail, one can always employ a sodium-potassium exchange resin such as sodium polystyrene sulfonate. In my experience, however, most patients have found this medication difficult to tolerate. In many patients, particularly those with only mild to moderate hyperkalemia, 5.0–5.6 mEq/liter, it is often best to institute no therapy and periodically check the plasma potassium concentration to ensure that the hyperkalemia has not reached dangerous levels. In all patients, drugs known to impair renal potassium excretion should be avoided (Table 8). Volume contraction, which decreases distal sodium delivery, also should be prevented.

A Speculative Thought

There are many other interesting features of this case, but rather than try to consider them all, I would like to end on a provocative note and propose still another explanation for the hyperkalemia in this patient. The patient recently succumbed at age 71 from a massive stroke. Postmortem examination of the kidneys revealed large glomeruli containing sickled red blood cells. An increase in mesangial cellularity and mesangial matrix was present, with thickening of the capillary loops, extensive interstitial fibrosis, and tubular atrophy. Electron microscopy revealed thickened glomerular basement membranes with electron-dense deposits and mesangial proliferative changes. Numerous electron-dense deposits within the tubular basement membranes were apparent also (Fig. 5). These pathologic findings are similar to those reported by Pardo et al., who studied seven patients with sickle cell disease and found renal tubular antigen-antibody complexes in the plasma and kidneys [96]. I wonder whether it is possible that this patient's impairment of renal tubular potassium secretion resulted from antibodies directed at the tubular basement membrane, as has been demonstrated in patients with systemic lupus erythematosus [97,98]?

Questions and Answers

Dr. James Melby *(Professor of Medicine, Boston University School of Medicine, Chief, Endocrinology Division, University Hospital, Boston, Massachusetts)*: As you suggested, it appears that at least some cases of hypoaldosteronism are due to a primary adrenocortical disorder. As you know, our own observations in collaboration with the Christlieb group at the Joslin Clinic suggest that at least two patients have had primary corticosterone methyl oxidase deficiencies [51]. One patient appeared to have corticosterone methyloxidase deficiency type 1 in which the precursor, corticosterone, was overabundant. In the other patient, who had corticosterone methyloxidase deficiency type II, the byproduct, 18-hydroxycorticosterone, appeared in excess. The defect can be amplified markedly by the administration of ACTH. We wondered whether the presence of big renin had anything to do with the biosynthetic defects we observed, but thus far we have been unable to relate circulating levels of big renin to inhibition of the enzymes involved in the oxidation of corticosterone to aldosterone.

The role of potassium is even more difficult to explain in patients with hypoaldosteronism. Potassium stimulates aldosterone byosynthesis at both an early and a late stage. There is also some suggestion that potassium stimulation of the conversion of cholesterol to aldosterone precursors is unimpaired in hypoaldosteronism but that potassium stimulation of corticosterone methyl oxidation is impaired.

Dr. DeFronzo: One of the ways to answer that question would be to culture zona glomerulosa cells in the presence of insulin to define whether potassium uptake is insulin dependent as it is in muscle and liver tissue. If it is, I think one could argue strongly that in the absence of insulin, a state of intracellular potassium depletion exists and that this depletion could account for the abnormalities in aldosterone biosynthesis observed in vivo [25,74].

Dr. Jordan J. Cohen: You stated that in studies with cultured zona glomerulosa cells, the low potassium concentration counteracted the stimulation of aldosterone secretion by angiotensin II and ACTH. Were those studies performed in the absence of insulin? If so, doesn't that suggest that the potassium entry step is not dependent on insulin?

Dr. DeFronzo: Yes, those studies were carried out in the absence of insulin. However, if one examines the dose-response curve, one finds that obtaining a maximum aldosterone response to angiotensin II and to ACTH requires concentrations of potassium greater than 5 mEq/liter [24,62]. Perhaps if insulin were added to the medium a maximum response could be achieved with concentrations in the physiologic range.

I would like to ask Dr. Melby a question. Do you think that prostaglandin deficiency plays any role in the impaired renin-aldosterone response in this heterogeneous group of patients? Recently, several reports have appeared that suggest a role for prostaglandin E deficiency in this syndrome [58,89,90]. What is known about the effects of prostaglandin on the enzymatic steps involved in steroidogenesis?

Dr Melby: We have found no evidence for this except in one paper by Saruta and Kaplan, who found that prostaglandins affect aldosterone secretion; in that study, superphysiologic amounts of PGE_2 were used [99]. I would like to suggest another explanation.

Recently, many papers have examined the regulation of adrenal

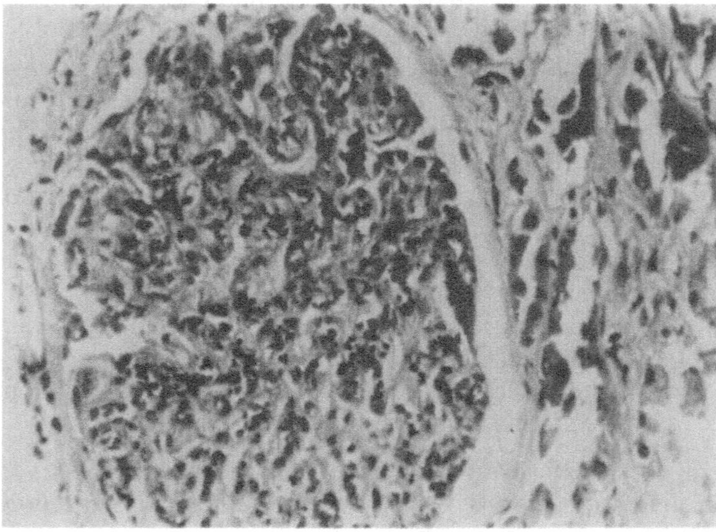

A

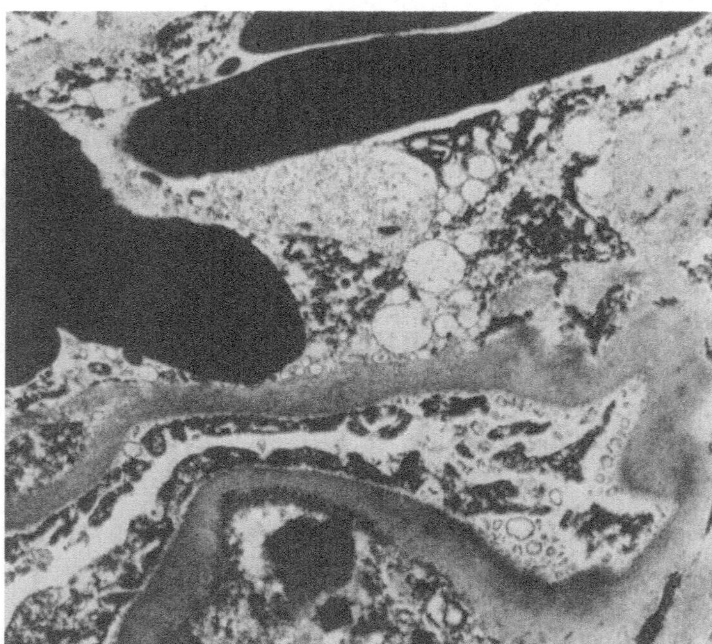

C

Fig. 5. Postmortem examination of the kidneys of the patient discussed here. **A** Light microscopy. The glomeruli are hypercellular with mesangial cell proliferation and an increase in mesangial matrix. **B** Light microscopy. The interstitium shows extensive scarring and tubular atrophy. Some postmortem auto-

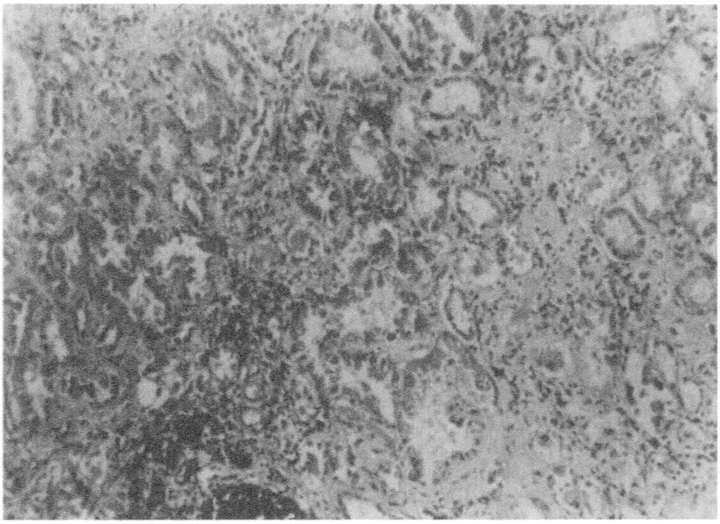

B

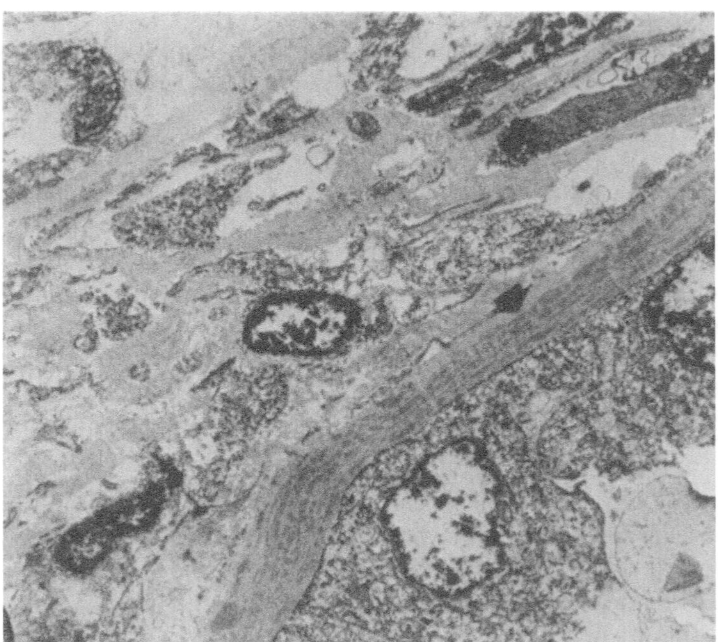

D

lysis also is present. **C** and **D** electron microscopy. There is thickening of the glomerular basement membrane by electron-dense deposits that extend into the mesangium *(arrows)*. The tubular basement membranes are extremely thickened by the diffuse deposition of electron-dense deposits *(arrows)*.

aldosterone secretion by dopamine. Dopamine tonically inhibits aldosterone secretion, and receptors for dopamine are present in the adrenal cortex. As a matter of fact, in some patients with autonomic insufficiency, the dopamine-to-norepinephrine ratio changes. Whether dopamine excess is involved in hypoaldosteronism I don't know, but it is tempting to speculate about it. The prostaglandin question is confusing. As I understand it, prostaglandin deficiency would probably lead to decreased renin secretion and not directly affect aldosterone secretion.

Dr. DeFronzo: I can't comment directly on the role of dopamine, but there is some additional new information on the effect of prostaglandins on the renin-angiotensin system. Tan and Mulrow examined the ability of furosemide to stimulate plasma renin activity and plasma aldosterone secretion in a group of normal volunteers before and after receiving indomethacin, a prostaglandin synthetase inhibitor [100]. A marked inhibition of both the renin and aldosterone response was found. On the basis of these studies, the authors postulated that prostaglandin deficiency plays an important role in the syndrome of hyporeninemic hypoaldosteronism. It is unclear, however, whether the changes were due to a vascular phenomenon or to inhibition of some enzymatic step in renin biosynthesis, aldosterone biosynthesis, or both.

Dr. Clark Sawin *(Chief, Endocrine-Diabetes Section, VA Hospital, Boston, Massachusetts)*: First, I thoroughly support your idea that many factors are involved in the pathogenesis of hyporeninemic hypoaldosteronism. I also concur with your observations that large doses of mineralocorticoids are often necessary in the treatment of these patients. As you pointed out, many patients get into difficulty because of sodium excess when treated indiscriminately with fludrocortisone, and the drug therefore must be used with great caution. Second, I would like to know whether there are sufficient data in normal individuals, especially data corrected for age, that enable one to interpret renin and aldosterone values under a variety of conditions. The published literature does not have a great deal of information on this.

Dr. DeFronzo: In answer to Dr. Sawin's question, I would like to note that the controls for all of the studies discussed today were age-matched. In our study of potassium homeostasis in patients with sickle cell disease, the mean age of the control population was 23 years and was similar to that of the sickle cell patients [19]. Furthermore, for all comparisons with the patient discussed today, a separate group of older individuals was used to establish control values. So, I think it is safe to say that renin levels decrease as a function of age but the values in this elderly patient were even lower than in age-matched controls.

Dr. Sawin: One final question—You pointed out that this patient had a substantial rise in his aldosterone level following volume contraction but that it did not rise as much as in normal controls. Did the serum potassium level change during that interval?

Dr. DeFronzo: The serum potassium level fell slightly, from 6.7 to 6.5 mEq/liter. This was probably due to the administration of furosemide, which was used to induce the volume contraction. In most of the reported cases of hyporeninemic hypoaldosteronism, plasma renin and aldosterone levels rose following volume contraction, but the rise is markedly blunted. In one study, the aldosterone level rose by two- to threefold and it was defined as a normal response [46]. However, since the basal plasma aldosterone level was very low, the absolute increase in plasma aldosterone concentration was significantly impaired as compared to normal controls. In this situation, I think it is misleading to look at the percentage increase in plasma aldosterone above the basal level rather than at the absolute values.

Dr. William B. Schwartz *(Professor of Medicine, Tufts University School of Medicine)*: How likely do you think it is that an atrophic adrenal gland might not respond to acute stimulation but might respond after several days of stimulation?

Dr. DeFronzo: I think this is a possibility that needs to be examined, as I tried to emphasize in my discussion. To prove that the aldosterone response to angiotensin II and to ACTH is blunted, those hormones should be given for at least 3 to 4 consecutive days. However, I would like to emphasize that the most potent stimulus to aldosterone secretion when present on a chronic basis is hyperkalemia. McCaa et al. have shown that if you increase the serum potassium level by as little as 0.3 to 0.5 mEq/liter, aldosterone levels will increase significantly and will remain elevated despite a return of the serum potassium concentration to normal [11]. The patient today had a serum potassium level that was persistently elevated to greater than 6 mEq/liter, yet his aldosterone response was still impaired.

Dr. Schwartz: Would you say therefore that it is extremely unlikely that even sustained ACTH or angiotensin II administration would produce an increase in aldosterone secretion?

Dr. DeFronzo: I think that in those patients in whom the defect lies in the adrenal gland, it will not make any difference how much ACTH or angiotensin II is given. However, one might expect a different result if the defect is secondary to impaired renin secretion. Here, chronic stimulation with angiotensin II or ACTH might be necessary to elicit a normal aldosterone response.

Dr. Cohen: That seems inconsistent to me. If the problem were at the level of secretion and if the adrenal glands were inherently normal, why wouldn't the persistent hyperkalemia stimulate aldosterone secretion?

Dr. DeFronzo: I don't know, unless, of course, multiple defects exist, as I suspect.

Dr. Melby: We are studying a large number of individuals from Amish families in Hershey, Pennsylvania. One infant of one of these families has clinically evident hypoaldosteronism with salt wasting and hyperkalemia [101]. He has an inherited cortocosterone methyloxidase deficiency type II, with elevated blood 18-hydroxycorticosterone levels and depressed plasma aldosterone levels. The defect is probably inherited in an autosomal recessive fashion. These patients might compensate for their deficiency by raising their renin activity. As these patients are only occasionally hyperkalemic, I believe that multiple defects must be involved because of this ability to compensate.

Dr. DeFronzo: Your findings are similar to what has been described in Iranian Jews, in whom a partial aldosterone biosynthetic defect also appears to be present [102]. Those patients have normal plasma aldosterone concentrations at the expense of markedly elevated plasma renin levels. They can excrete their daily intake of potassium normally but they require increased plasma potassium levels to do so.

Dr. Cohen: Hyponatremia is another potent stimulus to aldosterone secretion [103], which might in theory be used as a provocative test. Do you know whether anyone has ever attempted to use this stimulus to evaluate adrenal function?

Dr. DeFronzo: From a practical standpoint that would be difficult because one would have to decrease the serum sodium concentration by at least 10 mEq/liter to stimulate aldosterone secretion [104]. I think that this would be difficult to carry out without changing the volume status of the patient. As far as I know, hyponatremia has not been used as a provocative stimulus.

Dr. John T. Harrington: Were any abnormalities found in the adrenal gland at this patient's autopsy?

Dr. DeFronzo: Unfortunately, the adrenal glands from this patient were not recovered for examination post-mortem.

Dr. Harrington: Are there any systematic studies of adrenal gland morphology in patients with hyporeninemic hypoaldosteronism or sickle cell disease?

Dr. DeFronzo: Of the 81 patients reported with this syndrome, adrenal histology has been looked at in five. In one patient, the adrenal was described as atrophic, but in none were any significant histologic changes observed by light microscopy. I do not know of any reports describing abnormalities in adrenal pathology in patients with sickle cell disease, but this question has not been examined in a systematic fashion.

Dr. Mark Molitch *(Endocrinology Division, NEMC)*: You mentioned that impaired tubular potassium secretion might occur in patients with lupus nephritis. Have you seen any patients with lupus who had hyporeninemic hypoaldosteronism?

Dr. DeFronzo: No, the two patients that we reported previously both had normal renin and aldosterone responses. However, both had an impaired ability to augment potassium excretion in response to sodium sulfate and furosemide [98].

Dr. Molitch: We have been interested in a small number of patients who develop a modest hyperchloremic acidosis in the recovery phase following ketoacidosis. I wonder whether those patients have renal tubular disease or hyporeninemic hypoaldosteronism, perhaps due to volume overload in the recovery period.

Dr. DeFronzo: Oh et al. reported the frequent development of hyperchloremic acidosis during the treatment of 35 diabetic patients with ketoacidosis [105]. They did not directly examine renal acidification, however. One well-documented case of hyperkalemia and hyporeninemic hypoaldosteronism developing secondary to volume overload has been reported [106]. The patient consumed massive doses of sodium bicarbonate as baking soda for epigastric discomfort and developed hyperkalemia. When the sodium bicarbonate therapy was stopped, the plasma renin and aldosterone levels, which were low, rose and the hyperkalemia disappeared. The authors postulated that the chronic state of volume expansion was responsible for the aldosterone and renin suppression. I think this is an uncommon occurrence, however.

Dr. Jerome P. Kassirer: Long before the syndrome of hyporeninemic hypoaldosteronism was described, we recognized patients with mild renal insufficiency who had hyperchloremic acidosis and hyperkalemia. Typically these patients had some form of tubulointerstitial renal disease. What is your opinion of such patients, i.e., nondiabetics with mild renal insufficiency? Do some have renal tubular disease only and others have hyporeninemic hypoaldosteronism?

Dr. DeFronzo: I do think that these patients fall into two separate groups. In some, renal interstitial disease results in tubular injury and a permanent tubular defect in potassium and hydrogen ion secretion despite normal plasma renin and aldosterone levels. In others, a so-called type IV renal tubular acidosis is probably present. In this latter group, it has been postulated that an interstitial disease process injures the juxtaglomerular apparatus leading to hyporeninemia and eventually to hypoaldosteronism. The development of hypoaldosteronism is responsible, then, for the defect in both potassium and hydrogen ion secretion. In this context, the acid-base status of patients with hyporeninemic hypoaldosteronism is of interest. Of the published cases, approximately one-half have hyperchloremic metabolic acidosis. The data in the literature concerning the influence of aldosterone on renal acidification are somewhat controversial [57,107]. Sebastian et al. treated four such patients with fludricortisone and reported that renal acidification returned to normal and that the hyperchloremic acidosis was corrected [57].

Dr. Cohen: I think that study is hard to interpret. When those patients were given fludrocortisone, they were also ingesting a normal salt diet and hence almost certainly experienced positive sodium balance. We know from studies of chronic hydrochloric acid acidosis in the dog that DOCA-induced volume expansion stimulates acid excretion but that DOCA alone—i.e., without volume expansion—does not [108].

Dr. DeFronzo: A recent study by Hulter et al. has examined the role of aldosterone in renal acidification in a more controlled fashion utilizing the adrenalectomized dog model [109]. The authors conclude that a lack of aldosterone leads to an impairment in renal acidification and ammonia excretion.

Dr. Andrew Levey *(Renal Fellow, NEMC)*: Do you think that this patient's sympathectomy played any role in the genesis of the hyperkalemia?

Dr. DeFronzo: It is likely that the sympathetic nervous system is important in maintaining basal renin levels. Also, it is known that catecholamines are a provocative stimulus for renin secretion. Thus, I think the sympathectomy could have played some role in the development of the hyporeninemia. Although the sympathectomy was performed long before the hyperkalemia developed, nevertheless it may have been an underlying factor just as age was. The role of the sympathetic nervous system and decreased circulating epinephrine levels in the development of the hyporeninemic hypoaldosteronism syndrome clearly deserves to be examined in a more systematic pattern.

References

1. Malnic G, Klose RM, Giebisch G: Micropuncture study of renal potassium excretion in the rat. Am J. Physiol 206:674–686, 1974
2. Malnic G, Klose RM, Giebisch G: Micropuncture study of distal tubular potassium and sodium transport in rat nephron. Am J Physiol 211:529–547, 1966
3. Wright FS, Giebisch G: Renal potassium transport: contributions of individual nephron segments and populations. Am J Physiol 235:F515–F527, 1978
4. Reineck HF, Osgood RW, Stein JH: Net potassium addition beyond the superficial distal tubule of the rat. Am J Physiol 235:F104–F110, 1978

5. Hierholzer K: Secretion of potassium and acidification in collecting ducts of mammalian kidney. Am J Physiol 201:318–324, 1961
6. Finkelstein FO, Hayslett JP: Role of medullary structures in the functional adaptation of renal insufficiency. Kidney Int 6:419.-425, 1974
7. Silva P, Ross BD, Charney AN, Besarab A, Epstein FH: Potassium transport by the isolated perfused kidney. J Clin Invest 58:862–869, 1975
8. Giebisch G: The distal tubular potassium transport system. In New Aspects of Renal Function, Vol 6. Vogel HG, Ullrich KH, Amsterdam, Excerpta Medica, 1978, pp. 137–146
9. Good DW, Wright FS: Effects of sodium reabsorption, transepithelial voltage and flow rate on potassium secretion in renal distal tubule. Kidney Int 12:558, 1977
10. Irvine ROH, Dow J: Muscle cell pH and potassium movement in metabolic acidosis. Metabolism 17:563–570, 1968
11. McCaa RE, McCaa CS, Guyton AC: Role of angiotensin II and potassium in the long-term regulation of aldosterone secretion in intact conscious dogs. Circ Res 36–37 (Suppl. 1):157–167, 1975
12. DeFronzo RA, Sherwin RS, Dillingham M, Hendler R, Tamborlane WV, Felig P: Influence of basal insulin and glucagon secretion on potassium and sodium metabolism. J. Clin Invest 61:472–479, 1978
13. Kunau RT, Whinnery MA: Potassium transfer in distal tubule of normal and remnant kidneys. Am J Physiol 235:F186–F191, 1978
14. Schultze RG, Taggart DD, Shapiro H, Pennell JP, Caglar S, Bricker NS: On the adaptation in potassium excretion associated with nephron reduction in the dog. J Clin Invest 50:1061–1068, 1971
15. Hayslett J: Functional adaptation to reduction in renal mass. Physiol Rev 59:137–164, 1979
16. Hayes CP, McLeod ME, Robinson RR: An extrarenal mechanism for the maintenance of potassium balance in severe chronic renal failure. Trans Assoc Am Physicians 80:207–216, 1967
17. Alexander EA, Levinsky NG: An extrarenal mechanism of potassium adaptation. J. Clin Invest 47:740–748, 1968
18. Gonick HC, Kleeman CR, Rubini ME, Maxwell MH: Functional impairment in chronic renal disease. III. Studies of potassium excretion. Am J Med Sci 261:281–290, 1971
19. DeFronzo RA, Taufield PA, Black H, McPhedran P, Cooke CR: Impaired renal tubular potassium secretion in sickle cell disease. Ann Intern Med 90:310–316, 1979
20. Clapp JR, Rector FC, Seldin DW: Effect of unreabsorbed anions on proximal and distal transtubular potentials in the rat. Am J Physiol 202:781–786, 1962
21. Cade R, Shalhoub R: The effect of mineralocorticoids on renal handling of potassium. J Clin Invest 40:1028, 1961
22. Roseman MK, Sehy JT, Arruda JAL, Kurtzman NA: Studies on the mechanism of hyperkalemic distal renal tubular acidosis (dRTA): gradient type RTA in SC hemoglobinopathy. Kidney Int 12:473, 1977
23. Michelis MF, Murdaugh HV: Selective hypoaldosteronism. Am J Med 59:1–5, 1975
24. Fredlund P, Saltman S, Dando J, Douglas J, Catt KJ: Aldosterone produc-

tion by isolated glomerulosa cells: modulation of sensitivity to angiotensin II and ACTH by extracellular potassium concentration. Endocrinology 100:481–486, 1977
25. Haning R, Tait SAS, Tait JF: In vitro effects of ACTH, angiotensin, serotonin and potassium on steroid output and conversion of corticosterone to aldosterone by isolated adrenal cells. Endocrinology 87:1147–1167, 1975
26. Hudson J, Chobanian A, Relman A: Hypoaldosteronism. A clinical study of a patient with an isolated adrenal mineralocorticoid deficiency, resulting in hyperkalemia and Stokes-Adams attacks. N Engl J Med 257:529–536, 1957
27. Skanse B, Hokfelt B: Hypoaldosteronism with otherwise intact adrenocortical function, resulting in a characteristic clinical entity. Acta Endocrinol 28:29–36, 1958
28. Hill, S, Nickerson J, Chenault S, McNeil J, Starnes W, Gautney M: Studies in man on hyper- and hypoaldosteronism. Arch Intern Med. 104:982–994, 1959
29. Lambrew C, Carver S, Peterson R, Horwith M: Hypoaldosteronism as a cause of hyperkalemia and syncopal attacks in a patient with complete heart block. Am J Med 31:81–85, 1961
30. Ulick S, Gautier E, Vetter K, Markello J, Yaffe S, Lowe C: An aldosterone biosynthetic defect in a salt-losing disorder. J Clin Endocrinol Metab 24:669–672, 1964
31. Wilson I, Goetz F: Selective hypoaldosteronism after prolonged heparin administration. Am J Med 36:635–640, 1964
32. Posner J, Jacobs D: Isolated analdosteronism I. Clinical entity, with manifestations of persistent hyperkalemia, periodic paralysis, salt-losing tendency, and acidosis. Metabolism 13:513–521, 1964
33. Gerstein A, Kleeman C, Gold E, Franklin S, Maxwell M, Gonick H, Feffer M, Steinman T: Aldosterone deficiency in chronic renal failure. Nephron 5:90–105, 1968
34. Christlieb A, Hickler R, Lauler D, Williams G: Hypertension with inappropriate aldosterone stimulation. A syndrome. N Engl J Med 281:128–131, 1969
35. Vagnucci A: Selective aldosterone deficiency. J Clin Endocrinol Metab 29:279–289, 1969
36. Vagnucci A: Selective aldosterone deficiency in chronic pyelonephritis. Nephron 7:524–537, 1970
37. Ferrara E, Werk E, Hanenson I, Privitera P, Kenyon C: Selective hypoaldosteronism with blunted renin-activity responsiveness. Clin Res 18:602, 1970
38. McGiff J, Muzzarelli R, Duffy P, Gonzalez Y, Pierce C, Frawley T: Interrelationships of renin and aldosterone in a patient with hypoaldosteronism. Am J Med 48:247–252, 1970
39. Stockigt J, Collins R, Schambelan M, Brust N, Biglieri E: Subordinate hypoaldosteronism. Clin Res 19:174, 1971
40. Perez G, Siegel L, Schreiner G: Selective hypoaldosteronism with hyperkalemia. Ann Intern Med 76:757–763, 1972
41. Mellinger R, Petermann F, Jurgenson J: Hyponatremia with low urinary

aldosterone occurring in an old woman. J Clin Endocrinol Metab 34:85-91, 1972
42. Schambelan M, Stockigt J, Biglieri E: Isolated hypoaldosteronism in adults. A renin-deficiency syndrome. N Engl J Med 287:573-578, 1972
43. Brown J, Chinn R, Fraser R, Lever A, Morton J, Robertson J, Tree M, Waite M: Recurrent hyperkalemia due to selective adosterone deficiency: Correction by angiotensin infusion. Br Med J 1:650-654, 1973
44. Gossain V, Ferrara E, Werk E, Srivastava L, Privitera P, Hanenson I: Impaired renin responsiveness with secondary hypoaldosteronism. Arch Intern Med 132:885-890, 1973
45. Weidmann P, Reinhart R, Maxwell M, Rowe P, Coburn J, Massry S: Syndrome of hyporeninemic hypoaldosteronism and hyperkalemia in renal disease. J Clin Endocrinol Metab 36:965-977, 1973
46. Oh M, Carroll H, Clemmons J, Vagnucci A, Levinson S, Whang E; A mechanism for hyporeninemic hypoaldosteronism in chronic renal disease. Metabolism 23:1157-1166, 1974
47. Weidmann P, Maxwell M, Rowe P, Winer R, Massry S: Role of the renin-angiotensin-aldosterone system in the regulation of plasma potassium in chronic renal disease. Nephron 15:35-49, 1975
48. Goldfarb S, Cox M, Singer I, Goldberg M: Acute hyperkalemia induced by hyperglycemia: hormonal mechanisms. Ann Intern Med 84:426-432, 1976
49. Goldfarb S, Strunk B, Singer I, Goldberg M: Paradoxical glucose-induced hyperkalemia. Am J Med 59:744-750, 1975
50. Syzlman P, Better O, Chaimowit C, Rosler A: Role of hyperkalemia in the metabolic acidosis of isolated hypoaldosteronism. N Engl J Med 294:361-365, 1976
51. deLeiva A, Christlieb R, Melby J, Graham C, Day R, Luetscher J, Zager, P: Big renin and biosynthetic defect of aldosterone in diabetes mellitus. N Engl J Med 295:639-643, 1976
52. Perez G, Lespier L, Knowles R, Oster J, Vaamonde C: Hyporeninemia and hypoaldosteronism in diabetes mellitus. Arch Intern Med 137:852-855, 1977
53. Arora KK, Pfeifer MA, Wolter C, Melo J, Samols E: Hyperkalemia due to selective hypoaldosteronism. South Med J 70:634-636, 1977
54. Barbour GL, Keller AW: Distal renal tubular acidosis in selective hypoaldosteronism. South Med J 71:1397-1400, 1978
55. Perez GO, Lespier L, Knowles R, Oster JR, Vaamonde CA: Potassium homeostasis in chronic diabetes mellitus. Arch Intern Med 137:1018-1022, 1977
56. Brezis M, Litvin Y: Syndrome of hyporeninemic hypoaldosteronism. Isr J Med 13:1013-1021, 1977
57. Sebastian A, Schambelan M, Lindenfield S, Morris C: Amelioration of metabolic acidosis with fludrocortisone therapy in hyporeninemic hypoaldosteronism. N Engl J Med 297:576-583, 1977
58. Norby LH, Ramwell P, Weidig J, Slotkoff L, Flamenbaum W: Possible role for impaired renal prostaglandin production in pathogenesis of hyporeninaemic hypoaldosteronism. Lancet 2:1118-1122, 1978
59. Perez GO, Lespier LE, Oster JR, Vaamonde CA: Effect of alterations of

sodium intake in patients with hyporeninemic hypoaldosteronism. Nephron 18:259–265, 1977
60. Sparagana M: Hyporeninemic hypoaldosteronism with diabetic glomerulosclerosis. Biochem Med 14:93–103, 1975
61. Christlieb AR, Kaldany A, D'Elia JA, Williams GH: Aldosterone responsiveness in patients with diabetes mellitus. Diabetes 27:732–737, 1978
62. Tait JF, Tait SAS: The effect of changes in potassium concentration on the maximal steroidogenic response of purified zona glomerulosa cells to angiotensin II. J Steroid Biochem 7:687–690, 1976
63. Bayard F, Cooke CR, Tiller DJ, Beitins IS, Kowarski A, Walker GW, Migeon CJ: The regulation of aldosterone secretion in anephric man. J Clin Invest 50:1585–1595, 1970
64. Mitra S, Genuth SM, Berman LB, Vertes V: Aldosterone secretion in anephric patients. N Engl J Med 286:61–64, 1972
65. McCaa RE, McCaa CS, Read DG, Bower JD, Guyton AC: Increased plasma aldosterone concentration in response to hemodialysis in nephrectomized man. Circ Res 31:473–480, 1972
66. Brunner HR, Baer L, Sealey JE, Ledingham JGG, Laragh JH: The influence of potassium administration and of potassium deprivation on plasma renin in normal and hypertensive subjects. J Clin Invest 49:2128–2138, 1970
67. Schneider EG, Lynch RE, Willis LR, Knox FG: The effect of potassium infusion on proximal sodium reabsorption and renin release in the dog. Kidney Int 2:197–202, 1972
68. Sealey JE, Clark I, Bull MB, Laragh JH: Potassium balance and the control of renin secretion. J Clin Invest 49:2119–2127, 1970
69. Andres RM, Baltzan MA, Cader G, Zierler KL: Effect of insulin on carboyhydrate metabolism and on potassium in the forearm of man. J Clin Invest 41:108–115, 1962
70. Zierler KL: Effect of insulin on potassium efflux from rat muscle in the presence and absence of glucose. Am J Physiol 198:1066–1070, 1960
71. DeFronzo RA, Felig P, Ferrannini E, Wahren J: Sites and mechanism of insulin-mediated potassium metabolism in man. Clin Res 27:365A, 1979
72. Mortimore GE: Effect of insulin on potassium transfer in isolated rat liver. Am J Physiol 200:1315–1319, 1961
73. Kestens PJ, Haxhe JJ, Lambotte L, Lambotte C: The effect of insulin on the uptake of potassium and phosphate by the isolated perfused canine liver. Metabolism 12:941–950, 1963
74. Brown RD, Strott CA, Liddle GW: Site of stimulation of aldosterone biosynthesis by angiotensin and potassium. J Clin Invest 51:1413–1418, 1972
75. deChatel R, Weidmann P, Flammer J, Ziegler WH, Beretta-Piccoli C, Vetter W, Reubi FC: Sodium, renin, aldosterone, catecholamines, and blood pressure in diabetes mellitus. Kidney Int 12:412–421, 1977
76. Thomsen AC: The significance of renal biopsy for the diagnosis of pyelonephritis in diabetic patients, In Ciba Foundation Symposium on Renal Biopsy. Wolsten-Holme GEW, Cameron MP (eds.): Boston, Little, Brown, 1961, p. 281
77. Heptinstall RH: Pathology of the Kidney, 2nd ed. Boston, Little, Brown, 1974, pp. 940–941

78. Arieff AI: Kidney, water and electrolyte metabolism in diabetes mellitus. In Brenner BM, Rector FC (eds): The Kidney. Philadelphia, Saunders, 1976, pp. 1257–1296
79. Schindler AM, Sommers SC: Diabetic sclerosis of the renal juxtaglomerular apparatus. Lab Invest 15:877–884, 1966
80. Day RP, Leutscher JA, Gonzales CM: Occurrence of big renin in human plasma, amniotic fluid, and kidney extracts. J Clin Endocrinol Metab 40:1078–1084, 1975
81. Wagermark J, Ungersted U, Ljungquist A: Sympathetic innervation of the juxtaglomerular cells of the kidney. Circ Res 22:149–153, 1968
82. DeChamplain J, Genest J, Vegratt R: Factors controlling renin in man. Arch Intern Med 117:355–363, 1966
83. Christensen NJ: Plasma catecholamines in long-term diabetes with and without neuropathy and in hypophysectomized subjects. J Clin Invest 51:779–787, 1972
84. Tuck ML, Sambhi MP, Levin L: Hyporeninemic hypoaldosteronism in diabetes mellitus. Studies of the autonomic nervous system's control of renin release. Diabetes 28:237–241, 1978
85. Yun J, Kelly G, Bartter FC, Smith H: Role of prostaglandins in the control of renin secretion in the dog. Circ Res 40:459–464, 1977
86. Romero JC, Dunlap CL, Strong CG: The effect of indomethacin and other anti-inflammatory drugs on the renin-angiotensin system in man. J Clin Invest 58:282–288, 1976
87. Tan SY, Mulrow PJ: Inhibition of the renin-aldosterone response to furosemide by indomethacin. J Clin Endocrinol Metab 45:174–176, 1977
88. Saruta T, Kaplan NM: Adrenocortical steroid genesis: the effects of prostaglandins. J Clin Invest 51:2246–2251, 1972
89. Tan SY, Shapiro R, Franco R, Stockard H, Mulrow PJ: Indomethacin-induced prostaglandin inhibition with hyperkalemia. Ann Intern Med 90:783–785, 1979
90. Tan SY, Antonipillai I, Mulrow PJ: Inactive renin and impaired prostaglandin production in hyporeninemic hypoaldosteronism. Clin Res 29:452A, 1979
91. Hahn JA, Zipser RD, Zia PK, Horton R: Prostaglandins in hyporeninaemic hypoaldosteronism. Lancet 1:1379, 1978
92. Hahn JA, Zipser RD, Stone RA, Zia PK, Horton R: Vasoactive systems in hyporeninaemic hypoaldosteronism: deficiency of kallikrein. Clin Res 27:313A, 1979
93. Adler S: An extrarenal action of aldosterone on mammalian skeletal muscle. Am J Physiol 218:616–621, 1970
94. Bia M, Lee R, Jones A, DeFronzo RA: Role of insulin and adrenal hormones in acute potassium homeostasis. Clin Res 27:409A, 1979
95. DeFronzo RA, Goldberg M, Cooke CR, Barker C, Grossman RA, Agus ZS: Investigations into the mechanisms of hyperkalemia following renal transplantation. Kidney Int 11:357–365, 1977
96. Pardo V, Strauss J, Kramer H, Ozawa T, McIntosh RM: Nephropathy associated with sickle cell anemia. An autologous immune complex nephritis. II. Clinicopathologic study of seven patients. Am J Med 59:650–659, 1975

97. Brentjiens JR, Sepulveda M, Balliah T, Bentzel C, Erlanger BF, Elwood CL, Montes M, Hsu KC, Andres GA: Interstitial immune complex nephritis in patients with systemic lupus erythematosus. Kidney Int 7:342–350, 1975
98. DeFronzo RA, Cooke CR, Goldberg M, Cow M, Myers AR, Agus ZS: Inpaired renal tubular potassium secretion in systemic lupus erythematosus. Ann Intern Med 86:268–271, 1977
99. Saruta T, Kaplan NM: Adrenocortical steroidogenesis: The effects of prostaglandin. J Clin Invest 51:2246–2251, 1972
100. Tan SY, Mulrow PJ: Inhibition of the renin-aldosterone response to furosemide by indomethacin. J Clin Endocrinol Metab 45:174–176, 1977
101. Veldhuis JD, Kulin HE, Santen RJ, Wilson TE, Melby JC: Inborn error in the terminal step of aldosterone biosynthesis. N Engl J Med 303:117–121, 1980
102. Rosler A, Rabinowitz O, Theodor R, Ramirez LC, Vlick S: The nature of the defect in a salt wasting disorder in Jews in Iran. J Clin Endocrinol Metab 44:279–291, 1977
103. Cohen JJ, Hulter HN, Smithline NS, Melby, JC, Schwartz WB: The critical role of the adrenal gland in the renal regulation of acid-base equilibrium during chronic hypotonic expansion: evidence that chronic hyponatremia is a potent stimulus to aldosterone secretion. J Clin Invest 58:1201–1208, 1976
104. Walker WG, Cooke CR: Plasma aldosterone regulation in anephric man. Kidney Int 3:1–5, 1973
105. Oh MS, Carroll HJ, Goldstein DA, Fein IA: Hyperchloremic acidosis during the recovery phase of diabetic ketoacidosis. Ann Intern Med 89:925–927, 1978
106. Ostes JR, Perez GO, Rosen MS: Hyporeninemic hypoaldosteronism after chronic bicarbonate abuse. Arch Intern Med 136:1179–1181, 1976
107. Perez GO, Ostes JR, Vaamonde CA: Renal acidification in patients with mineralocorticoid deficiency. Nephron 17:461–473, 1976
108. Cohen JJ, Lyons H, Harrington JT, Schwartz WB: Total correction by DOCA of HCl-induced chronic metabolic acidosis. Clin Res 21:681, 1973
109. Hulter HN, Ilnocki LP, Harlottle JA, Sebastian A: Impaired renal H^+ secretion and NH_3 production in mineralocorticoid-deficient glucocorticoid-replete dogs. Am J Physiol 232:F136–F146, 1977

Ketosis

Principal Discussant
George F. Cahill, Jr.

Case Presentation

A 54-year-old man was admitted to the hospital in an obtunded state. A diagnosis of diabetes mellitus had been made at the age of 43, after he had experienced polydipsia, polyuria, and a 15-lb weight loss. In the 11 years after the diagnosis of diabetes was established, he was admitted to the hospital several times for acute and chronic alcoholism and cellulitis of the face. On one of these admissions, his blood glucose was 304 mg/dl and plasma bicarbonate was 14 mEq/liter. Treatment with 60 units of regular insulin and 3 liters of normal saline over an 8-h period restored the blood sugar and bicarbonate concentration to normal. The patient was discharged on 40 units of NPH insulin daily, but the physicians who examined him later in the clinic believed he was not complying with this therapeutic program.

Before admission, the patient had been drinking heavily, and on the morning of admission he was found in bed, incontinent, confused, and difficult to arouse. On admission he was grossly confused, unable to give a history, and combative. He was slightly obese and was taking 24 deep breaths/min. The blood was 110/70 mmHg, and the heart rate was 104 beats/min. The skin turgor was poor. His breath was fetid but acetone could not be detected. The neck veins were flat. There was a grade I/VI precordial systolic murmur. The lungs were clear except for scattered ronchi. The liver, which could be percussed four finger breadths below the right costal margin, seemed slightly tender. Ankle reflexes were absent, and pain sensation in the lower extremities was markedly decreased.

Laboratory findings included the following: hematocrit, 41% with normal indexes; white blood cell count, 8400/mm^3 with a normal differential; blood glucose, 193 mg/dl; BUN, 32 mg/dl; and serum creatinine, 1.6 mg/dl. Electrolyte values included sodium, 141 mEq/liter; potassium, 5.1 mEq/liter; chloride, 105 mEq/liter; and bicarbonate, 12 mEq/liter. The blood pH was 7.30 and the $PaCO_2$ was 25 mmHg. Ketones were positive in 1:4 dilution. Subsequent enzymatic analysis gave values of plasma acetoacetate, 1.2 mEq/liter; β-hydroxybutyrate, 9.0 mEq/liter; and lactate, 1.2 mEq/liter.

Treatment with intermittent small doses of regular insulin (10 units/h, three times) and with intravenous glucose and saline reversed the metabolic abnormalities within 8 h.

Discussion

Dr. George F. Cahill, Jr. *(Professor of Medicine, Harvard Medical School; Director of Research, Howard Hughes Medical Institute; and Physician, Brigham and Women's Hospital, Boston, Massachusetts)*: This man had a history of diabetes and the classic syndrome of weight loss, polydipsia, and polyuria 11 years prior to present admission. He was and is slightly obese. The relatively mild course of his metabolic disorder permitted him to stop insulin therapy without becoming ketotic. If not for the initial event and the current episode of ketosis, he would be classified as having typical non-insulin-dependent diabetes mellitus (NIDDM). The type of diabetes in this patient contrasts with the other common variety, insulin-dependent diabetes mellitus (IDDM), which is more frequent in youth and is associated with a progressive viral and/or autoimmune destruction of the beta cells. The latter form of the disease necessitates daily insulin injections to prevent gross metabolic decompensation and ketoacidosis because a total or nearly total lack of endogenous insulin production occurs within several years. Thus this patient is a non-insulin-dependent or "maturity-onset" diabetic, whose only overt symptom of diabetes was soft-tissue infection of the face, a problem probably also related to poor hygiene. Although the diabetes was reasonably well controlled, the patient did exhibit a neurologic deficit in his lower extremities. This condition also was probably exacerbated by his alcohol intake: alcohol and diabetes act synergistically in causing peripheral neuropathy.

On admission, the patient was somewhat hyperneic, and metabolic acidosis was discovered to be the cuase of the hyperventilation. Ketosis was the cause of the acidosis, as evidenced by the elevated values of β-hydroxybutyrate, 9 mM/liter, and acetoacetate (AcAc), 1.2 mM/liter. Plasma lactate was only 1.2 mM/liter. Thus he had moderate ketoacidosis but his blood glucose concentration was only 193 mg/dl. One might have expected a glucose value of 300 or 400 mg/dl, or even higher perhaps, especially in light of the slightly elevated blood urea and serum creatinine levels. He was treated appropriately with small doses of insulin, 5–10 units initially, and he was given both glucose and saline; the chemical abnormalities were corrected in several hours. Had the glucose levels been in the overtly diabetic range of 400 mg/dl or higher, it would have been appropriate to treat him with larger quantities of insulin given either intramuscularly or intravenously. Although the patient was somewhat hyperglycemic, he did not have bona fide diabetic ketoacidosis and thus he was appropriately treated with small doses of insulin, saline, and glucose from the start.

What was the pathogenesis of the metabolic disorder in this patient? He had not been eating, and the ketosis probably could be attributed partially to simple starvation. But it takes 1–2 weeks of total starvation to cause such a severe degree of ketosis [1,2]. In fact, in the fasting patient, increased excretion of ammonia by the kidney counterbalances the effect of the increased acid production, thus limiting the severity of acidosis. Another factor contributing to ketosis in this patient was the alcohol intake [3–5]. Alcohol is metabolized in the liver to form acetaldehyde and acetate, and the latter is released into the circulation for metabolism by other tissues. Flooding of the liver by acetate results in the production of ketoacids, especially β-hydroxybutyrate (BOHB) and this increased acetate load probably contributed to the ketoacidosis. In the presence of excessive alcohol metabolism, reduced NAD^+ (i.e., NADH) accumulates and leads to a preferential conversion of pyruvic acid to lactic acid. Although plasma lactate was nearly within the normal range when this patient was examined, the plasma lactate level might have been higher earlier. The slightly elevated BOHB/AcAc ratio (normal, 4/1) supports this contention because these two substrates, like lactate and pyruvate, are a redox couple. The lactate/pyruvate ratio represents the mean body cytosolic redox potential, and the BOHB/AcAc ratio refers to the mean of the mitochondrial redox potential. With anoxia or with an excessive production of reducing equivalents, as with alcohol metabolism, both ratios increase.

In sum, the patient had mild ketoacidosis that probably resulted from three processes, each leading to increased hepatic ketone production: starvation, alcohol consumption, and possibly diabetic decompensation.

Ketoacid Metabolism

The intermediary metabolism of the ketoacids has been reviewed in great detail in several recent articles. Hepatic ketogenesis was discussed extensively by McGarry, Mannaerts, and Foster [6–8], and the peripheral metabolism of the ketoacids and their effects on other substrates were reviewed by Robinson and Williamson [9]. Fenselau detailed the biochemical reactions involved in ketogenesis and ketoacid metabolism [10], and Liljenquist discussed ketoacid regulation [11] in Brownlee's series on diabetes mellitus [12]. These reviews permit

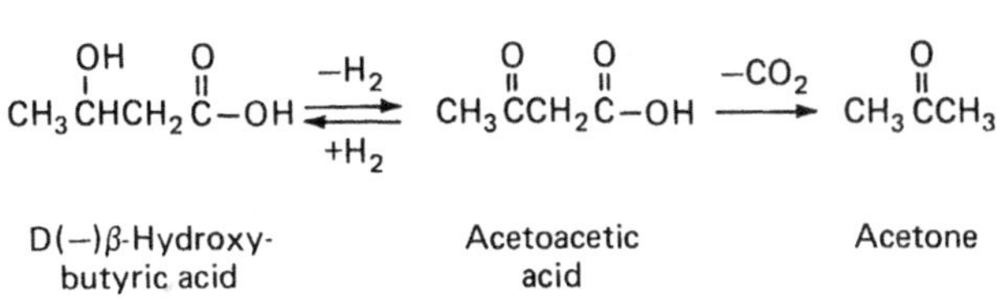

Fig. 1. Interrelationship between acetoacetate (AcAc) and β-hydroxybutyrate (BOHB), the reaction catalyzed by the enzyme β-hydroxybutyrate dehydrogenase with NAD^+ as acceptor to produce NADH plus H^+. Also shown is the nonenzymatic decarboxylation of AcAc to acetone, an irreversible step.

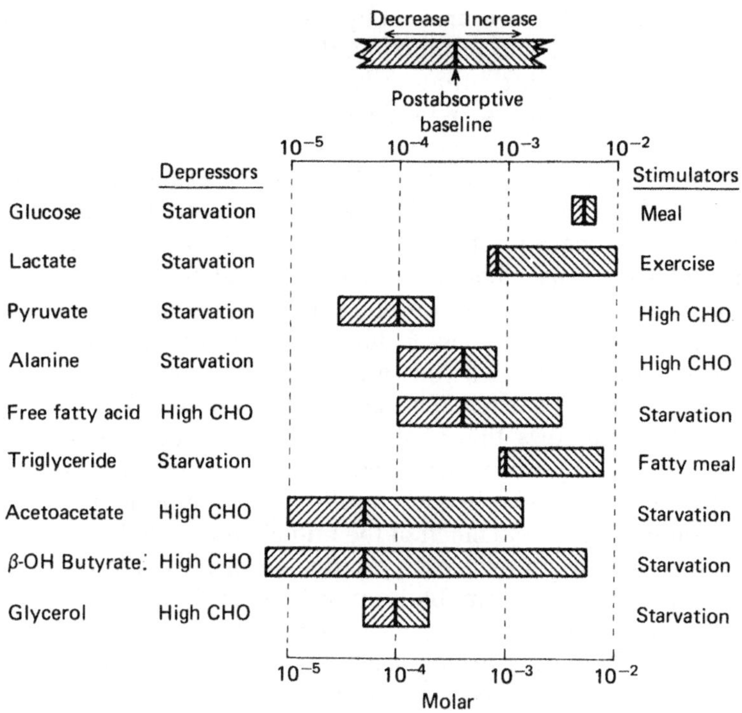

Fig. 2. Physiologic ranges of circulating substrates in normal humans expressed on a logarithmic scale. Of note is the narrow range of glucose concentrations and the three orders of magnitude variation in the concentration of BOHB.

me to concentrate on the pathways of ketogenesis, and I will emphasize the issues concerning substrate and sites of hormonal control.

Acetoacetate and β-hydroxybutyrate are the principal "ketone" products and are interconverted by a single step, an oxidation-reduction with NAD^+ and NADH as cofactors (Fig. 1). The enzyme for this interconversion, β-hydroxbutyrate dehydrogenase, is located primarily inside mitochondria, as compared with lactate dehydrogenase, which resides in the cytosol. Thus the BOHB/AcAc ratio reflects the mitochondrial $NADH/NAD^+$ ratio, and the lactate/pyruvate (L/P) ratio is indicative of the same ratio in the cytosol. The third "ketone," acetone, is thought to be the product of a nonenzymatic decarboxylation of AcAc, although its production still could be enzymatically catalyzed. Acetone production is, therefore, a function of the level of AcAc and the duration of its elevation; the presence of acetone is thus indicative of a sustained, severe ketoacidosis. Reichard et al. recently showed that about one-third of AcAc metabolically produced is decarboxylated to acetone and, surprisingly, about two-thirds of the acetone is recovered as glucose (13,14). This is a novel observation that disproves the old adage that fat cannot be converted into carbohydrate in humans. Although this route of conversion of fatty acids to acetate to acetoacetate to acetone to glucose is a circuitous one, it might play a very important role in prolonged fasting in humans.

Acetoacetate and β-hydroxybutyrate are produced in approximately equal amounts in humans and are made primarily by the liver [5]. No other tissue makes significant amounts of these ketones except muscle and kidney, which produce them only occasionally and in small amounts. Blood levels of AcAc and BOHB in the usual postabsorptive state are less than 0.1 mM/liter, and if large carbohydrate loads are administered, these levels can fall to as low as 0.010 mM/liter. Such low basal levels might consist of products of branched-chain amino acid catabolism instead of byproducts of hepatic acetate metabolism; thus, fat-derived ketogenesis under these circumstances is probably near zero. In fasting humans, AcAc and BOHB levels rise to 1.2–1.6 and 6–8 mM/liter, respectively, but it takes 1–2 weeks to reach this plateau. Thus the variation in their concentrations may be three orders of magnitude; this extreme range of concentration makes these compounds unique compared to all other metabolic fuels. For example, glucose levels vary between 4 and 6 mM; other fuels such as alanine, leucine, lactate, and fatty acids vary by less than one order of magnitude (Fig. 2).

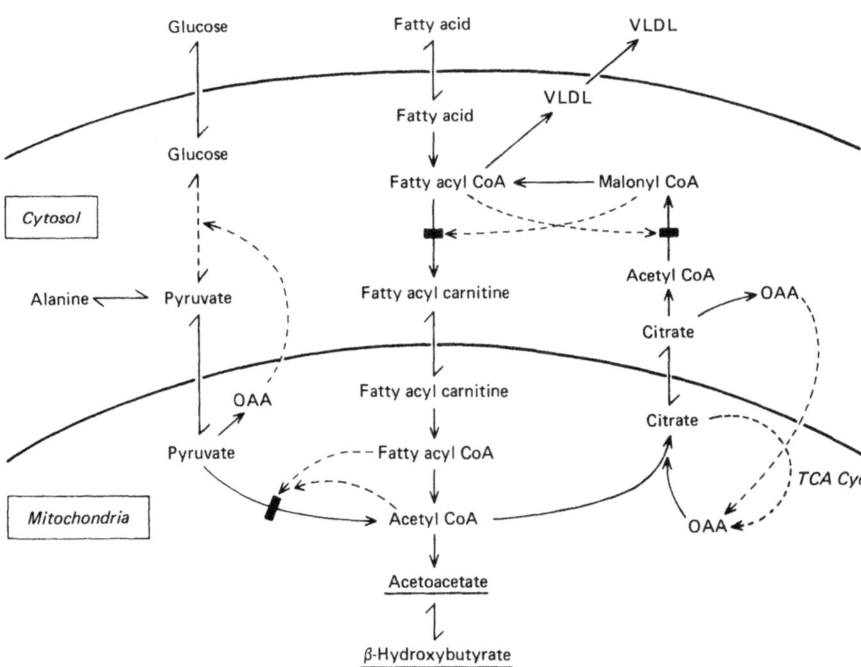

Fig. 3. Biochemical pathways in liver connecting carbohydrate metabolism on the left, fat oxidation in the center, and acetate oxidation to CO_2 or its incorporation into long-chain fatty acid on the right.

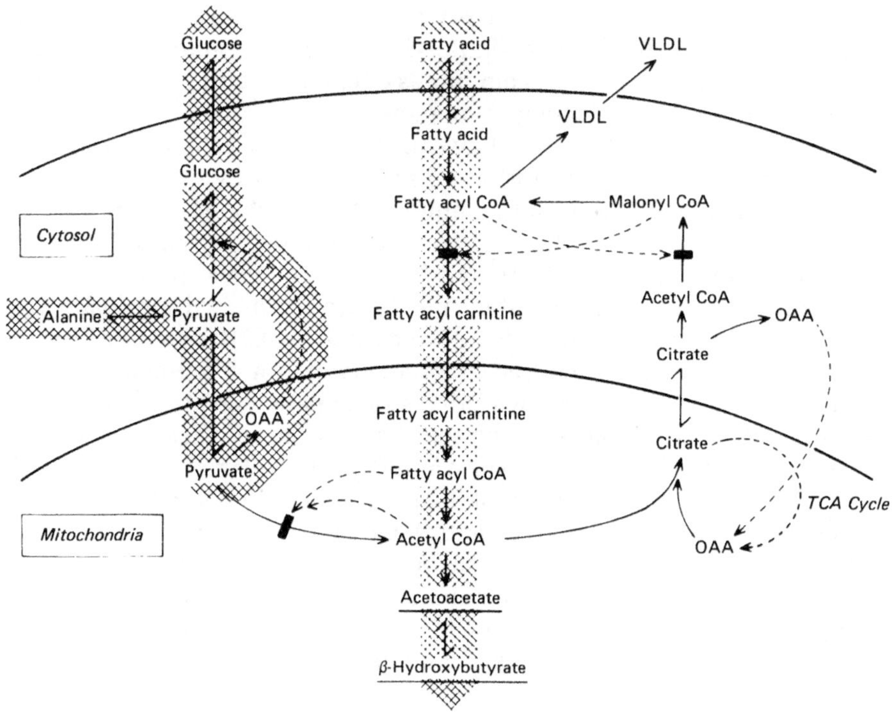

Fig. 4. Accentuation of gluconeogenesis from muscle-derived amino acid (alanine) and fatty acid oxidation to AcAc and BOHB in fasting, a state with low insulin and normal or elevated glucagon levels.

Acetoacetate and BOHB should be considered overflow products of the hepatic acetyl CoA pool. When CoA production surpasses its two routes of assimilation, ketoacid synthesis and release occur. As noted, the biochemical steps have been elucidated elsewhere [9,10]. Figure 3 summarizes hepatic metabolism; Fig. 4 contains a modified schema for the fasting (low-insulin) state. Free fatty acids released from adipose tissue are carried in plasma to the liver and by transport processes not yet clarified enter the liver cytosol where they are activated to their acyl CoA derivations. These derivatives are transacylated and the fatty acids are transported into the mitochondria as the carnitine ester. The acyl CoA ester is regenerated inside the mitochondria; then the classic "beta" oxidation of the long-chain fatty acyl CoA ester takes place, producing a number of acetyl CoAs and equal quantities of the reduced coenzymes NADH and FADH. These coenzymes donate their electrons to the mitochondrial energy chain, producing ATP and yielding their protons to oxygen to form water. One-third of the potential metabolic energy of a long-chain fatty acid is produced in this manner. When insulin levels are low and fatty acid levels are high, the metabolism of fat can supply all of the liver's energy needs. In a provocative theoretical discussion, Flatt pointed out that there must be a maximum rate for beta-oxidation of long-chain fatty acids and that this rate is determined by the liver's energy utilization, since ATP cannot be accumulated above basal amounts [16].

What are the two nonketogenic pathways of acetyl CoA utilization in liver? As in any other tissue, the most significant route is the condensation of acetyl CoA with oxaloacetate (OAA) in mitochondria to form citrate. Citrate formation is, of course, the first step in the primary energy-producing series of reactions known as the Krebs, tricarboxylic, or citric acid cycle. This cycle regenerates oxaloacetate and picks up the next acetyl CoA for the succeeding turn of the cycle. Only acetyl groups, not the recycling four-carbon acceptor, are oxidized by this process, although isotopic oxidation or exchange does take place. Sub-

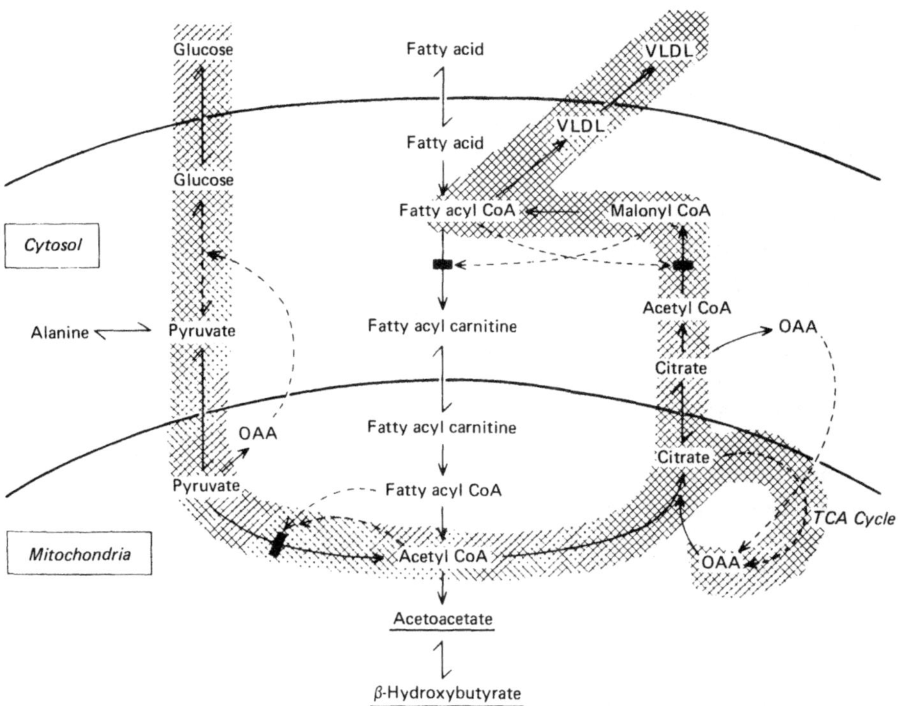

Fig. 5. The high-insulin–low-glucagon state in which there is glycolysis to pyruvate, then to acetyl CoA and oxidation of some of the acetate to CO_2 via the TCA cycle for energy. The remainder is used for fat synthesis via export from the mitochondria as citrate, cleavage to CoA, and subsequently fatty acyl CoA synthesis via the insulin-activated fatty acid synthetase system. The fatty acyl CoAs are used for triglyceride synthesis and then exported from the liver as very low density lipoprotein (VLDL).

Table 1. Acetate (acetyl CoA) metabolism.

Nutritional State	Source	Disposition
High insulin (feeding)	Pyruvate Amino acids Ethyl alcohol	Oxidation by tricarboxylic acid cycle Fatty acid synthesis
Low insulin (fasting)	Free fatty acids Amino acids Ethyl alcohol	Ketoacid export (± acetate export)

strates such as succinate α-ketoglutarate, or other amino acid analogs cannot be oxidized by the citric acid cycle but can be converted only to OAA. Oxaloacetate can exit from the mitochondrion only via phosphoenol pyruvate, which in turn can generate either glucose or pyruvate. In the latter case, acetyl CoA can be generated for eventual oxidation by the citric acid cycle. In summary, the citric acid cycle only oxidizes acetate as acetyl CoA and produces two molecules of carbon dioxide for each molecule of acetate.

The other route for acetyl CoA consumption is fat synthesis, a process that also requires mitochondrial formation of citrate (Fig. 5; Table 1). The citrate exits from the mitochondrion and is cleaved back to OAA and acetyl CoA in the cytosol. The acetyl CoA is carboxylated to malonyl CoA as the first step in long-chain fatty acid synthesis. Then, catalyzed by the fatty acid synthesis complex, the malonyl CoA units eventually form long-chain fatty acyl CoA molecules, which are incorporated into triglycerides. These triglycerides are exported by the liver as very low density lipoproteins (VLDL) to the periphery, especially adipose tissue; in adipose tissue, the triglyceride is stored in the oil vacuole at the center of the cell.

What are the controls of acetyl CoA disposition? Nature has devised a very simple cross-control system. When the liver is under the influence of large amounts of insulin but low levels of glucagon (e.g., after a carbohydrate meal), production of the enzyme catalyzing malonyl CoA synthesis is increased and levels of malonyl CoA increase (Fig. 5). McGarry, Mannaerts, and Foster have shown that the increased levels of malonyl CoA inhibit fatty acyl CoA entrance into mitochondria by decreasing the carnitine transferase step; thus the fatty acyl CoA moieties produced are spared from oxidation and ketone formation and are used instead for triglyceride synthesis [6–8]. By contrast, when insulin levels are low, for example during fasting, malonyl CoA production is decreased, and the fatty acyl CoA molecules coming from peripherally mobilized free fatty acids are available for ketoacid production (Fig. 4).

How do these biochemical controls relate to glucose consumption and production by the liver? Several substrates and hormonal controls are available to direct the net flux of substrate. When mitochondria are full of acetyl CoA in the low insulin state because of fatty acid release from the periphery, and with low levels of malonyl CoA and unchecked beta oxidation, then citrate formation is brisk, and large quantities of citrate exit from the mitochondria. In the cytosol, the enzyme that cleaves citrate is low when insulin levels are low. Thus, citrate levels increase and high levels of citrate inhibit the principal glycolytic enzyme, phosphofructokinase. With glycolysis dampened by these events, the stage is set for gluconeogenesis. Mitochondrial dehydrogenation of pyruvate also is inhibited because of inactivation as well as inhibition of the active moiety of the responsible enzyme. The pyruvate that comes to the liver from the periphery as alanine is spared oxidation to acetyl CoA and instead is carboxylated to OAA. Thus, the pyruvate is processed to phosphoenolpyruvate as the first step in "reverse glycolysis" or gluconeogenesis (Fig. 4). As a result of low insulin and probably also of normal or high glucagon levels, all systems are directed toward gluconeogenesis [17]. For several reasons, the hepatic citric acid cycle activity is reduced under these circumstances. Cycle activity is decreased first because ATP levels are ample, owing to fatty acid beta-

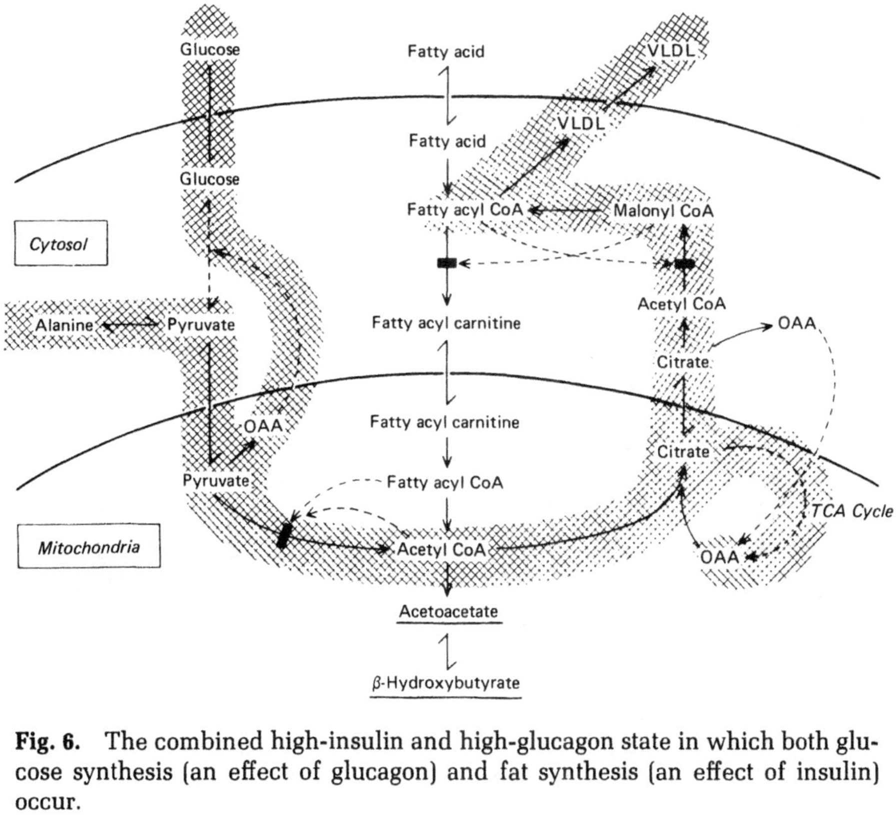

Fig. 6. The combined high-insulin and high-glucagon state in which both glucose synthesis (an effect of glucagon) and fat synthesis (an effect of insulin) occur.

oxidation, and OAA levels are decreased both because of augmented incorporation into phosphoenolpyruvate and the accumulated NADH that accelerates the formation of malate. Second, this reduced state also inhibits the cycle by providing less free NAD^+ at the various dehydrogenation steps. Finally, to return to the upper steps in glycolysis and gluconeogenesis, inhibition of phosphofructokinase allows glucose-6-phosphate to accumulate and results in glucose production in the liver via the critical and unique enzyme, glucose-6-phosphatase.

Thus we can think of the liver as working in any of two modes: a low-insulin state characterized by gluconeogenesis, lipolysis, and ketogenesis; and a high-insulin state characterized by glycolysis, lipogenesis, and fat export. In the former, the liver's energy is provided by beta oxidation of fatty acids; in the latter state, the tricarboxylic acid cycle produces the energy. The only exception to this rule occurs when protein is ingested without carbohydrate (Fig 6). When protein intake is high, gluconeogenesis occurs, probably because of high levels of glucagon. Yet there is little ketogenesis, and what little there is probably results from branched-chain amino acid metabolism. This metabolic state is probably explained by a high insulin as well as a high glucagon level [17,18]. Fatty acid synthesis can proceed in humans and carnivores when the diet consists of a high protein intake. A small amount of carbohydrate in the diet, however, suppresses glucagon production and inhibits gluconeogenesis (Fig. 7). This observation should not be taken to signify that insulin and glucagon are inhibitory of each other

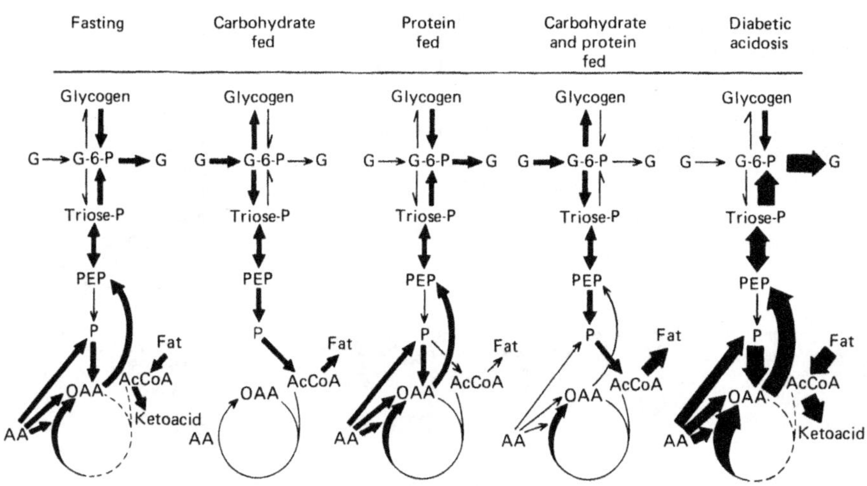

Fig. 7. Summary scheme of liver as in Figs. 3–6, but also containing a scheme of mixed carbohydrate-protein intake, in which glucagon is suppressed, and there is net glucose intake. On the right is the super-fasting state of diabetic ketoacidosis in which insulin-controlled processes are lacking.

in the liver, but that insulin also has secondary effects independent of glucagon levels. Recent research in phosphorylation of proteins in the liver after exposure to insulin, glucagon, or both shows that some proteins are uniquely phosphorylated by each of these hormones but at different sites and with differing metabolic effects [19]. These data support the separate messenger concept.

Ambient ketoacid levels are controlled by hepatic production and peripheral disposition. The latter is composed of two processes, renal excretion and oxidation by peripheral tissues, mainly muscle but also kidney. Evidence suggests that in prolonged ketoacidosis, renal conservation of ketoacids becomes more efficient [20]. Peripheral tissues, perhaps because of increased fatty acid utilization and thus a high NADH/NAD^+ ratio, decrease their utilization of ketoacids, as evidenced by production of 1 mole of BOHB for each mole of AcAc taken up [21,22]. Thus a major contribution to the ambient levels of ketoacids is their reduced peripheral metabolism.

The Physiology of Ketosis

The ketoacids are derived from the partial hepatic oxidation of long-chain fatty acids to 2-carbon fragments, or acetate, and then are exported to other tissues where they are oxidized. To a much lesser degree, the ketoacids are derived from the metabolism of the branched-chain amino acids and also can be formed from other sources of acetate, such as ethyl alcohol. In ruminants, a considerable quantity of acetate is produced in the rumen and in the liver from the large load of other short-chain fatty acids, such as butyrate, coming from the gut. In the fed state, ruminants can maintain appreciable levels of circulating ketoacids, which are utilized by skeletal muscle and mammary tissue for the synthesis of milk fat. Ketoacids also have another function in suckling mammalian young including humans [9]. The medium-chain fatty acids found in high proportion in milk enter mitochondria for oxidation more readily than do long-chain fatty acids because they bypass the carnitine transfer step and thus are not inhibited by high levels of malonyl CoA. Mild ketoacidosis therefore can occur in suckling animals, especially those consuming milk low in carbohydrates, such as the carnivores. In fact, porpoise and seal milk is almost devoid of lactose, and the pups are on a "ketogenic" diet very high in fat and protein. What purpose does this mild ketoacidosis serve? Increased ketoacids probably spare carbohydrates and in turn spare protein, but in these aquatic mammals, transfer of calories as extraaqueous lipid instead of water-soluble carbohydrate might be even more important as a water-conserving process.

Two events in human evolution have created a relatively unique metabolic predicament. The blood-brain barrier, shared by all vertebrates, prevents the extracellular fluid of the central nervous system from exchanging substances by simple diffusion with the blood [23]. Numerous tight junctions bridge and occlude the endothelial cells of the brain capillaries and preclude the flux of macromolecules; only simple, small, water-soluble molecules with specific transport processes can overcome this barrier. Lipoprotein complexes and the albumin-fatty acid complex are excluded from the adult human brain, and the only remaining fuel of significant concentration in the circulation that can provide calories is glucose. Glucose is thus the standard fuel for the central nervous system in all animals studied. At times amino acids can provide a small amount of energy, but use of this fuel requires disposition of their amino groups, usually as glutamine, so amino acid utilization is relatively trivial.

The second unique evolutionary component is the disproportionate size of the human brain and its relatively large fuel demand. In adults, the brain consumes one-fifth to one-quarter of the total calories; in children, the brain uses as much as one-half. Between meals, this energy demand relies on hepatic glycogen to provide blood glucose. At most, only one day's supply of glucose can be stored as liver glycogen, and fasting for a longer period necessitates gluconeogenesis. The adult brain consumes about 500 kcal daily, and that of a 5-year-old child uses only slightly less, perhaps 450 kcal. If these calories were derived solely from protein, about 0.5 kg of muscle would be consumed daily. It is obvious that such total reliance on protein would limit survival, especially in the child; but the brain's ability to utilize selectively the increased circulating ketoacids instead of glucose diminishes to one-fifth or one-fourth the otherwise obligatory rate of protein breakdown [24].

Of further assistance in gluconeogenesis is the glycerol from the lipolyzed adipose triglyceride [1,25]. About 10% of fat by weight is the glycerol moiety; thus, the 160–180 g of triglyceride metabolized daily by a fasting human provides about 16–18 g of glycerol. In addition, 10–15 g of glucose can be derived from acetoacetate via acetone [14]. Thus, the brain can even maintain some glucose utilization without relying on protein as a source. In fact, it is probably glycerol derived from triglyceride that provides glucose for the brain in the fasting black bear [26] and the nesting emperor penguin [27], both of which survive months of starvation without ketosis and without relying on gluconeogenesis. Also, their relatively small brains contribute to their ability to survive without exogenous protein.

The Fasting Human

In fasting ketosis, AcAc and BOHB serve as fat-derived, water-soluble fuel capable of crossing the blood-brain. Transport of these substances occurs via facilitated diffusion, a "downhill" process, and requires an adequate concentration of ketones in the circulation to provide the diffusion gradient. Fasting ketosis occurs after 1 to 2 weeks of starvation [1,2,24,25] and is produced by a rapid increase in hepatic production of ketones in the first few days [13–15], a diminished peripheral utilization of ketones [21], and more efficient renal conservation of these substances [20]. Thus with plasma levels of BOHB and AcAc of 6–8 and 1–2 mM, respectively, two-thirds or more of brain energy needs are supplied. Göttstein et al. have shown, by measurement of brain arteriovenous differences during ketoacid infusion, that the level of ketoacids determines their rate of utilization [28,29]. The brain's dependency on ketoacids was shown in humans by Drenick et al. [30] and Flatt et al. [31], and Müller et al. in dogs, in which glucose levels rapidly lowered with insulin produced no subjective or objective indexes of "hypoglycemia" [32]. I should point out that fasting ketosis evolves over several days in humans, and that this time period matches that required by the kidney to increase ammoniagenesis [33]. One might speculate that the primary function of renal ammoniagenesis is to conserve cations during fasting ketoacidosis; the parallel development of ketosis and ammoniagenesis in fasting supports this concept.

As ketosis becomes sufficient to provide the brain's energy needs, glucose utilization is diminished [24]. Ruderman et al. have shown that the mechanism of decreased glucose utilization is inhibition of phosphofructokinase by citrate, which dams up hexose phosphate and in turn inhibits brain hexokinase [34]. The net result is the sparing of gluconeogenesis and, pari passu, the sparing of muscle protein, extending survival time several-fold, from weeks to months.

How does muscle sense that it no longer should provide amino acids, primarily alanine and glutamine [35–40], for gluconeogenesis? It has been suggested that fat oxidation spares both ketoacid utilization [21] and perhaps the oxidation of the keto analogs of the branched-chain amino acids [41]. If so, resynthesis of muscle protein, inhibition of muscle breakdown, or both would be facilitated. This hypothesis is supported by the observation that administration of the keto analogs of the branched-chain amino acids in fasting humans reduces nitrogen excretion [42,43]. The ketoacids also might directly contribute to this diminished proteolysis by acting as direct inhibitors [44], but further characterization of this process is critical, because aberrations in the normal efficiency of this process are the basis of the hypercatabolic states associated with trauma, sepsis, denervation disuse, and diabetic ketosis.

In sumary, ketosis is a normal physiologic state in which fat-derived, water-soluble molecules capable of crossing the blood-brain barrier displace glucose as brain fuel. The primary signal for ketoacid production by the liver is a low insulin level, but ketoacid production is also modulated by formation of acetate both from long-chain fatty acids and from other sources such as ethyl alcohol, ketogenic amino acids, and medium- or short-chain fatty acids in the diet.

Questions and Answers

Dr. Jerome P. Kassirer: Dr. Cahill, what is the mechanism of the rapid reversal of the metabolic abnormalities in patients with alcoholic ketoacidosis? Typically small amounts of glucose, sodium chloride, and water are all that are needed to reverse ketosis and acidosis.

Dr. Cahill: When insulin levels are increased by glucose infusion, ketoacid production by the liver is terminated, and ketoacid levels fall to zero within a few hours. Also, if volume depletion occurs, insulin release may be suppressed by adrenergic nerve endings in the islets of Langerhans as well as by circulating catecholamines. Volume repletion thus is necessary to correct this inhibition of insulin release.

As ketoacid levels fall, plasma bicarbonate rises and pH returns to normal. This is why we are reluctant to use intravenous alkali. In fact, the same principle holds true in the therapy of diabetic ketoacidosis. We avoid using alkali unless it becomes absolutely necessary. Some consider a pH below 7.1 the indication for using alkali. I prefer to make a clinical judgment. If the patient's pulse is becoming weak, thready, and rapid, and blood pressure is falling, then I would administer alkali. Further, if the patient's P_{CO_2} is 20 mmHg or so, as a result of hyperventilation to compensate for the metabolic acidosis, I would be reluctant to use alkali. But if the patient is deteriorating rapidly because weakness is preventing hyperventilation, and the P_{CO_2} is rising as high as 35 mmHg, akali therapy is indicated.

Dr. Kassirer: Under what circumstances is it appropriate to use insulin to treat alcoholic ketoacidosis?

Dr. Cahill: These patients usually do not require insulin. Administering intravenous glucose is usually sufficient unless there is concomitant volume depletion; if so, dextrose and saline should be used.

Dr. Jordan J. Cohen: It seems clear from the literature as well as from our own experience that some individuals are particularly susceptible to the development of alcoholic ketoacidosis. This is evidenced by numerous reports of recurrent episodes in the same person and by the relatively small percentage of alcoholics who manifest the condition. Is there a metabolic explanation for this susceptibility?

Dr. Cahill: I can't explain this susceptibility but I do wonder why it's so relatively rare. Despite the millions of alcoholics who fast for days while ingesting large amounts of ethanol, very few of these individuals appear at the hospital.

Dr. John T. Harrington: Is there any direct quantitative relationship between blood ethanol levels and the severity of the acidosis in patients who have repeated episodes of alcoholic ketoacidosis? Secondly, can ketoacidosis be induced in normal fasting individuals simply by infusing ethanol?

Dr. Cahill: I don't know, nor do I know whether anyone has tried inducing ketoacidosis by giving alcohol experimentally to fasting people.

Dr. Harrington: Does one ever see ketoacidosis in association with hypoglycemia?

Dr. Cahill: Yes, especially when hypoglycemia is severe. A large reducing load to the liver such as alcohol will reduce oxaloacetate to malate, making this substrate unavailable for gluconeogenesis. These circumstances may lead to alcoholic ketoacidosis complicated by severe hypoglycemia, i.e., with a blood sugar of 20 or 30 mg/dl. In this instance the most acute problem is to treat hypoglycemia.

Dr. Kassirer: I would like to return to the question of alkali therapy in severe diabetic ketoacidosis and alcohol ketoacidosis. Although it is true that patients with severe acidosis may recover uneventfully merely by treatment of ketosis, I have serious reservations about withholding alkali therapy when acidosis is extreme. Even with robust respiratory adaptation, patients with plasma bicarbonate concentrations of 2–3 mEq/liter typically have blood pH values less than 7.0, a state that in itself impairs the function of many organs and threatens life. When plasma bicarbonate concentration is this low, a further reduction of only 1 mEq/liter, consequent to a delay in initiation of therapy or a slight delay in response to therapy, will result in lethal acidosis. For this reason I believe that bicarbonate therapy is warranted in severe acidosis. The amount to give however, is the critical issue. I would advocate giving enough to raise plasma bicarbonate only 4–5 mEq/liter: this increase should raise blood pH only modestly and protect the patient. A greater increase in plasma bicarbonate is to be avoided. Given the propensity of hyperventilation to persist during the early phase of correction of acidosis, a large increase in plasma bicarbonate induced by alkali therapy can yield remarkable alkalemia. I know that opinions differ on this issue, but do you disagree with me?

Dr. Cahill: No, I agree with your view. But I would not allow alkali therapy to supplant or delay attempts to expand volume. Diabetic ketoacidosis is one of the few conditions in medicine in which expedience is critical. It is important to insert a large-bore needle in a large vein promptly and to administer isotonic saline rapidly. The only other crucial factor is the serum potassium concentration. If serum potassium is low or even normal, potassium should be given as soon as therapy with insulin has begun.

Dr. Nicolaos Madias (*Renal Service, NEMC*): Dr. Lemieux and co-workers have shown that ketone bodies depress renal ammoniagenesis [45,46]. Do you have any thoughts about this?

Dr. Cahill: No, I don't. I believe that the mechanisms that control ammoniagenesis by the kidney are still an open area for research. The controls and rate-limiting steps of ammonia production and even the pathway for ammonia production remain controversial.

Dr. Cohen: Dr. Cahill, you noted that this patient had a relatively low blood sugar given the degree of ketosis he had. Some investigators claim that a small percentage of patients with classic diabetic ketoacidosis are euglycemic [47]. Do you agree?

Dr. Cahill: One can't have euglycemia and diabetes; it's a matter of semantics. After a week of fasting it is possible to have ketosis with normal blood sugar, with plasma ketone levels as high as 6 mEq/liter. But there must be a net negative carbohydrate loss from the body to produce more ketosis. Let me illustrate by a small clinical "pearl": If a patient calls me in the evening to report that her urine tests strongly for sugar, that she cannot remember having taken her insulin in the morning, and that she is worried about developing ketoacidosis, the dietary history alone usually suffices to determine whether there are grounds for concern. If the patient has eaten her usual lunch and dinner, the chance of her having ketoacidosis is virtually zero. In fact, she may be insulin deficient but her glycosuria is the result of dietary "spillage": i.e., her hyperglycemia is not endogenous. If, on the other hand, the patient failed to eat lunch and ate little at dinner, there is a considerable probability that she is ketotic. She has sustained a net carbohydrate loss associated with gluconeogenesis and its accompanying ketosis. In other words, one can draw a parallel between the net negative carbohydrate balance and the degree of ketosis. Thus, I do not believe diabetic ketoacidosis can develop without copious urinary spillage of endogenously derived glucose.

Dr. Madias: It has been suggested that hypophosphatemia can cause insulin resistance and glucose intolerance [48]. In your opinion, does hypophosphatemia have important pathogenetic and/or therapeutic implications for the patient with diabetic ketoacidosis?

Dr. Cahill: If the patient has had chronic ketoacidosis with substantial lean tissue loss, phosphate depletion is almost certainly a concommitant feature. Once one gives insulin, phosphate moves into cells. For this reason potassium should be given as the phosphate salt. I am not convinced that administering phosphate ordinarily is critical, but if the individual is debilitated, I prefer to give potassium as phosphate rather than as chloride.

Dr. Cohen: The starving person who uses ketone bodies instead of glucose to fuel the brain must, as a consequence, develop some degree of acidosis. Is there any metabolic advantage to the acidosis per se?

Dr. Cahill: That is an important question, because ketosis is the basis of the protein-sparing effect of modified fast. Namely, if one completely deprives people of food and then gives them a little bit of protein, they maintain nitrogen balance. But the process is very inefficient. One has to administer approximately 80–100 g of protein to spare about 20 g. This 20 g would be lost if no protein were given.

Dr. Cohen: There is no reason, I gather, to think that the inevitable acidosis is advantageous.

Dr. Cahill: No, but there are normal people in the world who are chronically acidotic. The blubber-eating Eskimo is the prototype.

Dr. Cohen: As illustrated by today's patient, the ratio of β-hydroxybutyric acid to acetoacetic acid is unusually high in alcoholic ketoacidosis. This circumstance often poses a diagnostic problem on the wards because the nitroprusside reaction does not detect β-hydroxybutyrate. Is there any convenient way for the clinician or, for that matter, the routine clinical laboratory to estimate the concentration of this substance?

Dr. Cahill: The best approach is to measure plasma bicarbonate concentration and obtain a rough estimation of acetoacetate using one of the crude bedside tests. A positive acetoacetate level and a very low plasma bicarbonate concentration suggest ketosis with a high level of β -hydroxybutyrate. The combination of a barely positive acetoacetate test and a very low plasma bicarbonate concentration signifies either a very reduced state with high concentrations of β-hydroxybutyrate or else a coincidental lactic acidosis. Fortunately, as far as treatment is concerned, it does not make too much difference because therapy is directed at correcting volume deficiency, at returning blood sugar toward normal with insulin, and at correcting acidosis with alkali if the situation is life threatening.

References

1. Cahill GF, Herrera MG, Morgan AP, Soeldner JS, Steinke J, Levy AL, Reichard GA Jr, Kipnis DM: Hormone-fuel interrelationships during fasting. J Clin Invest 45:1751–1769, 1966
2. Cahill FG: Starvation in man. N Engl J Med 282:668–675, 1970
3. Jenkins DW, Eckel RE, Craig JW: Alcoholic ketoacidosis. JAMA 217:177–183, 1971

4. Levy LV, Duga V, Girgin M, Gordon EE: Ketoacidosis associated with alcoholism in nondiabetic subjects. Ann Intern Med 78:213–219, 1973
5. Cooperman MT, Davidoff F, Spark R, Pallotta V: Critical studies of alcoholic ketoacidosis. Diabetes 23:433–439, 1974
6. McGarry JD, Mannaerts GP, Foster DW: A possible role for malonyl CoA in the regulation of hepatic fatty acid oxidation and ketogenesis. J Clin Invest 60:265–270, 1977
7. McGarry JD, Foster DW: Hormonal control of ketogenesis. Biochemical considerations. Ann Intern Med 137:495–501, 1977
8. McGarry JD, Foster DW: Diabetic ketoacidosis. In Rifkin H, Raskin B (eds.): Diabetes Mellitus, Vol. 5. New York, American Diabetes Association, 1981, pp. 185–194
9. Robinson AM, Williamson DH: Physiological roles of ketone bodies as substrates and signals in mammalian tissues. Physiol Rev 60:143–187, 1980
10. Fenselau A: Ketone body metabolism in normal and diabetic man. In Brownlee M (ed.): Handbook of Diabetes Mellitus, Vol. 3. New York, Garland STPM Press, 1981, pp. 143–208
11. Liljenquist JE: Ketogenesis and its regulation. In Brownlee M (ed.): Handbook of Diabetes Mellitus, Vol. 3. New York, Garland STPM Press, 1981, pp. 119–142.
12. Brownlee M: *Handbook of Diabetes Mellitus*, Vols. 1–5. New York, Garland STPM Press, 1981
13. Reichard GA Jr, Owen OE, Haff AC, Paul P. Bortz WM: Ketone-body production and oxidation in fasting obese humans. J Clin Invest 53:508–515, 1974
14. Reichard GA, Haff AC, Skutches CL, Paul P. Holroyde CP, Owen OE: Plasma acetone metabolism in the fasting human. J Clin Invest 63:619–626, 1979
15. Garber AJ, Menzel PH, Boden G, Owen OE: Hepatic ketogenesis and gluconeogenesis in humans. J Clin Invest 54:981–989, 1974
16. Flatt JP: On the maximal possible rate of ketogenesis. Diabetes 21:50–53, 1972
17. Cherrington AD: Gluconeogenesis: Its regulation by insulin and glucagon. In Brownlee M, (ed.): Handbook of Diabetes Mellitus, Vol 3. New York, Garland STPM Press, 1981, pp. 49–117
18. Exton JH: Gluconeogenesis. Metabolism 21:945–990, 1972
19. Avruch J, Witters LA, Alexander MC, Bush MA: The effects of insulin and glucagon on the phosphorylation of hepatic cytoplasmic peptides. J Biol Chem 253:4754–4761, 1978
20. Sapir DG, Owen OE: Renal conservation of ketone bodies during starvation. Metabolism 24:23–33, 1975
21. Owen OE, Reichard GA Jr: Human forearm metabolism during progressive starvation. J Clin Invest 50:1536–1545, 1971
22. Owen OE, Reichard GA Jr, Boden G, Patel MS, Trapp VE: Interrelationships among key tissues on the utilization of metabolic substrates. In Katzen HM, Mahler RI, (eds.): Advances in Modern Nutrition, Vol. 2. New York, Wiley, 1978, pp. 517–550.
23. Raporport SI: Blood-Brain Barrier in Physiology and Medicine. New York, Raven Press, 1976

24. Owen OE, Morgan AP, Kemp HG, Sullivan JM, Herrera MG, Cahill GF: Brain metabolism during fasting. J Clin Invest 46:1589–1595, 1967
25. Owen OE, Felig P, Morgan AP, Wahren J, Cahill GF Jr: Liver and kidney metabolism during prolonged starvation. J Clin Invest 48:574–583, 1969
26. Nelson RA, Wahner HW, Jones JD, Ellefson RD, Zollman PE: Metabolism of bears before, during, and after winter sleep. Am J Physiol 224:491–496, 1973
27. LeMaho Y: The Emperor Penguin: A strategy to live and breed in the cold. Am Sci 65:679–693, 1977
28. Göttstein U, Müller W, Berghoff W, Goartner H, Held K: Zur utilisation von nicht-veresterten fettsauren und ketonkorpen im gehirn des menschen. Klin Wochenschr 49:406–411, 1971
29. Göttstein U, Held K, Müller W, Berghoff W: Utilization of ketone bodies by the human brain. In Meyer JS, Reivich M, Lechner H, Eichhorn O, (eds.): Research on the Cerebral Circulation, Fifth International Salzburg Conference, 1970. Springfield, Ill., Thomas, 1972, pp. 137–145
30. Drenick EJ, Alvarez LC, Tamasi GC, Brichman AJ: Resistance of symptomatic insulin reactions after fasting. J Clin Invest 51:2757–2762, 1972
31. Flatt JP, Blackburn GL, Randerg G, Stanburg JB: Effects of ketone body infusion on hypoglycemic reaction in postabsorptive dogs. Metabolism 23:151–158, 1974
32. Müller WA, Aoki TT, Flatt JP, Blackburn GL, Egdahl RH, Cahill GF Jr: Effects of β-hydroxybutyrate, glycerol and free fatty acid infusions on glucagon and epinephrine secretion in dogs during acute hypoglycemia. Metabolism 25:1077–1086, 1976
33. Madison, LL, Seldin DW: Ammonia excretion and renal enzymatic adaptation in human subjects, as disclosed by administration of precursor amino acids. J Clin Invest 37:1615–1627, 1958
34. Ruderman NB, Ross PS, Berger M, Goodman MN: Regulation of glucose and ketone-body metabolism in brain of anaesthetized rats. Biochem J 138:1–10, 1974
35. Felig P, Owen OE, Wahren J, Cahill GF Jr: Amino acid metabolism during prolonged starvation. J Clin Invest 48:584–594, 1969
36. Pozefsky T, Felig P, Tobin J, Soeldner JS, Cahill GR Jr: Amino acid balance across tissues of the forearm in post-absorptive man. Effects of insulin at two dose levels. J Clin Invest 48:2273–2282, 1969
37. Marliss EB, Aoki TT, Pozefsky T, Most AS, Cahill GF Jr: Muscle and splanchnic glutamine and glutamate metabolism in post-operative and starved man. J Clin Invest 50:824–817, 1971
38. Felig P: Amino acid metabolism in man. Annu Rev Biochem 44:933–955, 1975
39. Aoki TT, Toews CV, Rossini AA, Ruderman NB, Cahill GF Jr: Gluconeogenic substrate levels in fasting man. Adv Enzyme Regul 13:329–336, 1976
40. Sherwin RS: Amino acid and protein metabolism in normal and diabetic humans. In Brownlee M (ed.): Handbook of Diabetes Mellitus, Vol. 3, New York, Garland STPM Press, 1981, pp. 1–47
41. Aoki TT, Finley RJ, Cahill GF Jr: The redox state and regulation of amino acid metabolism in man. Biochem Soc Symp 43:17–29, 1978
42. Sapir DG, Owen OE, Pozefsky T, Walser M: Nitrogen sparing induced by

a mixture of essential amino acids given chiefly as their ketoanalogues during prolonged starvation in obese subjects. *J. Clin Invest* 54:974–980, 1974
43. Sapir DG, Walser M: Nitrogen sparing induced early in starvation by infusion of branched-chain ketoacids. Metabolism 26:304–308, 1977
44. Sherwin RS, Hendler RG, Felig P: Effect of ketone infusions on amino acid and nitrogen metabolism in man. J Clin Invest 55:1382–1390, 1975
45. Lemieux G, Vinay P, Robitaille P, Plante GE, Lussier Y, Martin P: The effect of ketone bodies on renal ammoniagenesis. J Clin Invest 50:1781–1791, 1971
46. Lemieux G, Pichette C, Vinay P, Gougoux A: Cellular mechanisms of the antiammoniagenic effect of ketone bodies in the dog. Am J Physiol 239:F420–F426, 1980
47. Munro JF, Campbell IW, McCuisk AC, Duncan LJP: Euglycemic diabetic ketoacidosis. Br Med J 2:578, 1973
48. DeFronzo RA, Lang R; Hypophosphatemia and glucose intolerance: Evidence for tissue insensitivity to insulin. N Engl J Med 303:1259–1263, 1980

Part III

Disturbances in Calcium and Phosphorus Metabolism

Introduction

This section includes four Forums devoted to disordered calcium and phosphorus metabolism. Dr. Francis P. Muldowney leads off the section with an illuminating discussion of a case of surgically proven hyperparathyroidism in a woman with recurrent renal colic, nephrocalcinosis, and repeatedly normal values for serum calcium. He employs this case deftly to illustrate the usefulness of his recommended scheme for the differential diagnosis of renal stone disease. He presents his opinion of the potential value of the ionized serum calcium measurement as a supplement to other tests, especially in distinguishing between mild hyperparathyroidism and idiopathic hypercalciuria. Dr. Muldowney, Research Professor of Medicine at St. Vincent's Hospital, Dublin, Ireland, has earned an international reputation as a clinical scholar and investigator. His erudite review of hypercalciuric states is amplified not only by the penetrating questions posed by those gathered in Dublin for this Forum but by an accompanying Forum commentary prepared by Dr. Fredric L. Coe. Dr. Coe, a noted American authority on renal stone disease, considers the difficulties often encountered in the differential diagnosis of hypercalciuria that stem from the imprecision inherent in certain of the laboratory measurements upon which we rely.

Dr. Samuel O. Thier discusses a case of chronic renal insufficiency in a young woman who also manifested hypercalcemia. His discussion incorporates several instructive elements: a review of the pathophysiology of secondary hyperparathyroidism in patients with renal insufficiency; a summary of the characteristic features of primary hyperparathyroidism; a reminder of the large variety of ways whereby hypercalcemia can damage the kidney; and a carefully reasoned reconstruction of the sequence of events that likely resulted in the findings in the case presented. Dr. Thier is Chairman of the Department of Medicine at the Yale University School of Medicine and is renowned for his gifts as a clinician-teacher; these gifts are fully in evidence in this Forum.

Dr. Jack W. Coburn, a leading authority on metabolic bone disease, presents a case of severe renal osteodystrophy occurring in a man with end-stage renal disease. This perplexing and often disabling complication of chronic renal failure is known to be multifactorial in origin and to require thoughtful analysis in each instance to pinpoint the most appropriate therapy. His Forum contains new information about the role of altered vitamin D metabolism and about the influence of secondary hyperparathyroidism in the pathogenesis of renal osteodystrophy. Dr. Coburn, Professor of Medicine at the UCLA School of Medicine, fields a number of difficult questions during the ensuing open discussion and his answers serve to elaborate on the many troublesome features of this important condition.

Dr. Eberhard Ritz, Head of the Division of Nephrology at the University of Heidelberg in the Federal Republic of Germany, presents a fascinating discussion of acute hypophosphatemia occurring after the initiation of parenteral hyperalimentation in a patient with longstanding Crohn's disease and malnutrition. Dr. Ritz uses this case as a springboard for a review of the pathophysiology of phosphate depletion and of the widely divergent clinical manifestations of this serious electrolyte disturbance. He also offers recommendations regarding the prevention of this complication. This Forum, held in Heidelberg, offered an opportunity for many local experts to participate in the informative discussion.

Diagnostic Approach to Hypercalciuria

Principal Discussant
Francis P. Muldowney

Case Presentation

A 40-year-old woman was admitted to the metabolic ward of St. Vincent's Hospital in Dublin. Two years previously, she had been admitted to the genitourinary ward because of left renal colic. At that time, an i.v. urogram showed bilateral spotty nephrocalcinosis in kidneys of normal size, and a solitary renal cyst was visible on the right side. Laboratory findings disclosed the following: hematocrit, 47%; blood urea nitrogen (BUN), 10 mg/100 ml; serum sodium, 141 mEq; serum potassium, 4.4 mEq; serum chloride, 104 mEq; serum bicarbonate, 26 mEq/liter; serum uric acid, 3.8 mg; total calcium concentration from a single sample of serum, 10.7 mg (normal, 9.0–10.6 mg, 95% limits), and ionized serum calcium, 5.5 mg/100 ml (normal, 4.1–5.3 mg/100 ml, 95% limits); urine calcium, 262 mg/24 h (normal < 250 mg/24 h); the urine sediment was unremarkable, and a culture of the urine was sterile.

One year later, the patient entered the outpatient clinic with an episode of right renal colic. On this occasion, total serum calcium concentration was 10.3 mg and ionized serum calcium was 5.5 mg/100 ml; a simultaneous parathyroid hormone (iPTH) level was 0.18 ng/ml as measured by radioimmunoassay using the Slatopolsky carboxy-terminal specific antiserum (normal range 0.0–0.33 ng/ml). The findings of a second i.v. urogram indicated no change in kidney status; there was no evidence of pelvic-ureteric dilation. The patient was admitted subsequently to the metabolic ward for investigation of hypercalciuria, nephrocalcinosis, and marginal hypercalcemia, although iPTH level was apparently normal.

On admission the patient had no history of excessive ingestion of milk, oral alkali preparations, or vitamin supplements. Her mother and brother each had had one episode of renal colic in the past. Physical examination was unremarkable with blood pressure of 110/70 mmHg. Laboratory findings revealed the following: hematocrit, 43%; white blood cell count, 6700/mm^3; sedimentation rate, 1 mm/h; urine protein was absent; EKG was normal; chest radiogram showed healed tuberculous foci; radiograms of the hands were normal; BUN, 12 mg/100 ml; serum sodium, 142 mEq; serum potassium, 4 mEq; serum chloride, 107 *mEq; serum bicarbonate, 23.5 mEq/liter; total protein, 7.2 g; serum albumin, 4.6 g/100 ml; alkaline phosphatase, 7.4 King-Armstrong U; serum creatinine, 0.9 mg/100 ml. For 4 days, a fixed diet that contained 500 mg of calcium and 1 g of phosphorus was given to the patient; laboratory values for serum taken on the morning of days 3 and 4 were total calcium, 9.9 and 10.0 mg:ionized calcium, 5.2 and 5.1 mg: prosphate was 2.7 mg/100 ml on both mornings (normal 2.6–4.2 mg/100 ml). The following additional laboratory values were obtained on mornings 3 and 4: urinary calcium, 323 and 289 mg/24 h; percent of tubular reabsorption of phosphate, 74.5 and 76.8% (normal, 83–87%). Serum iPTH levels were 0.57, 0.35, and 0.55 ng/ml. The serum level of 25-hydroxy vitamin D was 6.9 ng/ml (normal, 11.8 ± 4.0 ng/ml).*

In spite of five normal values for total serum calcium obtained in the fasting state (mean, 10 mg/100 ml), it was decided to refer the patient for surgical exploration of the neck because her mean ionized serum calcium concentration of 5.4 mg/100 ml was at the upper 95% limit of normal, and because three of four iPTH values were elevated. Serum taken on the morning of parathyroid surgery showed total serum calcium concentration to be 10.5 mg and ionized serum calcium, 5.7 mg/100 ml. The 24-h urinary calcium excretion was 349 mg. The surgical procedure revealed an enlarged parathyroid gland. The gland, weighing 360 mg, was removed; the tissue was adenomatous on histologic examination. Two other parathyroid glands were biopsied and proved to be normal. The patient's postoperative course was uneventful. Review after 5 months revealed a total serum calcium concentration of 8.8 mg, an ionized serum calcium concentration of 5 mg/100 ml, a urinary calcium excretion of 184 mg/day, and a serum iPTH level of 0.14 ng/ml.

Discussion

Dr. Francis P. Muldowney *(Research Professor of Medicine, University College, and Physician-in-Charge, Metabolism and Renal Unit, St. Vincent's Hospital, Dublin, Ireland)*: I believe the diagnostic problem of renal stone disease is best approached, not by a long and learned list of causes, but by remembering the relative frequency of the most important ones. In 1970 Yendt [1] provided a most helpful breakdown of his series of 439 patients with renal stone disease: he showed that 42% had idiopathic hypercalciuria, 11% had primary hyperparathyroidism, 8% had urinary infection, 5% had uric acid stone, and 2% had cystinuria; no cause was found in 24%. This is a convenient list to remember at the bedside and puts into perspective the relative importance of, for example, infection/obstruction, which is a minor cause, and idiopathic hypercalciuria, which is a major cause of renal stone disease. One may note that more sophisticated renal tubular disease, such as classical renal tubular acidosis or medullary sponge kidney, scarcely deserve mention. Nevertheless, a systematic approach to the diagnosis in each patient must attempt to be reasonably comprehensive as well as crudely practical; one must know each horse in the race as well as the betting odds. Idiopathic hypercalciuria may be the "favorite;" but it may just occasionally take second place to an outsider such as milk-alkali syndrome!

With this in mind, Fig. 1 sets out a sequence of diagnostic steps using certain key techniques in the order best calculated to give weight to the major causes, while allowing necessary consideration to the minor ones. The first question is whether hypercalciuria is present. If not, we move into a minor pathway to consider causes such as infection/obstruction, urate stone, or cystinuria. Patients with either of the latter two conditions frequently have a familial history that is helpful, and laboratory data such as serum uric acid concentration and results of urinary amino acid chromatography enable one to make the diagnosis. Infection, obstruction, urate stone, or cystinuria are causal factors in some 15 to 20% of all patients with renal stone disease [1].

The presence of hypercalciuria may be documented in a number of ways. The standard indicator is 24-h urinary calcium excretion—upper limits of normal are 300 mg in the male and 250 mg in the female [2]. The patient under discussion today, a female, had a 24-h urinary calcium excretion in excess of 250 mg on 2 successive days while receiving a diet that contained 500 mg of calcium. An additional index of hypercalciuria is the fasting morning "spot" urine calcium concentration as

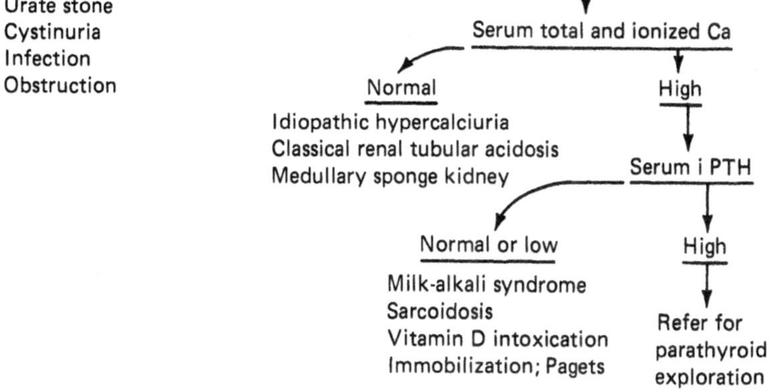

Fig. 1. Suggested scheme of approach to diagnosis in renal stone disease based on presence or absence of hypercalciuria, hypercalcemia, and serum parathyroid hormone (iPTH) elevation.

Table 1. Urinary and serum calcium (Ca) in the fasting state and following oral loading with Ca, 30 mg/kg of body weight.

		Control (n = 9)	Idiopathic Hypercalciuria (n = 18)	Control vs. Idiopathic Hypercalciuria
Creatinine (Cr) clearance (ml/min)		106 ± 16	103 ± 17	NS
Total serum Ca (mg/100 ml)	Fasting	9.25 ± 0.41	9.35 ± 0.36	NS
	Postload[a]	10.0 ± 0.52	10.24 ± 0.48	NS
		<0.02	<0.001	
Ionized serum Ca (mg/100 ml)	Fasting	5.02 ± 0.29	4.86 ± 0.21	NS
	Postload	5.24 ± 0.24	5.16 ± 0.31	NS
		<0.2	<0.005	
Urine Ca (mg/100 ml GF)	Fasting	0.07 ± 0.051	0.149 ± 0.078	<0.01
	Postload	0.241 ± 0.069	0.355 ± 0.084	<0.005
		<0.001	<0.001	
Urine Ca/Cr ratio	Fasting	0.068 ± 0.044	0.149 ± 0.076	<0.001
	Postload	0.233 ± 0.077	0.354 ± 0.069	<0.001
		<0.001	<0.001	
Urine Ca as percentage filtered ionized Ca	Fasting	1.87 ± 0.87	3.23 ± 1.48	<0.05
	Postload	4.45 ± 1.27	7.04 ± 1.69	<0.001
		<0.01	<0.001	

[a]Postload data refer to the collection period 3 to 4 h following ingestion of the calcium.
Note: n, number of patients; GF, glomerular filtrate.

it relates to filtered calcium load (Table 1). This measurement has the great advantage of avoiding the cumbersome collection of total 24-h volume, which is prone to collection errors and the consequent variability of results. For instance, a fasting urinary calcium-to-creatinine concentration ratio or a urinary calcium per 100 ml of glomerular filtrate that exceeds 0.11 is likely to represent hypercalciuria. The "spot" urine calcium-to-creatinine concentration ratio provides a useful screening test for the busy nephrologist and may be repeated as often as desired.

If hypercalciuria is present as in our patient today, the next question is whether the *serum* calcium concentration is elevated. If the serum calcium concentration appears to be normal, and if no other demonstrable cause is apparent, the diagnosis of idiopathic hypercalciuria can be made with some assurance. If the serum calcium concentration is elevated, however, the alternate pathway of investigation should be taken using iPTH level as a main determinant of management. Note that this pathway ends with surgical neck exploration for a parathyroid adenoma, or with evaluation directed toward nonparathyroid causes of hypercalcemia, most of which are reversible, such as milk-alkali syndrome. Before proceeding along either route, one must be reasonably certain that hypercalcemia does or does not exist. If the wrong route is taken because of incorrect or inadequate laboratory evaluation, the patient may receive inappropriate therapy. There are two classic examples of this problem: administration of thiazide therapy for supposed idiopathic hypercalciuria that is really undocumented primary hyperparathyroidism, and fruitless neck exploration and biopsy in a patient with normal parathyroid glands. I should mention one further unfortunate consequence of the wrong decision at this critical juncture. The definition and subsequent investigation and classification of patients who are predisposed to the formation of renal stones may be unintentionally obscured, and incorrect assumptions may be made concerning etiology and pathophysiology for each subgroup, unless clear lines of distinction and definition are seen and agreed to by all workers in the field. The techniques that are available today were not available 10, 15, or 30 years ago when many of the standard investigations were made, [3,4,5]. At that time, conclusions were based on values for total serum calcium or perhaps ultrafilterable calcium concentration only. It is now possible to measure the ionized fraction of the calcium concentration by ion-specific electrodes and the iPTH level by a sensitive radioimmunoassay; thus, the onus is on us to assess the value of these data in the same critical fashion as was done for the less revealing data relied on in the past.

Idiopathic hypercalciuria accounts for 42% of all cases of renal stone disease [1]. Unfortunately, it resembles the next most common cause, primary hyperparathyroidism, in many ways. The critical distinguishing feature between the two disorders is the presence or absence of hypercalcemia: Both frequently show hypercalciuria; both may show hypophosphatemia with lowered tubular phosphate reabsorption; and to make difficulty doubly defiant, Coe et al, [6] have demonstrated that both may show elevated immunoreactive serum iPTH levels. Our immediate problem in this patient, therefore, is one familiar to all nephrologists, that of differentiating between idiopathic hypercalciuria and primary hyperparathyroidism. Since such differentiation is achieved classically by the presence or absence of hypercalcemia, we must devote some time to that particular point.

Florid hypercalcemia is, of course, identified easily—i.e., a serum calcium concentration above 11 mg/100 ml, which corresponds to 99% confidence limit (+3 SD) of the normal range. Our control studies show that serum calcium values between 10.9 and 10.6 mg/100 ml correspond to the 99 and 95% confidence limits, respectively, and thus would be expected to occur in 2.5% of the normal population; values between 10.5 and 10.2 mg/100 ml (+1 SD) would be expected in about one-sixth of the population. "Hypercalcemia" or "normocalcemia" are, therefore, inappropriately absolutist terms that should be defined rather by the levels of confidence or degrees of doubt! We prefer not to use the term "normclacemia" and consider all values above 10 mg and below 11 mg/100 ml to be indicative of marginal hypercalcemia. These values immediately suggest to us the following tactics: (1) repeated, careful laboratory examination of samples taken in the fasting state and with minimal venous stasis and (2) further corroboration by measuring the ionized serum calcium concentration with an ion-specific, flow-through electrode. In the patient discussed today, the grand mean value for total calcium concentration was 10.0 mg/100 ml—less than 1 SD above the average normal level—whereas the ionized serum calcium concentration was more clearly elevated at 5.3 mg/100 ml, or 2 SD above the average normal value. This comparison reflects accurately the relative values of the two techniques in our experience [7]. In short, a marginal finding for total serum calcium concentration in primary hyperparathyroidism appears to be more easily defined, and with greater statistical confidence, by measuring the ionized fraction of the serum calcium concentration.

If significant hypercalcemia can be confirmed, the next question is whether it is of parathyroid or nonparathyroid origin. The logical sequence leads to measurement of serum iPTH level. We have used Slatopolsky's excellent antiserum for some years, and the results in the important group of patients who have marginal primary hyperparathyroidism are illustrated in Fig. 2. In 1975 and 1976, we originally defined the limits above which neck exploration should be advised. At that time, we felt that an ionized serum calcium concentration above 5.6 mg/100 ml, i.e., +3 SD, with a serum iPTH level above the upper limit of normal, 0.33 ng/ml, should be the proper conservative guidelines, which would avoid inappropriate surgery in patients who did not have primary hyperparathyroidism [7]. With accumulating experience, we have now lowered the limit to 5.3 mg/100 ml, i.e., +2 SD, for ionized serum calcium concentration, provided that the iPTH level is elevated. Twelve patients with values for total serum calcium of 10.9 mg/100 ml or less—six with 10.4 mg/100 ml or less—and ionized serum calcium of 5.3 mg/100 ml or more have been referred for neck exploration. In ten patients, iPTH level was available, and it was elevated in nine. In each patient, the presence of primary hyperparathyroidism was confirmed at surgery: adenoma was found in ten patients, and multiple hyperplasia was found in two.

It should be noted further that seven of the patients with idiopathic hypercalciuria continue to show ionized serum calcium values at or above the +1 SD level. Although iPTH levels are normal or low in the group, one must accept the possibility that these may represent primary

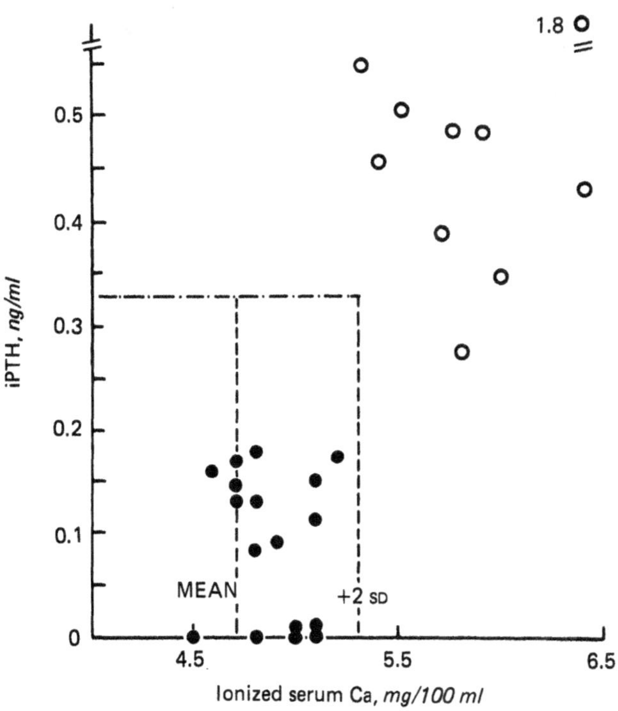

Fig. 2. Relationship in renal stone disease of serum parathyroid hormone (iPTH) to ionized serum calcium (Ca) values in patients with marginal primary hyperparathyroidism (*open circles*) and idiopathic hypercalciuria (*closed circles*). Mean +2 SD indicated for ionized Ca. Total normal range indicated for iPTH. "Marginal" refers to proven primary hyperparathyroidism with serum total Ca between 10 and 10.9 mg/100 ml.

Table 2. Urinary calcium (Ca) in relation to serum Ca concentration and parathyroid hormone (iPTH) level in primary hyperparathyroidism and in idiopathic hypercalciuria.

		Urine		Serum		
		C_{cr} (ml/min)	Ca (mg/24 h)	Total Ca (mg/100 ml)	Ionized Ca (mg/100 ml)	iPTH (ng/ml)
Hypercalcemic hyperparathyroidism	Mean	72.9	434	12.4	6.8	0.81
	SD	23.2	210	1.5	1.2	0.22
	N	11	11	11	11	11
Marginal hyperparathyroidism	Mean	94.6	329	10.5	5.7	0.71
	SD	25.4	98	0.2	0.3	0.34
	N	12	14	14	14	12
Idiopathic hypercalciuria	Mean	103	372	9.4	4.9	0.09
	SD	17	63	0.4	0.2	.07
	N	18	18	18	18	17
Normal			<300 (male) <250 (female)	9.8 ± 0.9	4.7 ± 0.6 (±2 SD)	0.15 ± 0.06

Note: Urinary Ca is seen to be elevated in all, including those patients with hyperparathyroidism who have minimal elevation of serum Ca concentration (marginal hyperparathyroidism). C_{cr}, creatinine clearance; N, number of patients.

hyperparathyroidism of mild degree, which is undetectable by current immunoassay techniques. Thus, it is possible that all patients with idiopathic hypercalciuria reflect a spectrum of mild but currently undetectable hyperparathyroidism. We do not, however, advocate neck surgery in this group since hypercalciuria can be easily controlled by oral chlorthalidone in the majority of patients.

In the case of hypercalcemia that is not associated with hyperparathyroidism, as shown by normal or low iPTH levels (Fig. 1), the clinical history and routine investigation should carefully exclude known causes such as milk-alkali syndrome, Paget's disease, prolonged immobilization, vitamin D intoxication, and sarcoidosis. All of these may be associated with hypercalcemia, which is often rather fleeting and mild in character. Milk-alkali syndrome represents a form of calcium-induced renal tubular alkalosis with a high tubular bicarbonate threshold [8,9]. Vitamin D ingestion, like milk-alkali intake, may not be admitted or even realized by the patient, and measurements of serum 25-hydroxy vitamin D concentration may be necessary [10]. Both vitamin D and milk-alkali ingestion are associated with systemic alkalosis in contrast with the acidosis and hyperchloremia that may be seen in hyperparathyroidism [11]. The patient under discussion today showed a mild hyperchloremic acidosis, which was a helpful diagnostic indicator.

The mechanism of hypercalciuria in hypercalcemia is thought to be a simple increase in filtered calcium load. An exception to this general rule would be provided if glomerular filtration rate (GFR) had decreased, as commonly happens in chronic cases. Some have taken the view that primary hyperparathyroidism is also an exception because the effect of PTH-induced hypercalcemia to increase the filtered load of calcium is thought to be offset by a direct stimulating effect of the hormone on tubular reabsorption [12]. It is difficult, however, to find convincing data to support this conclusion in the clinical sphere. In the patients studied by us, shown in Table 2, hypercalciuria was visible even in those patients with primary hyperparathyroidism in whom serum calcium concentration and filtered load were minimally elevated. This finding held true both for the data derived from 24-h urine collections and for the data derived from fasting morning urine specimens [13]. Thus, even if the filtered calcium load is elevated to a minimal degree, it is not compensated for by increased tubular calcium reabsorption despite high circulating iPTH levels. Primary hyperparathyroidism therefore remains an important cause of hypercalciuria even in patients with minimal hypercalcemia. Whether hypercalciuria in primary hyperparathyroidism at any given calcium concentration is less than in other causes of hypercalcemia may require further documentation. At this point, however, the argument becomes somewhat academic and scarcely relevant to the differential diagnosis of clinical hypercalciuria. Genuinely relevant, however, is the close resemblance of so called "resorptive" hypercalciuria due to primary hyperparathyroidism and "renal" hypercalciuria in the sense that both clearly show increased fractional calcium excretion. Thus a renal calcium "leak" becomes yet another point of similarity between primary hyperparathyroidism and its great simulator, idiopathic hypercalciuria.

If hypercalcemia is excluded, our diagnostic scheme (Fig. 1) leads to the category of normocalcemic hypercalciuria of which idiopathic hypercalciuria is the most important member. Other causes, such as classical or distal renal tubular acidosis and medullary sponge kidney, are readily excluded by serum and urine acid-base measurements or by careful i.v. urographic examination for caliectasis. The etiology of idiopathic hypercalciuria has been a favorite topic of argument for some years because the intestinal calcium hyperabsorption theory [5,14,15] has been opposed to the renal calcium "leak" theory supported by Coe et al. [6]. Based on our recent measurements of fractional excretion of filtered ionized calcium, we have concluded that all patients with iodiopathic hypercalciuria can be shown to have a renal calcium leak [13]. Table 1 lists urine calcium expressed in three different ways in relation to GFR or filtered calcium load. Compared with normal control patients, the group of patients with idiopathic hypercalciuria excrete a higher proportion of filtered calcium. Most patients show excessive fractional excretion even in the fasting state. Almost all patients show this characteristic in the period following oral calcium loading. We have recently confirmed this postload tubular "leak" pattern even in those patients with hypercalciuria who have the mildest degree of calcium leak, as indicated by normal fasting urinary calcium-to-creatinine concentration rations [13]. This latter group had previously been designated to be "absorptive" by Pak et al. [15].

I should like to stress that we have looked carefully in our patients with idiopathic hypercalciuria at serum calcium concentration following calcium loading. The earlier data of Peacock et al. [5] had suggested a greater increment in serum calcium concentration in patients with idiopathic hypercalciuria compared with control patients. This indeed has been one of the major arguments adduced in favor of the intestinal hyperabsorption theory [14,15]. We have not, however, found any difference in postabsorptive serum calcium concentration between our two groups; both control patients and patients with idiopathic hypercalciuria reached exactly similar concentrations of total and, in particular, of ionized serum calcium [13]. Thus, the sequence postulated by Pak et al. [15]—calcium hyperabsorption causing hypercalcemia, which suppresses PTH and thereby diminishes tubular calcium reabsorption—cannot be sustained in view of the essential absence of relative postabsorptive hypercalcemia. Neither can normal or low values for serum iPTH (Table 2) obtained 12 h after the last meal in fasting patients with hypercalciuria be reasonably related to a theoretical postprandial hypercalcemia. In retrospect, the patients thought to have idiopathic hypercalciuria by Peacock et al. [5] included several who initially were suspiciously hypercalcemic compared with controls and indeed overlapped the range of 10 to 10.5 mg/100 ml, which includes many of our patients with marginal primary hyperparathyroidism (Table 2). It does not therefore seem surprising that following oral calcium loading the serum levels of such patients should show an inordinate increase, as indeed our own data in similar patients with marginal hyperparathyroidism amply confirm [13]. Once again, one must stress the importance of careful preliminary exclusion of masked primary hyperparathyroidism with marginal hypercalcemia from any apparent idiopathic hypercalciuria grouping before proceeding to make deductions concerning intestinal or renal tubular function. Of course, some degree of intestinal hyperabsorption does exist, and this has indeed been demonstrated in external balance studies [16]. Dr. John Ryan of our department (Ryan, personal communication, 1979) has confirmed such a pattern using ^{45}Ca in five of our patients with idiopathic hypercalciuria. Hyperabsorption may, however, be a compensation for renal calcium loss rather than an initiating stimulus, as was pointed out by Jackson and Doncaster in 1959 [17]. Our data are consistent with this veiw.

To summarize so far, our data suggest strongly that hypercalciuria in the idiopathic syndrome is due to diminished renal tubular calcium reabsorption, or a renal "leak." We therefore agree essentially with the concept supported by Coe et al. [6], with the important exception that we do not confirm their postulate that such a leak gives rise to secondary hyperparathyroidism. In our experience to date, all patients with genuniely normal calcium concentration who had stone formation and hypercalciuria—i.e., idiopathic hypercalciuria carefully defined—showed normal serum iPTH levels. Those of our patients with hypercalciuria who showed elevated iPTH levels also showed significantly elevated serum concentration of ionized calcium and were later shown at neck surgery to have primary hyperparathyroidism.

Indeed, one must question seriously the assumption that a mild chronic increase in urinary calcium excretion causes a decrease in ionized serum calcium concentration with a resulting increase in serum iPTH levels [6]. McCarron et al, [18] have recently demonstrated that an increase in urinary calcium to 300 mg/day on a chronic basis by oral sodium loading does not result in a decrease in ionized serum calcium concentration or an increase in iPTH level. The earlier study of Coe et al, [6] had demonstrated that an increase in urinary calcium concentration could be induced by daily furosemide administration for 1 week. Under these circumstances, iPTH levels increased, but it is not clear that the increase in urinary calcium excretion was the responsible factor or even that hypocalcemia resulted. A decrease in extracellular fluid volume, for instance, may have been important. Rosenbaum et al, [19] have shown that an increase in antidiuretic hormone excretion, such as might be expected following furosemide administration, is accompanied by increasing iPTH plasma levels. The data of McCarron et al, [18] are important because they showed that an increase in urinary calcium excretion produced by sodium loading with *increased* extracellular fluid volume resulted in no change in ionized serum calcium concentration and a slight decrease in iPTH level.

The mechanism of the renal tubular "leak" of calcium in idiopathic hypercalciuria must at present remain open to speculation. Elevated serum concentrations of 1,25-dihydroxy vitamin D have been reported [20] and may represent either a primary defect or one generated by the phosphate depletion that results from the well-described defect in tubular phosphate reabsorption. Alternatively, as mentioned earlier, a spectrum of underlying primary hyperparathyroidism of varying mildness or severity may induce both renal phosphate loss and excess generation of 1,25-dihydroxy vitamin D in renal parenchyma. Whatever the ultimate defect may be, the net effect appears as hypercalciuria apparently due to diminished tubular calcium reabsorption, with intestinal hyperabsorption acting in a compensatory fashion only. In discussing this patient for the *Nephrology Forum,* it seems appropriate to rescue idiopathic hypercalciuria from its status as a plaything of the gastroenterologists and bring it back firmly to the kidney where it surely belongs!

Questions and Answers

Dr. John Donohoe *(Consultant Nephrologist, Mater Misericordiae Hospital, Dublin, Ireland)*: Thank you very much Dr. Muldowney for the eloquent discussion. Your stirring conclusion is dear to the heart of any nephrologist! I should like to begin the question and answer period by asking a general question. As you know, urinary calcium excretion is diminished by administration of thiazides in patients with idiopathic hypercalciuria. Coe has shown that serum iPTH levels, which are significantly higher than controls prior to thiazide therapy, return virtually to normal with thiazides [6]. He interpreted these findings to be consistent with secondary hyperparathyroidism consequent to a primary renal leak of calcium. In regard to the patient presented today, I wonder if you might have considered carrying out a therapeutic trial of thiazides to delineate further the mechanism of the hypercalciuria?

In addition, do you know of any studies that focus on "autonomy" of the parathyroid glands in idiopathic hypercalciuria? Have there been any efforts, for example, to determine by calcium infusion whether hyperparathyroidism is primary or secondary in such patients?

Dr. Muldowney: The difficulty about suppression tests is that not only can secondary hyperparathyroidism be suppressed, but many patients with primary hyperparathyroidism can ultimately be suppressed as well. Potts et al, [21] have shown that many patients with adenomatous parathyroid tissue have decreased plasma iPTH levels following calcium infusion, and we have confirmed that finding [7]. We have shown that, both in patients with secondary hyperparathyroidism of intestinal malabsorption and in those with adenomas or primary hyperparathyroidism, a calcium infusion will suppress iPTH levels. For that reason, it has always seemed to me to be unsatisfactory to use suppressibility as an index to determine whether a given patient has primary or secondary hyperparathyroidism. The data obtained by Coe et al, [6], I feel, can be interpreted as indicating primary hyperparathyroidism as easily as secondary hyperparathyroidism, although the latter was the chosen interpretation of the study. The same rationale applies to the recent data of Bordier et al, [22] in which sufficient 25-hydroxy vitamin D was given orally to raise serum calcium concentration. They found that in approximately one-half of the patients the iPTH level was suppressible by that technique; in the other half it was not, but the significance of this finding is not really clear.

Dr. John T. Harrington: Dr. Muldowney, I have a problem in understanding the precise reasons for hypercalciuria in patients with so-called normocalcemic hyperparathyroidism. It has been argued that patients with primary hyperparathyroidism are hypercalciuric because of the hypercalcemia and the consequent increased filtered load of calcium; the latter is thought to override the direct tubular effect of parathyroid hormone, namely, to increase distal calcium reabsorption. The patient presented today had a normal ionized serum calcium concentration at times, yet she was still hypercalciuric. How do you explain this?

Dr. Muldowney: This is an important point. As I mentioned earlier, we do know from micropuncture studies that the effect of PTH on the kidney is to promote the tubular reabsorption of calcium. This effect has been widely extrapolated in the clinical sphere to suggest that those patients who are hypercalcemic from hyperparathyroidism have a lower urinary calcium excretion than those who are hypercalcemic to the same degree from other causes. The data to support this hypothesis are amazingly scanty, so scanty that I cannot find any. Our population is in many ways an ideal group in which to conduct such a study because primary hyperparathyroidism is being defined in a group whose excess filtered load is very small because their degree of hypercalcemia is very minor (Table 2); if the effect of a high PTH level in promoting tubular reabsorption were ever going to overcome the effect of a high filtered load, it should do it in this group. In fact, hypercalciuria is a feature in a significant number of patients in the group; thus, they are hypercalciuric even at a time when the increase in the filtered load is minimal. I think this indicates that even in the very marginal, minimally hypercalcemic patient with primary hyperparathyroidism, hypercalciuria is still a feature. Therefore, the general rule holds that hypercalcemia from any cause, including primary hyperparathyroidism, is associated with hypercalciuria. The only exception to that would be a patient who has a significant reduction in GFR.

Dr. Brendan Duffy *(Consultant Nephrologist, Regional Hospital, Galway, Ireland)*: *First,* could you comment on the level of serum phosphate in your patients with idiopathic hypercalciuria? As you know, phosphate depletion produces a marked hypercalciuria. *Second,* is there any evidence of "incomplete" renal tubular acidosis in these patients and if so, what is its relationship to PTH?

Dr. Muldowney: The presence of phosphate depletion in idiopathic hypercalciuria is interesting because, as I mentioned earlier, this condition resembles primary hyperparathyroidism. Indeed, phosphate depletion may be the primary defect in idiopathic hypercalciuria. As you noted, it tends to cause hypercalciuria, perhaps directly or perhaps because it promotes the metabolism of vitamin D rapidly from 25-hydroxy to 1,25-dihydroxy vitamin D. Phosphate depletion is a stimulator of the 1-hydroxylase system in the kidney. As a result, you would expect to find a high concentration of 1,25-dihydroxy vitamin D in the serum, and indeed this has been found in the syndrome of idiopathic hypercalciuria [20]. On the other hand, it may be that 1,25-dihydroxy vitamin D itself causes hypercalciuria, and this may be the reason why many of these patients have a mild compensatory gastrointestinal calcium hyperabsorption. To answer your second question, we have shown renal tubular acidosis in patients with marginal hyperparathyroidism [7], and we think this is due to the excess circulating PTH levels. In the group of patients with idiopathic hypercalciuria, we have not seen a significant systemic acidosis except with a few patients who had a rather low serum bicarbonate concentration and a slight lowering of the bicarbonate reabsorption threshold. We didn't attempt bicarbonate loading in the patient under discussion because I didn't think we stood to gain much from it.

Dr. Dermot Murnaghan *(Consultant Nephrologist, Regional Hospital, Cork, Ireland)*: Could you review your thoughts regarding your patients in whom hypercalciuria persisted postoperatively? This finding suggests that there is a primary renal calcium leak in at least those patients.

Dr. Muldowney: Dr. Murnaghan's point is well taken; to what extent does the hypercalciuria persist in patients thought to have primary hyperparathyroidism despite removal of the adenoma? If it persists, it might lead one to believe that the primary calcium leak was the first event that gave rise to secondary hyperparathyroidism, which ultimately became autonomous and primary. Fair enough. In our group of 15 patients, 12 patients did in fact become normocalciuric and three remained hypercalciuric following removal of the adenoma. Perhaps your question recalls the data of Bordier in which he demonstrated persistence of hypercalciuria in patients following removal of the adenoma. But he had loaded all of the patients with sufficient 25-hydroxy vitamin D prior to surgery to produce further hypercalcemia and undoubtedly hypercalciuria. I feel that such loading is really a gentle intoxication and I suspect that the patients in our group would have reacted with persistent hypercalciuria. Whether the hypercalciuria would have been due to the intrinsic defect or to the vitamin D intoxication is impossible to determine.

Dr. David Powell *(Consultant Endocrinologist, Mater Misericordiae Hospital, Dublin, Ireland)*: We are concerned with the difficulty in distinguishing idiopathic hypercalciuria from mild primary hyperparathyroidism because of the substantial therapeutic implications. We anticipate a low total serum calcium concentration in patients with idiopathic hypercalciuria, but a relatively elevated total serum calcium concentration, at least in the upper range of normal, in patients with mild hyperparathyroidism. You have shown that the mean total serum calcium concentration is low in your patients with idiopathic hypercalciuria but the ionized fraction is high. It appears that the total serum calcium concentration is not a good reflection of the ionized serum calcium concentration in patients with idiopathic hypercalciuria; there seems to be a slightly greater proportion of total serum calcium in ionized form in patients with idiopathic hypercalciuria than in control patients. I wonder if you could explain this in physicochemical terms?

Dr. Muldowney: We wonder how to explain it too. There is no doubt that the patients with idiopathic hypercalciuria [13] have a total serum calcium concentration—9.4 $\pm$ 0.4 mg/100 ml—that appears to be below the normal mean—9.8 $\pm$ 0.4 mg/100 ml—whereas the ionized serum calcium concentration is above it. Whether this is a PTH-induced effect or some totally unknown effect is not clear, but the phenomenon is there and it is an important one.

Dr. Brian Keogh *(Consultant Nephrologist, Meath Hospital, Dublin, Ireland)*: What are your thoughts on screening for other factors that might be involved in calcium stone formation, such as increased urinary uric acid concentration or oxalate excretion?

Dr. Muldowney: In screening patients we do include the serum uric acid concentration, although urinary uric acid concentration is not sought. I am aware of the theory discussed by Coe [23] that high urinary excretion of uric acid may tend to "inhibit the inhibitors" of calcium crystalization in the urine. The phenomenon appears to be true but I have not yet found the information to be meaningful in a diagnostic situation.

Dr. Harrington: You place a great deal of weight on the results of the ionized serum calcium determination in your evaluation of patients with idiopathic hypercalciuria. In its absence would you use parathyroid venous drainage localization studies either in primary hyperparathyroidism or in patients being reoperated?

Dr. Muldowney: We have used the localization studies—i.e., putting a catheter into the venous drainage of the thyroid and parathyroid areas—in a few situations. The patients in whom we have used it are those in whom we have genuine doubts whether hypercalcemia is of parathyroid origin or neoplastic origin. That is, of course, a totally different situation than defining the origins of kidney stones. Fortunately, hypercalcemia induced by a PTH or PTH-like substance secreted from a tumor does not usually last long enough to produce a renal stone. I am a little worried about the venous catheterization studies because they are rather complex maneuvers in themselves. An excellent radiologist and a catheterizer are required to do them, and the procedure is rather lengthy. Surgical exploration for parathyroid adenoma would seem to be as practical. With the catheterization studies, it is not always clear what might be the gradient in the venous effluent from a normal parathyroid gland compared with a drainage of the venous effluent from, say, the thyroid. Perhaps Dr. Powell would comment on this technique.

Dr. Powell: In patients with cancer-induced hypercalcemia, we do not find high iPTH levels [24], although we have performed catheter studies to diagnose coincident hyperparathyroidism in a patient with cancer [25]. In patients with hyperparathyroidism, thyroid vein catheterization is a little complex, certainly, and requires special radiologic skill. It is performed in the awake patient, is not painful, causes no morbidity, and is a useful preoperative procedure for many patients with overactive parathyroid glands.

To answer the query raised, we studied parathyroid gradients in thyroid veins in patients with parathyroid disorders [26] and also in patients without any calcium disorder [27]. Comparable gradients were found in both groups, although of course absolute values were higher in those with overactive parathyroids. So the size of the gradient is not diagnostic but depends on the size of the vein catheterized, and the degree of dilution of the gland effluent. The major worth of the technique as a diagnostic tool is in patients with hyperparathyroidism in whom bilateral thyroid vein gradients indicate four-gland hyperplasia, whereas a unilateral gradient—i.e., no gradient on the other side and thus a value the same as the peripheral level—indicates a single source of secretion, an adenoma, on the side of the gradient. This is the information the surgeon needs.

Dr. Donohoe: Dr. Muldowney, could you comment on the present thinking regarding the importance of "inhibitors" of stone formation in the genesis and treatment of calcium stones? Also, could you comment on the use of phosphate either as sodium cellulose phosphate or orthophosphate in the treatment of hypercalciuria?

Dr. Muldowney: Inhibitors of urinary stone formation may act either at the point of crystal formation or subsequently to prevent aggregation of these crystals. The subject has been discussed recently and placed in perspective by Fleisch [28], who has emphasized the in vitro character of the evidence, and the important methodologic problems, not the least being the difficulty of repeating with whole urine the data previously derived from dilute solutions. The topic remains a theoretical one, as yet difficult to transfer from bench research to clinical evaluation or application. The simple fact remains that supersaturation of the urine is determined in the main by calcuim concentration and secondarily by oxalate concentration [28].

Since urinary pyrophosphate is regarded as an inhibitor of stone formation, and since oral ingestion of orthophosphate increases its excretion, this mode of therapy has been employed by a number of workers with varying interpretations [28]. Opinions also vary concerning the important hazard of developing extraskeletal calcification [29,30].

Dr. Harrington: Dr. Muldowney, what are your thoughts on the importance of dietary manipulation in the treatment of idiopathic hypercalciuria?

Dr. Muldowney: Dietary restriction of calcium is indicated in idiopathic hypercalciuria because urinary calcium may be reduced to values found in control patients when dietary calcium is restricted to 400 to 500 mg/day [31]. In practice, this is readily achieved by avoiding dairy products such as milk and cheese. The possible importance of sodium intake remains to be fully assessed, but recently we have studied the effect of changing sodium intake from 60 to 200 mEq in two consecutive 3-day periods. On this regimen, six stone-forming patients with previous inconstant hypercalciuria with a random diet showed 24-h urinary calcium excretion to be in the range of 100 to 280 mg with an intake of 60 mEq of sodium per day; this increased to 260 to 550 mg with an intake of 200 mEq of sodium per day on the third day. Clearly dietary sodium restriction may prove to be important. Carbohydrate intake has been shown to affect urinary calcium in acute studies by Lemann et al, [32], but more study is needed before carbohydrate restriction should be added to the growing number of dietary prohibitions in stone disease.

Dr. Powell: Dr. Muldowney, could you comment on the alleged link between medullary sponge kidney and hyperparathyroidism?

Dr. Muldowney: It is difficult to assign importance to an association between two diseases reported to coincide on relatively few occasions [33–35]. If there is a causal relationship, the primary event might be primary hyperparathyroidism leading to nephrocalcinosis and interstitial nephritis with tubular ectasia, or alternatively a renal calcium leak of sufficient severity to induce secondary hyperparathyroidism, ultimately going on to an autonomous or primary form.

Dr. Harrington: What are the indications for surgery in patients with proven but marginal hyperparathyroidism? If such a patient has had only one or two episodes of stone formation, are we justified in recommending surgery? Is there a role for thiazides in this situation?

Dr. Muldowney: The patients with marginal hyperparathyroidism whom I have discussed have had considerable difficulty with recurrent renal colic and stones. In general, for this group of patients, I think it is best to remove the source of the problem surgically, if one is sure of the diagnosis. A strong point against the use of thiazides under these circumstances is that more severe hypercalcemia may result, and this may go unrecognized if the patient escapes medical supervision. If one could rely on adequate follow-up—perhaps three or four times a year—this approach might be acceptable. But, in my experience, such patients tend not to return for follow-up, so I think it is safer to advise surgery. On the other hand, patients with marginal hyperparathyroidism who have not had recurrent stones or renal colic can be managed conservatively—i.e., without surgery or thiazides.

Forum Commentary

Dr. Fredric L. Coe *(Director, Division of Renal Medicine, Michael Reese Hospital and Medical Center, Chicago, Illinois)*: Naturally, we are delighted that Dr. Muldowney has found elevated fractional excretion of calcium in most cases of idiopathic hypercalciuria. This need not be primary evidence, however, for a renal leak in the sense that intestinal calcium hyperabsorption could be thought of as leading to chronic suppression of PTH secretion. If increased fractional excretion of calcium can be found to correlate with normal or high levels of serum iPTH, then it seems difficult to escape the conclusion that a renal leak must be present.

Although it has not been described in detail, many published case series provide examples of mild hypercalcemia in primary hyperparathyroidism associated with marked hypercalciuria. The patient presented at this Forum appears to be an example of this phenomenon. Even though the increase in apparent filtered load is not marked, it is quite possible to have hypercalciuria, despite increased rather than decreased calcium reabsorption. Fractional excretion of calcium is of course the total urine calcium excretion divided by the product of GFR and the ultrafilterable calcium concentration. Since the ultrafilterable calcium concentration in primary hyperparathyroidism is commonly slightly above normal, the value for fractional calcium excretion tends to be lower than the value obtained by merely dividing calcium excretion by GFR. In other words, it is possible to have marked hypercalciuria with minimal hypercalcemia even in the presence of slightly increased renal tubular calcium reabsorption, and the increased calcium reabsorption is perfectly consistent with the known physiologic action of parathyroid hormone.

The problem of serum parathyroid hormone levels in idiopathic hypercalciuria has vexed many of us. The actual prevalence of "high" values has varied markedly with the immunoassay used. Perhaps it is time that other criteria than the presence or absence of high serum iPTH levels be used to define "renal" hypercalciuria. Although a renal leak theory tends to lead to the prediction of secondary hyperparathyroidism, might it not be worthwhile to try to find more direct ways of diagnosing a renal leak and then see what the iPTH levels are in patients who clearly have this abnormality?

As to the point raised by Dr. Muldowney that the patients from my laboratory could have had primary hyperparathyroidism, I have some reservations. The serum calcium concentrations for these patients were included in the original report. Virtually no values exceeded 10 mg/100 ml, and every patient was studied at least in triplicate; most had quadruplicate samples. If we are to presume that the patients we described had primary hyperparathyroidism, then we are back to the old problem of "normocalcemic" primary hyperparathyroidism, something that Dr. Muldowney probably does not endorse and I find rather unsatisfactory as a concept. Unlike 1,25-dihydroxy vitamin D, PTH certainly does not augment urinary calcium excretion when the serum calcium concentration is below 10 mg/100 ml; it does in fact raise the fractional reabsorption of calcium. For this reason, one would have great difficulty explaining truly normocalcemic hypercalciuria as a consequence of a primary increase in PTH secretion. It is more likely that some immunoassays tend to reflect higher values of serum iPTH in idiopathic hypercalciuria than do others.

References

1. Yendt ER: Renal calculi. Can Med Assoc J 102:479–489, 1970
2. Hodgkinson A, Pyrak LN: The urinary excretion of calcium and inorganic

phosphate in 344 patients with calcium stone of renal origin. Br J Surg 46:10–18, 1959
3. Albright F, Henneman PH, Benedict PH, Forbes AP: Idiopathic hypercalciuria—(a preliminary report). Proc Roy Soc Med 46:1077–1081, 1953
4. Henneman PH, Benedict PH, Forbes AP, Dudley HR: Idiopathic hypercalciuria. N Engl J Med 259:802–807, 1958
5. Peacock M, Knowles F, Nordin BEC: Effect of calcium administration and deprivation on serum and urine calcium in stone-forming and control subjects. Br Med J 2:729–731, 1968
6. Coe FL, Canterbury FM, Firpo JJ, Reiss E: Evidence for secondary hyperparathyroidism in idiopathic hypercalciuria. J Clin Invest 52:134–142, 1973
7. Muldowney FP, Freaney R, McMullin JP, Towers RP, Spillane A, O'Connor P, O'Donoghue P, Moloney M: Serum ionised calcium and parathyroid hormone in renal stone disease. Q J Med 45:75–86, 1976
8. Muldowney FP: Black D (ed.): Renal Acidosis, Renal Disease. London, Blackwell, 1979
9. Muldowney FP, Williams P: Parathyroid hormone, renal tubular acidosis and renal tubular alkalosis. In: Proc 5th Int Cong Nephrol. Basel, Karger, 1974, pp. 158–164
10. Davies M, Adams PH: The continuing risk of vitamin D intoxication. Lancet 2:621–623, 1978
11. Martin K, O'Connor P, Muldowney FP, McDullin JP, McDowell D, Towers RP: Primary hyperparathyroidism: A review of 35 cases. Irish J Med Sci 147:62–69, 1978
12. Smith LH: Calcium-containing renal stones. Kidney Int 13:383–389, 1978
13. Muldowney FP, Freaney R, Ryan JG: The pathogenesis of idiopathic hypercalciuria: evidence of renal tubular calcium leak. Q J Med 49:87–94, 1980
14. Nordin BEC: Hypercalciuria. Clin Sci Molec Med 52:1–8, 1977
15. Pak CYC, Ohata M, Laurence EC, Synder W: The hypercalciurias: causes, parathyroid function and diagnostic criteria. J Clin Invest 54:387–399, 1974
16. Edwards NA, Hodgkinson A: Metabolic studies in patients with idiopathic hypercalciuria. Clin Sci 29:143–157, 1965
17. Jackson WPU, Doncaster C: A consideration of the hypercalciuria in sarcoidosis, idiopathic hypercalciuria and that produced by vitamin D. A new suggestion regarding calcium metabolism. J Clin Endocrinol Metab 19:658–680, 1959
18. McCarron DA, Luft F, Krutzik S, Rankin L, McClung MR, Bennett WM: Ionized calcium, $U_{ca}V$ and PTH response to chronic Na loading. Clin Res 27:424a, 1979
19. Rosenbaum R, Greenwalt A, Lewis J, Klahr S, Slatopolsky E: Evidence that ADH does not increase the release of parathyroid hormone directly. Clin Res 27:428a, 1979
20. Sken SH, Baylink BJ, Neilsen RL: Increased serum 1,25-dihydroxy vitamin D in idiopathic hypercalciuria. J Lab Clin Med 90:955–962, 1977
21. Potts JT, Murray TM, Peacock M, Niall MD, Tregear GW, Keutmann HT, Powell D, Deftos LJ: Parathyroid hormone: Sequence, synthesis, immunoassay studies. Am J Med 50:639–649, 1971
22. Bordier P. Ryckewart A, Gueris J, Rasmussen H: On the pathogenesis of so-called idiopathic hypercalciuria. Am J Med 63:398–409, 1977

23. Coe FL: Treated and untreated recurrent calcium nephrolithiasis in patients with idiopathic hypercalciuria, hyperuricosuria, or no metabolic disorder. Ann Intern Med 87:404–410, 1977
24. Powell D, Singer FR, Murray TM, Minken C, Potts JT Jr: Non-parathyroid humoral hypercalcemia in patients with neoplastic diseases. N Engl J Med 289:176–181, 1973
25. Powell D: Case records of the Massachusetts General Hospital, case 34, 1972. N Engl J Med 287:401–406, 1972
26. Powell D, Shimken PM, Doppman JL, Wells S, Marx SJ, Aurbach GD, Ketcham AS, Potts JT Jr: Primary hyperparathyroidism. Preoperative tumor localization and differentiation between adenoma and hyperplasia. N Engl J Med 286:1169–1175, 1972
27. Shimkin PM, Powell D: Parathyroid hormone levels in thyroid-vein blood of patients without abnormalities of calcium metabolism. Ann Intern Med 78:714–716, 1973
28. Fleisch H: Inhibitors and promoters of stone formation Kidney Int 13:361–371, 1978
29. Thomas WC: Use of phosphates in patients with calcareous renal calculi. Kidney Int 13:390–396, 1978
30. Dudley FJ, Blackburn CRB: Extraskeletal calcification complicating oral phosphate therapy. Lancet 2:628–630, 1970
31. Peacock M, Hodgkinson A, Nordin BEC: Importance of dietary calcium in definition of hypercalciuria. Br Med J 3:469–471, 1967
32. Lemann J, Peiring WF, Lennon EJ: Possible role of carbohydrate-induced calciuria in calcium oxalate kidney stone formation. N Engl J Med 280:232–237, 1969
33. Gremillion DH, Kee JW, McIntosh DA: Hyperparathyroidism and medullary sponge kidney: A chance relationship? JAMA 237:799–800, 1977
34. Rao DS, Frame B, Block MA, et al.: Primary hyperparethyroidism: A cause of hypercalciuria and renal stones. JAMA 237:1353, 1977
35. Rao DS, Frame B, Block MA: Hyperparathyroidism and medullary sponge kidney, JAMA 238:1912–1913, 1977

Renal Insufficiency and Hypercalcemia

Principal Discussant
Samuel O. Thier

Case Presentation

A 32-year-old woman was admitted to New England Medical Center (NEMC) for the first time for evaluation and management of renal failure.

The patient was first noted to have persistent proteinuria at age 9. She was well until age 18 when she rapidly gained weight (11.4 kg) and developed marked edema. An i.v. urogram was normal, and she was treated with bed rest, salt restriction, and diuretics. During the next several years, she had several transient episodes of edema and weight increase.

At age 21 during her first pregnancy, she was hospitalized for evaluation of progressive dyspnea, edema, and headaches. Examination disclosed a blood pressure of 160/90 mmHg and minimal peripheral edema. Laboratory findings were as follows: hemoglobin, 10.1 g; blood urea nitrogen (BUN), 13 mg; serum creatinine, 1.2 mg; and serum albumin, 3.7 g/100 ml. Results of urinalysis revealed proteinuria (2+) and an occasional white blood cell. The blood pressure was controlled, and the pregnancy was uneventful.

At age 28, laboratory findings disclosed the following: BUN, 52 mg; serum albumin, 2.5 g; serum calcium, 9.7 mg; and serum phosphorus, 3 mg/100 ml. One year later, hypercalcemia was first noted when the serum concentrations for calcium and phosphorus were 12.3 and 3.4 mg/100 ml, respectively; the BUN was 49 mg/100 ml.

Nine months later, the patient developed nausea and vomiting and was hospitalized. Laboratory findings at that time were BUN, 50 mg; serum calcium, 13.5 mg; serum phosphorus, 4.4 mg; serum uric acid, 11.5 mg; and serum albumin, 3.3 g/100 ml. Results of urinalysis revealed proteinuria (4+). The patient was treated with i.v. fluids, prednisone, allopurinol, and mithramycin and subsequently discharged. One month later, laboratory findings were BUN, 63 mg; serum creatinine, 3.1 mg; serum uric acid, 9.7 mg; serum calcium, 13.3 mg; serum phosphorus, 4.6 mg; and serum albumin, 3.1 g/100 ml. Despite treatment with prednisone, diuretics, and allopurinol, the patient developed recurrent episodes of nausea, vomiting, diarrhea, bone pain, arthralgias, and muscle weakness.

Six months later, laboratory findings disclosed the following: serum calcium, 15.4 mg; serum phosphorus, 6.8 mg; serum albumin, 2.8 g; BUN, 68 mg; and serum creatinine, 4.8 mg/100 ml. An abdominal plain film was allegedly normal, and a bone survey was normal except for the skull, which showed "salt and pepper" porosity. A subtotal parathyroidectomy was performed; three large glands and part of the fourth gland were removed. The histologic diagnosis was chief cell hyperplasia; no adenoma was found. Postoperatively, the serum creatinine level fell to 3.5 mg, and the serum calcium fell to 7.2 mg/100 ml. The serum phosphorus concentration was 6.1 mg/100 ml, and the alkaline phosphatase was 2.6 Bodansky U. The patient was discharged on a regimen of vitamin D (100,000 U/day), calcium lactate, ethacrynic acid, and methyldopa.

Nine months later while receiving the same medications, the serum calcium concentration was 8 mg; the serum phosphorus was 6.8 mg; and the BUN was 85 mg/100 ml. Seven months later, the serum calcium concentration was 9.1 mg; the serum phosphorus was 7.6 mg; and the BUN was 85 mg/100 ml.

Eight months later (1 month prior to admission to NEMC), the patient developed anorexia, pruritus, and progressive fatigue. Because of emotional stress and depression, she omitted her medications and, shortly thereafter, was admitted to a hospital. On admission, physical examination revealed a blood pressure of 220/140 mmHg and a grade II hypertensive retinopathy. Laboratory findings at that time were serum calcium, 8 mg; serum phosphorus, 12 mg; BUN, 164 mg; and serum creatinine, 12.5 mg/100 ml. Results of urinalysis revealed proteinuria (4+); 15–20 red blood cells; and 0–2 white blood cells/high power field. She was treated with methyldopa and i.v. fluids and transferred to NEMC.

On admission, the patient was somnolent. Physical examination disclosed the following findings: blood pressure, 150/100 mmHg; pulse, 80 and regular; respirations, 22/min; temperature, 36 °C; no band keratopathy; arteriolar narrowing and arteriovenous nicking in the optic fundi; diffuse bone tenderness, most markedly over the ribs; no costovertebral angle tenderness; and no presacral or peripheral edema. Cardiac examination revealed a grade II/VI systolic ejection murmur at the lower left sternal border and apex. Laboratory findings revealed the following: hemoglobin, 9.5 g/100 ml; white blood cell count, 7400/mm^3; platelet count, 312,000/mm^3; serum sodium, 133 mEq; serum potassium, 3.4 mEq; serum chloride, 95 mEq; total carbon dioxide, 19 mEq/liter; BUN, 147 mg; serum creatinine, 9.7 mg; serum calcium, 9.2 mg; serum phosphorus, 12 mg; total serum protein, 5.6 g; and serum albumin, 3.1 g/100 ml. Results of urinalysis revealed pH, 6; proteinuria (3+); 4–5 red blood cells; 5–7 white blood cells; and several coarse granular casts; the urine culture was sterile. A chest radiogram was normal. Abdominal plain film (Fig. 1) revealed the following: kidneys with normal contours;

right kidney, 13.2 cm in length; left kidney, 12.2 cm in length; a diffuse increase in density of both kidneys with focal areas of calcification consistent with nephrocalcinosis; and a slight increase in the bone density of the pelvis, lower ribs, and in spine. Initially, the patient was treated with oral phosphate binders, antihypertensive medications, diuretics, and a low-protein diet. Progressive impairment of renal function ensued, and 2 months later hemodialysis was begun.

Discussion

Dr. Samuel O. Thier *(Chairman, Department of Medicine, Yale University School of Medicine, New Haven, Connecticut)*: In summary, a 32-year-old woman with a history of proteinuria since age 9 developed edema and a picture that sounds like nephrotic syndrome at age 18. At that time, an i.v. urogram was said to be normal. Episodes of edema punctuated the rest of her clinical course.

During the patient's first pregnancy at age 21, she developed hyper-

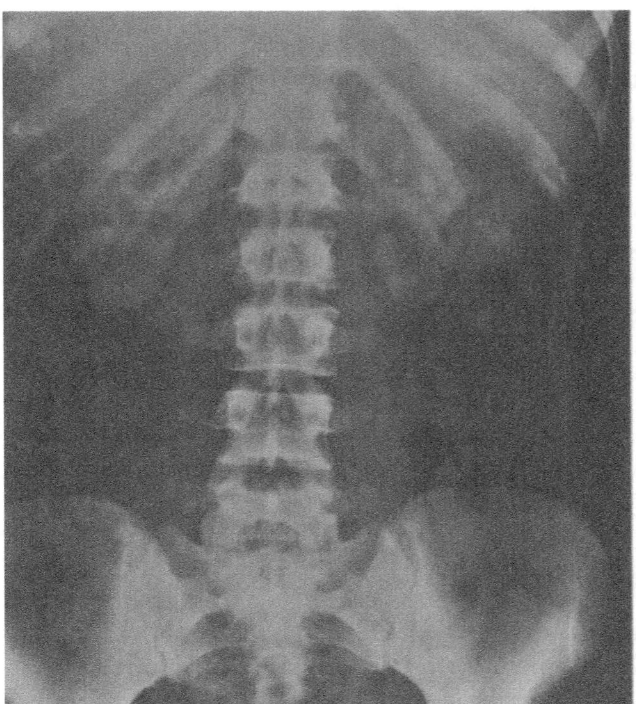

Fig. 1. Abdominal plain film showing bilateral nephrocalcinosis. Calcification is both diffuse and spotty in nature.

tension for the first time. Proteinuria was again present, and her serum albumin concentration was normal. Her blood urea nitrogen (BUN) concentration was 13 mg, and her serum creatinine concentration was 1.2 mg/100 ml. Since her serum creatinine concentration might well have been expected to be in the range of 0.5 ± 0.6 mg/100 ml as a result of the physiologic hyperfusion of the kidneys during pregnancy, it is reasonable to assume that the serum creatinine concentration of 1.2 mg/100 ml represents early evidence of renal dysfunction [1].

There is no further information to evaluate this possibility and, in fact, no further information at all until laboratory findings at age 28 disclosed a BUN concentration of 52 mg, a serum albumin of 2.5 g, a serum calcium of 9.7 mg, and a serum phosphorus of 3 mg/100 ml. Recognizing that approximately half of the serum calcium is bound to protein, and the majority of that to albumin, we can correct the calcium for the low albumin concentration (assuming that for each 1 g/100 ml decrement in the concentration of albumin, the total serum calcium concentration would be reduced by 0.8 to 1.0 mg/100 ml). With this correction, her total serum calcium concentration can be estimated to be in the 10.5–10.7 mg/100 ml range. Thus, she may very well have had an elevated serum ionized calcium concentration at age 28. One year later, her BUN concentration was 49 mg/100 ml. She had unequivocal hypercalcemia with a serum calcium concentration of 12.3 mg and a serum phosphorus concentration of 3.4 mg/100 ml.

Nine months later, her serum calcium concentration was up to 13.5 mg, and her serum phosphorus was up to 4.4 mg/100 ml. Her serum concentration of albumin was 3.3 g, and her BUN was 50 mg/100 ml. Treatment at that time with prednisone, allopurinol, and mithramycin could not have been expected to produce any permanent reduction in the serum calcium concentration; in point of fact, 1 month later the BUN was 63 mg/100 ml, and the patient's hypercalcemia was unchanged. Diuretics were added to her therapy.

Six months later, her serum calcium concentration reached its peak at 15.4 mg/100 ml, and hyperphosphatemia was present for the first time. She also had a serum creatinine concentration of 4.8 mg/100 ml. X-ray films of her abdomen and bones were said to be normal, but films of her skull were consistent with hyperparathyroidism. Surgical removal of three parathyroid glands and a portion of the fourth gland was performed. Pathologic examination revealed chief cell hyperplasia; no adenoma was found. Her serum calcium concentration fell into the normal range and was never again elevated. Her serum creatinine level fell transiently, but then began to rise again, and she was treated with vitamin D, calcium lactate, ethacrynic acid, and alpha-methyldopa.

Over the next 1.5 years, the patient remained hyperphosphatemic and became clinically uremic. She was transferred to this institution with severe hyperphosphatemia (12 mg/100 ml) and a serum creatinine concentration of 12.5 mg/100 ml. At that time, the patient showed evidence of nephrocalcinosis on abdominal films (Fig. 1) and was admitted for management of her chronic renal failure.

This patient appears to have chronic renal disease, most likely chronic glomerulonephritis complicated by hypercalcemia. It would not be profitable to second guess her management when she was 18 since we do not have enough information about her underlying renal disease or the reasoning behind her treatment. It is worth noting that she may have had nephrotic syndrome at that time. More than a decade later, we still await the results of good controlled studies to define more accurately the best modes of therapy for the various histologic types of nephrotic syndrome.

There do seem to be a few key questions relative to this patient's course that I think we should try to answer. First, and most important, was this patient's hypercalcemia a complication of her underlying renal disease, or was it a second primary disorder? In either case, the presence of the hypercalcemia unquestionably complicated her renal disease and probably accelerated the deterioration in renal function. Second, what should have been done about her hypercalcemia?

To belabor the differential diagnoses when the diagnosis is obvious seems gratuitous. Therefore, I will state unequivocally that this patient had autonomous hyperparathyroidism. The question is whether it was primary or tertiary. I will take the position that her hypercalcemia was the result of primary hyperparathyroidism. I will explain why I believe this to be the case, and then I will attack my own premise, before you can, to see if other reconstructions of the events are tenable.

That this patient had hyperparathyroidism seems unquestionable. She had hypercalcemia associated with a normal or slightly low serum phosphorus concentration; she had hyperplasia of her parathyroid glands, and her serum calcium concentration returned to normal after a subtotal parathyroidectomy. If measures had been made of her immunoreactive parathyroid hormone or of nephrogenous cyclic AMP [2], which is a more sensitive measure of parathyroid function, they would undoubtedly have been elevated early in the course of her illness. If she had had a single, clear-cell adenoma, my argument would be simple; the pathologic examination of her parathyroid glands, however, showed chief cell hyperplasia, which is more typical of secondary hyperparathyroidism and some cases of autonomous tertiary hyperparathyroidism. Chief cell hyperplasia may be found in patients with the multiple endocrine adenoma syndrome, and it has become clear in recent years that chief cell hyperplasia may be found in as many as 10% or more of patients with primary hyperparathyroidism [3]. Nonetheless, such hyperplasia is found most commonly in secondary hyperparathyroidism, and therefore it is important to examine the patient's course for evidence of stimuli that would have produced secondary parathyroid hyperplasia.

Pathologically, there are said to be changes characteristic of a stimulated hyperplastic parathyroid gland, which include vacuolation of chief cells and an increased number of transitional oxyphil cells [3]. There is nothing in the record to indicate whether these histologic changes were found in this patient's glands, but it would be worth reviewing the pathology to assess this possibility. Whether it is possible to distinguish between secondary hyperplasia stimulated by hypocalcemia and primary chief cell hyperplasia on the basis of these pathologic findings is questionable. I certainly would not be comfortable assessing primary versus secondary hyperparathyroidism on the basis of histology alone. In a recent study of cell suspensions obtained from human parathyroid glands, a different response was observed in cells from primary hyperplastic versus adenomatous glands [4]. It was claimed that release of parathyroid hormone is more easily suppressed in hyperplastic tissue than in adenomatous tissue as the calcium concentration in the incubation medium is raised. Although differences in the performance of these parathyroid cells *in vitro* are statistically significant, the differences are small. Furthermore, both hyperplastic and adenomatous gland cells may exhibit suppressibility or lack of suppressibility. Thus, this approach *in vitro* is physiologic, but does not yield a separation clean enough to help us answer our question. In all fairness, the approach has not been applied to the question of secondary versus primary or tertiary hyperparathyroidism.

Physiologically, parathyroid gland hyperplasia and parathyroid hormone synthesis are stimulated by a reduction in the concentration of serum ionized calcium. In renal insufficiency, as the glomerular filtration rate (GFR) falls, there is a transient retention of phorphorus if the phosphorus intake is unchanged. The retained phosphorus has at least two important effects: first, it directly lowers serium ionized calcium; and, second, it inhibits the production of 1,25-dihydroxy vitamin D by the proximal renal tubular cell. This metabolite of vitamin D plays an important role in stimulating intestinal absorption of calcium, and a reduction in its activity leads to a reduced calcium absorption. Thus, for at least two reasons an increased serum phosphorus concentration lowers the concentration of serum ionized calcium and stimulates the synthesis of parathyroid hormone. The stimulation of parathyroid hormone synthesis reduces phosphorus reabsorption in the proximal tubule of the kidney and enhances calcium reabsorption in the distal tubule. These effects result in a lowering of serum phosphorus concentration, a rise in serum calcium concentration, a return of the production of 1,25-dihydroxy vitamin D toward normal, and a new steady state at which the serum parathyroid hormone level is slightly elevated. With further reduction in GFR, this series of events is reproduced, and the parathyroid hormone level rises progressively [5]. This process seems capable of maintaining the serum phosphorus concentration within the normal range until the GFR falls below 25% of normal. For reasons that are not clear, at glomerular filtration rates below this level, further reductions in tubular reabsorption of phosphate are not proportional to the reduction in filtration rate, and the serum phorphorus concentration rises. In any event, nothing in this simple scheme can account for serum calcium concentrations rising above normal. In fact, whenever the serum calcium concentration reaches a high normal range, parathyroid hormone production is suppressed, and a new steady state is achieved. The parathyroid glands in such patients show chief cell hyperplasia and the evidence of stimulation indicated earlier. For the glands to become autonomous, as has been reported in some patients with prolonged hypocalcemia, either from intestinal malabsorption or renal failure, it is necessary to postulate a prolonged period of stimulation without appropriate feedback inhibition. That is, there must be evidence of prolonged phosphate retention, or prolonged reductions in serum ionized calcium concentration, or both. Such prolonged and continuous stimulation of the parathyroid glands may result in autonomous function. In the patient under discussion, there is no evidence for hypocalcemia at all, and certainly none for a prolonged period of hypocalcemia. Nor is there any evidence of even a high normal serum phosphorus concentration, let alone an elevated concentration, prior to the development of hypercalcemia. Therefore, there is no evidence of ongoing stimulation of the parathyroid glands. A comparison of this patient's blood chemistries with those of 195 patients with renal failure reported in a series several years ago highlights the fact that patients who develop renal failure over prolonged periods of time rarely develop hypercalcemia prior to dialysis or transplantation [6]. Only one of the 195 patients developed clinically important hypercalcemia prior to dialysis or transplantation. Seven patients in the series had occasional elevations of their serum calcium concentration, but their mean calcium concentrations were not elevated, Similarly, only one of the 195 patients had a serum phosphorus concentration below normal. Thus, our patient had neither a stimulus for the development of hypercalcemia, nor a pattern of chemical abnormality of serum calcium and phosphorus consistent with the usual patient with renal failure.

What other events might have led to parathyroid stimulation early in her renal failure? In a recent study by Bordier et al., the evidence suggests that administration of 1,25-dihydroxy vitamin D or 25-hydroxy vitamin D to patients with renal osteodystrophy can effect an increase in serum calcium concentrations and a lowering of parathyroid hormone levels [7]. These data are consistent with previous evidence which indicated that 1,25-dihydroxy vitamin D suppressed parathyroid hormone production. As far as I can discern, the suppression of parathyroid hormone production is related to an increase in serum calcium concentrations and is not a direct effect of the vitamin *per se*. To postulate that a reduction in 1,25-dihydroxy vitamin D early in a long course of renal failure leads to an increase in parathyroid hormone production requires evidence of a reduced serum calcium concentration. As I have said repeatedly, there is no such evidence in this patient. There is additional evidence, however, that the less-studied vitamin D metabolite, 24,25-dihydroxy vitamin D, may inhibit parathyroid hormone production directly, i.e., independently of the serum concentration of calcium ions [8]. If this is true, reduced production of this metabolite may directly increase parathyroid hormone level. For this increase to be important, it is necessary to postulate either a disproportionate reduction in 24,25-dihydroxy vitamin D in this patient or an inordinate sensitivity to its absence. These are highly speculative possibilities and seem unlikely to serve as strong affirmations that we are dealing with secondary and ultimately tertiary hyperparathyroidism in this instance.

Because this patient had serum calcium and phosphorus concentrations out of line with virtually all patients developing renal failure, no evidence of phosphate retention or prolonged hypocalcemia, and hypercalcemia antedating major renal insufficiency, I believe that the parathyroid hormone excess was primary and initially unrelated to her renal disease. The pathologic findings of chief cell hyperplasia give me pause in putting this formulation forward, but they do not override the rest of the evidence.

Viewing this patient's problem from several standpoints for the sake of completeness, let me suggest that she may have had primary hyperparathyroidism for a long time, and that primary hyperparathyroidism produced all of the clinical findings. With a little imagination, we could argue that because calcium phosphate was being deposited in the loop of Henle and collecting duct cells, as occurs with hypercalcemia, tubular injury occurred and led to the release of an antigen that stimulated an immunologic response. The immunologic response of antibody and antigen produced glomerular damage and proteinuria. Due to fluctuating degrees of hypercalcemia, tubular injury was intermittent, and episodes of glomerular damage recurred. In time, the process became more persistent and produced greater injury. This sequence of tubular injury leading to glomerular damage has been postulated in other predominantly interstitial diseases, such as sickle cell disease, and has also been postulated as the basis of the proteinuria seen in experimental models of renal failure. In a recent study of the effects of phosphate restriction in preventing renal injury, it has been demonstrated that phosphate restriction leads to a reduction in proteinuria [9]. The authors postulate that the phosphate administration may lead to deposition of calcium phosphate, tubular injury, and antibodies to tubular antigens producing proteinuria. I will grant that this formulation is rather far-fetched, but I offer it as a counterweight to the 24,25-dihydroxy vitamin D speculation.

From a more practical standpoint, the important question in this patient is, What processes might have been slowed or prevented by effective treatment of her hypercalcemia when it first appeared? There are numerous ways of treating hypercalcemia, but there is no really effective substitute for parathyroidectomy when hypercalcemia is secondary to hyperparathyroidism in a patient with renal insufficiency. Therefore, the form of therapy that should have been instituted in this patient is not really in question. My concern is, Which aspects of her problem might have been prevented? Hypercalcemia leads to functional and anatomic lesions of the kidney [10]. Functionally, hypercalcemia interfers with antidiuretic hormone action, which leads to a nephrogenic diabetes insipidus-like picture. Hypercalcemia also produces interference with sodium reabsorption in the tubule, which leads to a saline diuresis and possibly a very significant hypovolemic state. Higher concentrations of serum calcium produce increased afferent arteriolar resistance in the glomeruli and increased arteriolar resistance throughout the body. The result at the renal level is a reduction in GFR, and the result at the systemic level is the potential for the development of hypertension. Acute hypercalcemia may lead to stimulation of hydrogen ion secretion and a transient alkalemia, but the chronic effects of hypercalcemia on acid-base regulation are more likely related to the deposition of calcium in the collecting duct, causing impairment of hydrogen ion secretion and the development of acidemia. Of perhaps greater importance is the fact that deposition of calcium phosphate in the tubular cells and interstitium may initiate interstitial injury and fibrosis, a process that may persist and progress even after the hypercalcemia is corrected.

Thus, it is clear that the physiologic effects of hypercalcemia are capable of accelerating and complicating many of the key problems of renal insufficiency, particularly the difficulties in volume homeostasis, hydrogen ion balance, and blood pressure regulation. The failure to treat hypercalcemia in its early phases increases the possibility of renal injury in every patient; in the patient with underlying renal disease, this may sharply accelerate the rate of functional deterioration.

In this patient, all of the functional changes might have occurred at the same time that anatomic injury was initiated. Calcium phosphate was deposited in the cells of the loop of Henle and the collecting duct, which led to injury of those cells and the deposition of calcium phosphate in the tubular and interstitial areas. The establishment of these deposits of calcium initiated a fibrosing process, which might very easily have progressed even after correction of hypercalcemia. Thus, the hypercalcemia was capable of producing an intrinsic anatomic renal injury and a functional abnormality in the kidney, which added to the difficulties of hydrogen ion secretion, maintenance of volume homeostasis, and regulation of blood pressure in chronic renal failure.

Questions and Answers

Dr. Jerome P. Kassirer: Does the maintenance of a normal serum calcium concentration without supplementary vitamin D in a patient who has undergone subtotal parathyroidectomy for the secondary hyperparathyroidism of uremia imply that the patient has continued hyperparathyroidism?

Dr. Thier: Following subtotal parathyroidectomy, if the remaining parathyroid tissue is adequate to maintain a normal serum calcium concentration, then the desired effect of the manuever has been achieved. It seems to me the next question is, Can parathyroid activity be suppressed or not? If it can't be suppressed, I would be somewhat concerned that hyperparathyroidism might still pose a problem. I doubt that I would do anything further however as long as the serum calcium concentration remains within the normal range.

Dr. Kassirer: Of course, if the serum calcium concentration is 9 mg/100 ml and the phosphorus is 12 mg/100 ml, as it was in this patient, the risk for further calcification is probably rather high.

Dr. Thier: It is not clear what would happen in this type of patient if the phosphate concentration decreased to say 6.0 mg/100 ml: Would the serum calcium concentration increase above normal with incomplete suppression of the parathyroid gland, or would it increase and completely suppress what was left of the parathyroid gland? I think one would have to see which response occurs before deciding on the next step.

Dr. Jordan J. Cohen: Dr. Thier, is your routine practice to restrict dietary phosphate or administrater a phosphate binder in the early stages of renal failure?

Dr. Thier: That is still a personal decision that each nephrologist has to make. Unfortunately, I don't think we have any solid data presently on which to base that decision. The experimental evidence from animal models indicating that the rate of renal insufficiency may be retarded by phosphate restriction is suggestive, but a controlled study in humans is yet to be reported.

Dr. Cohen: We are confronted daily with the decision of whether to advise phosphate restriction in patients with mild renal insufficiency. Not only the benefits but the risks remain unclear. Although the risks of administering phosphate binders over the short run seem to be pretty low, we really don't know what the risks are of long-term treatment. There may be other problems.

Dr. Thier: We have good data based on careful balance studies in experimental animals showing that serum phosphorus can be maintained at a normal level by reducing phosphate intake in proportion to the reduction in GFR. Unfortunately, we can't measure whether the phosphate intake is being reduced proportionately when we give a patient a set dose of a phosphate binder. The question is whether we are giving the right amount or overshooting the mark and taking the risk of developing a phosphate-depletion syndrome over a period of time. Until we really have some way of estimating the risk, I think it will remain a difficult clinical situation. Parathyroid hormone determinations are not quite accurate enough for this purpose; nephrogenous cyclic AMP might prove to be a more reasonable way to measure parathyroid activity clinically. At present, I usually wait until the serum creatinine is 3 or 4 mg/100 ml, and then I prescribe phosphate binders. Perhaps I ought to use phosphate binders before that degree of renal function impairment is reached. Theoretically, by preventing the hyperphosphatemia from ever occurring, one could prevent the parathyroid hormone levels from ever increasing; that would be very good preventive medicine. I am too nervous to attempt that just yet.

References

1. Ferris TF: Renal disease. In Burrow GN, Ferris TF (eds.): Medical Complications During Pregnancy. Philadelphia, Saunders, 1975. p. 1
2. Broadus AE, Mahaffey JE, Bartter FC, Neer RM: Nephrogenous cyclic adenosine monophosphate as a parathyroid function test. J Clin Invest 60:771–783, 1977
3. Roth SI, Marshall RB: Pathology and ultrastructure of the human parathyroid glands in chronic renal failure. Arch Intern Med 124:397–407, 1969
4. Brown ED, Brennan MF, Hurwitz S, Windeck R, Marx, SJ, Spiegel AM, Koehler JO, Gardner DG, Aurbach GD: Dispersed cells prepared from human parathyroid glands: Distinct calcium sensitivity of adenomas versus primary hyperplasia. J Clin Endocrinol Metab. 46(2):267-275, 1978
5. Slatopolsky E, Caglar S, Pennell JP, Jaggart DD, Canterbury JM, Reiss E, Bricker NS: On the pathogenesis of hyperparathyroidism in chronic renal disease. J Clin Invest 50:492, 1971
6. Katz AI, Hampers CL, Merrill, JP: Secondary hyperparathyroidism and renal osteodystrophy in chronic renal failure: Analysis of 195 patients with observations on the effects of chronic dialysis, kidney transplantation, and subtotal parathyroidectomy. Medicine 48:333–374, 1969
7. Bordier P, Zingraff J, Gueris J, Jungers P, Marie P, Pechet M, Rasmussen H: The effect of $1\alpha(OH)D_3$ and $1\alpha,25(OH)_2D_3$ on the bone in patients with renal osteodystrophy. Am J Med 64:101–107, 1978

8. Care AD, Pickard DW, Peacock M, Mawer B, Taylor CM, Ledel J, Norman AW: Reduction of parathyroid hormone secretion by 24,25-dihydroxy cholecalciferol. In Norman AW, Schaffer K, Coburn JW, DeLuca HF, Fraser D, Grigoleit HG, Von Herrath D, Vitamin D: Biochemical, Chemical, and Chemical Aspects Related to Calcium Metabolism. (eds.): Berlin, Walter de Gruyter, 1977
9. Ibels LS, Alfrey AC, Haut L, Huffer WE: Preservation of function in experimental renal disease by dietary restriction of phosphate. N Engl J Med 298:122–125, 1978
10. Massry SG, Coburn JW: Divalent ions and the kidney. In Kurtzman NA, Martinez-Maldonado M, (eds.): Pathophysiology of the Kidney. Springfield, Ill., Thomas, 1977, p. 596

Renal Osteodystrophy

Principal Discussant
Jack W. Coburn

Case Presentation

A 66-year-old man with chronic renal failure was admitted to the Wadsworth VA Medical Center for evaluation of bone pain and severe muscle weakness. Approximately 3 years prior to admission, an elevated serum creatinine of 6 mg/dl was first detected. Evaluation at that time included an intravenous pyelogram, which revealed bilateral scarred and shrunken kidneys without evidence of obstruction. The 24-h urine protein excretion was 1.5 g; serum calcium, 8.6 mg/dl; serum phorphorus, 6.5 mg/dl; and alkaline phosphatase, 90 IU. One urine culture was sterile and the antinuclear antibody was negative.

Renal failure progressed and 18 months prior to admission the patient was started on maintenance hemodialysis. He did well on dialysis except for the development of bone pain and severe muscle weakness.

Medications at the time of admission included: digoxin, 0.125 mg every other day; Dilantin, 300 mg daily; aluminum hydroxide, 3 tabs three times daily. Physical examination revealed blood pressure, 140/70; pulse, 80/min; respiration, 12/min; temperature, 37.5°C. A grade I/VI systolic murmur was heard at the left sternal border. A functioning arteriovenous fistula was present in the right arm. The remainder of the physical examination was unremarkable. Laboratory data revealed the following: hematocrit, 34%; WBC, 7500/mm^3; BUN, 85 mg/dl; creatinine, 10.7 mg/dl; serum calcium, 10.2 mg/dl; and serum phosphorus, 3.6 mg/dl. The serum magnesium was 2.9 mEq; serum sodium, 138 mEq; serum potassium, 5.4 mEq; serum chloride, 97 mEq; and serum bicarbonate, 18 mEq/liter. The alkaline phosphatase was 217 units; serum albumin, 3.8 g/dl; total protein, 8 g/dl; serum immunoreactive parathyroid hormone (iPTH), 1.55 ng/ml (normal less than 0.4 ng/ml); and 25-hydroxycholecalciferol, 19 ng/ml (normal, 12–60 ng/ml). Roentgenograms revealed subperiosteal resorption of both hands and distal clavicles. One day after admission, an ileal crest bone biopsy was performed.

The biopsy showed increased resorbing and forming surface, increased osteoid (18.3% unmineralized bone), and severe marrow-space fibrosis (4.8%) (Fig. 1). These findings were interpreted as consistent with osteomalacia and osteitis fibrosa with osteitis fibrosis predominating.

Treatment with 1,25-dihydroxycholecalciferol [$1,25(OH)_2D_3$] was initiated at a dose of 1 μg/day, and aluminum hydroxide was continued at a dose of 3 tabs three times daily. Within 1 month of initiation of treatment, the patient's muscle weakness improved dramatically and his bone pain diminished. By 2 months, when the serum calcium was 10.0 mg/dl and the serum phosphorus was 3.0 mg/dl, the alkaline phosphatase had declined slightly to 180 units and the PTH had fallen to 0.95 ng/ml. By 6 months, the serum alkaline phosphatase had fallen further to 105 units, serum calcium was then 12 mg/dl, and serum phosphorus was 7 mg/dl. The serum calcium continued to rise to 13.2 mg/dl and the $1,25(OH)_2D_3$ was discontinued. One month later a repeat bone biopsy was performed. Serum calcium at the time of biopsy was 10.4 mg/dl; serum phosphorus, 4.4 mg/dl; alkaline phosphatase, 95 units; and serum PTH 0.22 ng/ml. The patient's clinical course is shown in Fig. 2.

The repeat biopsy showed an increase in the forming surface, a slight decrease in the resorbing surface, and a marked reduction in marrow-space fibrosis (1%)(Fig. 3). Percentage minerilization had improved to 95.1%.

Discussion

Dr. Jack W. Coburn *(Director, Nephrology Training Program, VA Wadsworth Medical Center, and Professor of Medicine, UCLA School of Medicine, Los Angeles, California)*: This patient presents a number of features characteristic of symptomatic renal osteodystrophy. I will use this term in a broad, generic sense to include all skeletal abnormalities in uremia, i.e., osteitis fibrosa, osteomalacia, osteosclerosis, and growth failure in children. On the basis of the radiographic findings of increased subperiosteal resorption and elevated levels of serum immunoreactive parathyroid hormone (iPTH), there is little doubt that our patient has significant secondary hyperparathyroidism.

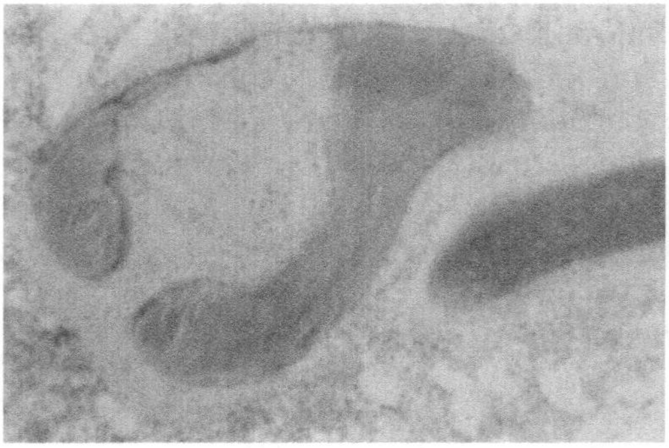

Fig. 1. Pretreatment bone biopsy showing extensive marrow fibrosis. There is an increase in unmineralized osteoid (*small dark bodies*) underlying rows of osteoblasts. (The mineralized bone appears as large dark bodies.) Goldner's modification of Masson's trichrome stain. (Photomicrograph supplied courtesy of Dr. Donald J. Sherrard, VA Hospital, Seattle, Washington.)

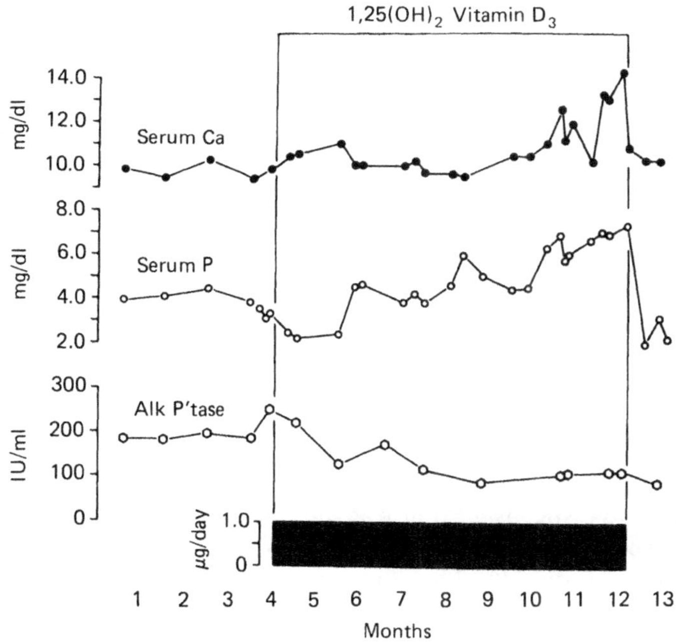

Fig. 2. Serial levels of serum calcium, phosphorus, and alkaline phosphatase during treatment with 1,25(OH)$_2$D$_3$. The early fall in serum phosphorus level and the later rise in both serum calcium and phosphorus are apparent. The latter events occurred after alkaline phosphatase had fallen toward normal. The prompt decreases in both serum calcium and phosphorus following the withdrawal of 1,25(OH)$_2$D$_3$ are evident. (Reproduced from Ref. 74, © Walter de Gruyter.)

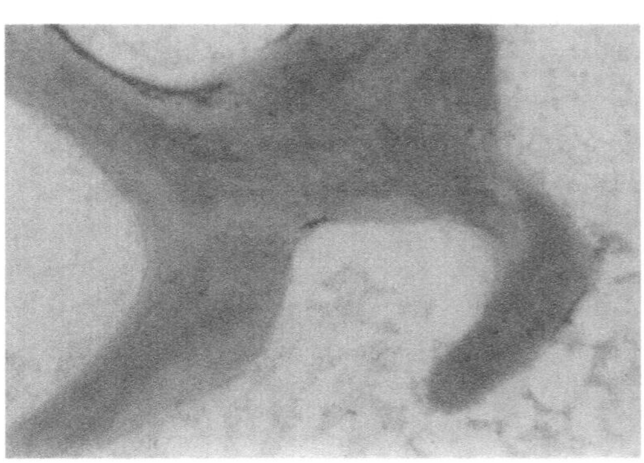

Fig. 3. Biopsy obtained after 9 months of treatment with 1,25(OH)$_2$D$_3$. 1.0 µg/day. There is a marked reduction in marrow fibrosis and improvement in mineralization, although an increase in unmineralized osteoid persists. Goldner's modification of Masson's trichrome stain. (Photomicrograph supplied courtesy of Dr. Donald J. Sherrard, VA Hospital, Seattle, Washington.)

Pathogenesis of Secondary Hyperparathyroidism

Before discussing the clinical features of this patient, I will review factors thought to produce secondary hyperparathyroidism in uremia. These pathogenetic factors, believed to originate early in the course of renal disease, presumably are operative for many years before the patient manifests overt bone disease in the late stages of advanced renal insufficiency [1]. A decrease in ionized calcium in the blood is probably the only important factor that increases the secretion of parathyroid hormone (PTH) and leads to the consequent parathyroid hyperplasia. Major factors leading to hypocalcemia in renal failure include phosphate retention, abnormalities of vitamin D metabolism, and a reduced skeletal response to the calcemic action of PTH. Other conditions, listed in Table 1, also might be contributory.

Phosphate Retention

Slatopolsky et al. have suggested that transient and even undetectable increments in serum phosphorus levels occur as GFR decreases early in the course of renal failure [2]. They argued that such transient hyperphosphatemia lowers blood calcium and increases PTH secretion, which in turn reduces the tubular reabsorption of phosphate and leads

Table 1. Conditions that might contribute to altered calcium homeostasis and bone disease in renal failure.

I. Hypocalcemia and secondary hyperparathyroidism
   1. Retention of phosphate
   2. Altered bioactivation of vitamin D
   3. Skeletal resistance to PTH
   4. Reduced degradation of PTH

II. Defective mineralization of bone
   1. Abnormal collagen synthesis (possibly related to vitamin D)
   2. Abnormal crystal growth and maturation
   3. Accumulation of pyrophosphate and/or magnesium in bone
   4. Reduced carbonate content of bone

III. Factors of variable and uncertain role
   1. Heparin administration
   2. Acidosis
   3. Phosphate deficiency
   4. Vitamin D loss with nephrotic syndrome
   5. Skeletal accumulation of trace elements (e.g., fluoride, aluminum)
   6. Modification by treatment
      a. Anticonvulsants, other drugs
      b. Parathyroidectomy
      c. Vitamin D
      d. Dialysate Ca, Mg, etc.

Source: Adapted from Ref. 91.

to phosphaturia. Thus, serum phosphorus and calcium levels return toward normal, but only at the expense of inducing a higher circulating level of PTH. Considerable evidence, primarily derived from studies in dogs with reduced renal function, supports the view that phosphate retention plays a primary role in the pathogenesis of secondary hyperparathyroidism in renal failure [3,4,5]. A notable problem with this theory is that such increments in serum phosphorus levels have not been identified, and in fact, serum phosphorus levels are often low or normal in patients with mild renal insufficiency [6,7]. When renal function falls below 25% of normal, overt hyperphosphatemia frequently develops, and this elevation of serum phosphorus clearly can be an important factor in the development of secondary hyperparathyroidism at this stage of renal failure [8].

Abnormalities of Vitamin D Metabolism

Strong evidence indicates that disorders in vitamin D metabolism alter the regulation of calcium and phosphorus in uremic patients [9]. It is now apparent that vitamin D itself, although largely inactive, is a precursor of more active sterols. Thus, either endogenous or exogenous vitamin D_3 first is converted in the liver to 25-hydroxy-vitamin D_3 [10], the major circulating form of vitamin D [11]. This sterol then undergoes 1-hydroxylation in the cortex of the kidney [12] to form 1,25-dihydroxy-vitamin D_3 [$1{,}25(OH)_2D_3$]. The latter sterol provides a more potent stimulus to intestinal calcium absorption than do any of the other forms of the vitamin [13].

The renal generation of $1{,}25(OH)_2D_3$ is subject to physiologic regulation: it is stimulated by a diet low in calcium [14], increased levels of PTH [15,16], and hypophosphatemia [17]. It can be inhibited by a high-calcium diet, hyperphosphatemia [17], and $1{,}25(OH)_2D_3$ itself [18]. Given the central regulatory role of the kidney in calcium and phosphorus metabolism, it is not surprising that vitamin D metabolism is altered in patients with renal insufficiency.

When does this abnormality of vitamin D metabolism develop during the course of progressive renal insufficiency? A decrease in the generation of $1{,}25(OH)_2D_3$ early in the course of the disease could lead to both decreased calcium absorption and decreased action of PTH on the bone, processes that in turn would lead to hypocalcemia. Hypocalcemia would stimulate PTH secretion, which would be expected to increase the renal generation of $1{,}25(OH)_2D_2$ and to restore serum levels of $1{,}25(OH)_2D_3$, intestinal calcium absorption, and serum calcium to normal; all of these changes would occur at the expense of an increased level of serum PTH. The data bearing on the question are not conclusive; however, the intestinal absorption of calcium is normal in most patients with mild to moderate renal insufficiency [7,19]. Preliminary studies of blood levels of serum $1{,}25(OH)_2D$ in patients with early renal insufficiency have yielded conflicting results. Slatopolsky et al, reported normal or slightly increased levels of 1,25$(OH)_2D_3$ in adults with creatinine clearances above 30 ml/min [20], whereas Portale et al, found reduced levels in children with an average GFR of 41 ml/min [21]. It is possible that high PTH levels maintain the serum levels of 1,25$(OH)_2D_3$ near normal in azotemic patients until renal insufficiency becomes marked. The mechanism of reduced renal generation of 1,25$(OH)_2D_3$ in patients with mild to moderate renal insufficiency is uncertain; phosphate retention and diminished tubular reabsorption of phosphate, both of which occur early in the course of renal insufficiency, could reduce the generation of 1,25$(OH)_2D_3$ for any given level of PTH secretion. Preliminary data of Llach et al. suggest that in patients with mild renal insufficiency, dietary phosphate restriction in proportion to the degree of reduction in GFR is associated with an increase in intestinal calcium absorption and a fall in serum iPTH [22].

Although we are still uncertain whether vitamin D metabolism is altered early in the course of renal insufficiency, most data indicate that the blood levels of 1,25$(OH)_2D_3$ are low or undetectable in end-stage uremia [23,24]. In advanced renal disease, the lack of 1,25$(OH)_2D_3$ probably contributes importantly to the reduced intestinal absorption of both calcium and phosphorus, the impaired calcemic response to PTH, and retarded growth in children. Moreover, many of these abnormalities can be restored to normal after treatment with doses of 1,25$(OH)_2D_3$ that are presumably in the physiologic range [25–29].

Deficiency of 1,25$(OH)_2D_3$ also could lead to secondary hyperparathyroidism by virtue of a direct effect of this sterol on the parathyroid gland. Brumbaugh et al. have described specific cytoplasmic receptors, similar to those found in known target tissues for vitamin D_3, for 1,25$(OH)_2D_3$ in the parathyroid glands [30]. Moreover, certain data suggest that 1,25$(OH)_2D_3$ can directly inhibit PTH secretion [31], although such data have not invariably been confirmed [32,33]. Oldham et al. suggested that 1,25$(OH)_2D_3$ might modulate PTH secretion at any given level of blood calcium; data supporting this view appear in Fig. 4 [34]. In the absence of 1,25$(OH)_2D_3$, a higher level of serum calcium might be needed to produce a similar degree of suppression of PTH secretion. At this point, such a suggestion is speculative and further studies are needed to clarify this possible action of vitamin D.

Despite the low levels of 1,25$(OH)_2D_3$ found in patients with advanced renal failure, many uremic patients lack features of vitamin D deficiency. Intestinal calcium absorption is not uniformly reduced [7,35] and osteomalacia occurs in only a small fraction of such patients [36,37]. Moreover, even in anephric patients bone biopsies often show no histologic evidence of osteomalacia [38]. Why such patients fail to develop evidence of vitamin D deficiency is not clear. The persistence of normal or even elevated serum phosphorus levels might protect uremic patients from osteomalacia; this hypothesis is suggested by the finding that the degree of osteomalacia is inversely related to serum phosphorus levels in end-stage renal failure [39].

Reduced Skeletal Response to PTH

Skeletal resistance to the calcemic action of PTH also contributes to hypocalcemia in patients with renal insufficiency. The calcemic response to a standardized infusion of parathyroid extract is subnormal in patients with moderate to advanced renal insufficiency, and in those undergoing dialysis [40]. Recovery from induced hypocalcemia in patients with creatinine clearances of 35–90 ml/min is delayed as compared to results in normal individuals; this phenomenon occurs despite a greater augmentation in serum iPTH levels in the patients with mild renal insufficiency. These observations indicate that skeletal resistance to PTH appears early in the course of renal insufficiency [6]. Although the mechanisms responsible for the impaired calcemic response to PTH

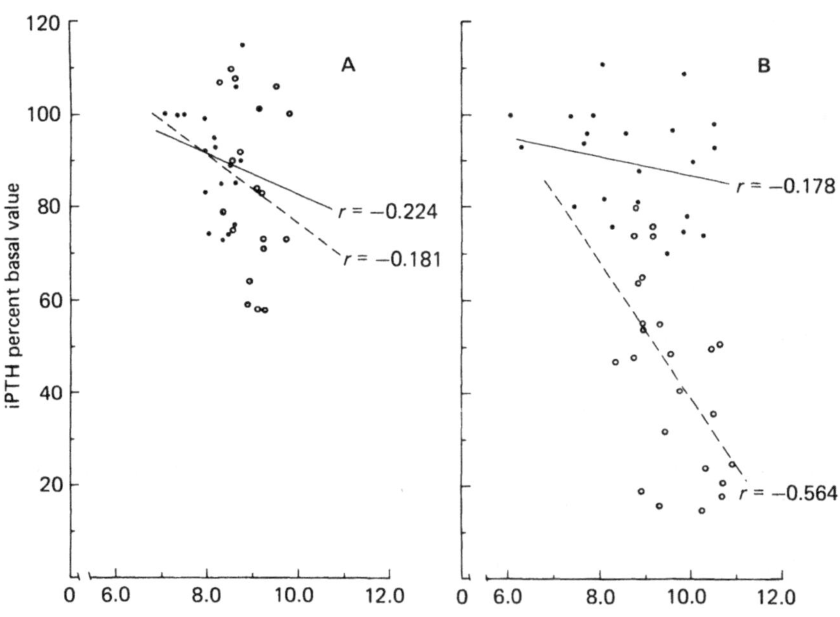

Fig. 4. Correlation between serum iPTH and serum calcium concentrations during the slow intravenous calcium infusion in ricketic puppies. The animals were injected with either vehicle alone (**A**) or 1 μg of 1,25(OH)$_2$D$_3$ (**B**) 4 h before the initiation of calcium infusion. Samples collected during the initial 90 min of infusion, shown as solid circles, have a continuous regression line, whereas samples obtained between 90 min and 180–200 min of the calcium infusion are shown by open circles and an interrupted line. (Reproduced from Ref. 34 with permission of The Endocrine Society.)

remain uncertain, alterations in vitamin D metabolism have been incriminated [41,42].

Effect of Anticonvulsant Drugs

Treatment with phenytoin (Dilantin) also might contribute to bone disease in the patient we are discussing here. The long-term ingestion of phenytoin, phenobarbital, or both is associated with a high incidence of osteomalacia in nonuremic patients treated for seizure disorders [43,44]. Jubiz et al. found low serum levels of $25(OH)D_3$ but normal levels of $1,25(OH)_2D_3$ in patients treated with anticonvulsant drugs who had clinical evidence of osteomalacia [45]. Hahn et al. have suggested that these drugs might activate a hepatic microsomal P-450 enzyme, and that this activation might lead to abnormal hydroxylation, changing vitamin D and $25(OH)D_3$ to biologically inactive sterols [46]. Pierides et al. reported a higher incidence of symptomatic bone disease in dialysis patients treated with barbiturates and phenytoin than in patients not receiving such treatment [47,48]. Because of the normal serum level of $25(OH)D_3$ in our patient, phenytoin treatment probably did not contribute significantly to his bone disease. His serum level of $25(OH)D_3$, however, is lower than that observed in most residents of southern California, where sunlight exposure is usually substantial.

Clinical Manifestations of Renal Osteodystrophy

Now I should like to examine the clinical manifestations in this patient. Bone pain that develops with renal osteodystrophy is often subtle and insidious in onset; the axial skeleton—back, hips, and ribs—is most commonly involved, but pain can involve the knees, heels, and shoulders. Symptoms are often aggravated by sudden changes in position, e.g., when the ptient turns over in bed or sits up. Because the pain is related to motion, patients often become sedentary and sometimes even bedridden. Symptoms can be independent of the specific type of skeletal pathology present. Pain might be worse at night, but little relationship exists between the bone pain and temperature or climate. Physical findings usually are absent; consequently, the symptoms commonly are attributed to minor trauma or a psychosomatic cause. The degree of pain does not necessarily correlate with the extent of radiographic abnormalities; thus, patients with severe lesions can be free of symptoms, although it is somewhat unusual for patients to be symptomatic in the absence of radiographic abnormalities. Many other signs and symptoms have been associated with high levels of PTH [Table 2]. Massry and Goldstein recently suggested that PTH might even be a uremic toxin [49].

I believe that the patient's muscle weakness deserves some attention, because this symptom is commonly overlooked despite the fact that myopathy occurring in conjunction with renal osteodystrophy is very common. We recently presented our experience with seven uremic patients who had severe proximal muscle weakness [50]; all but one had been treated with long-term maintenance dialysis, and the slowly progressive symptoms had existed for an average of 24 months before treatment. Abnormalities of gait were present in all patients; three patients exhibited a waddling, "penguin" gait that is characteristic of the proximal myopathy of vitamin D deficiency [51]. Two patients had weakness when they elevated their arms, and they experienced difficulty in combing or setting their hair. Of the seven patients, six had difficulty rising from a chair and were unable to climb stairs. Despite evidence of proximal weakness, distal muscle strength, e.g., strength of the hand grip, frequently was normal. The myopathy is associated with normal serum enzymes, creatinine phosphokinase, and transminase; electromyographic changes are usually nonspecific.

Because of its slow, insidious nature, the myopathy often is overlooked or attributed to debility in dialysis patients who have other evidence of chronic illness. Although the pathogenesis of proximal myopathy in patients with chronic renal failure remains uncertain, muscle weakness has been attributed to hyperparathyroidism [52], phosphate depletion [53], and abnormal vitamin D metabolism [51,53]. We and others have observed significant prompt improvement in muscular weakness during treatment with $1{,}25(OH)_2D_3$ [27]. Our finding of such muscle weakness in patients who have markedly elevated, normal, or even undetectable levels of serum iPTH suggests that factors other than PTH play a pathogenetic role. We have noted serum calcium levels of 8.1–11.3 mg/dl and serum phosphorus levels of 2.9–5.5 mg/dl in patients with myopathy. Moreover, myopathy has improved during treatment with $1{,}25(OH)_2D_3$ even without a change in serum levels of calcium or phosphorus. In two patients, muscle strength improved while serum iPTH levels remained unchanged. Moreover, bone biopsies from five patients revealed divergent results: we found osteomalacia in two,

Table 2. Clinical manifestations of calcium and phosphorus abnormalities in renal failure.

Bone pain	Acute periarthritis
Myopathy	Hypertension
Pruritus	Spontaneous tendon rupture
Muscle cramps	Calciphylaxis
Fractures	Neuropathy
Retardation of growth	Altered mentation
Skeletal deformities	Impotence
Pseudogout	Pancytopenia

Source: Adapted from Nortman DF, Coburn JW: *Postgraduate Medicine*, vol. 64, no. 5, Nov. 1978 © McGraw-Hill, Inc.

marked osteitis fibrosa in one, and "mixed" lesions in two others. In one patient, a muscle biopsy revealed atrophy of type-2 fibers, a finding typical of the myopathy associated with vitamin D deficiency [54]. Electron microscopic examination of muscle biopsies in uremic patients has revealed severe degenerative changes, with disorganization of myofibrils and dispersion of Z-band material; these abnormalities reverted to normal following treatment with $25(OH)D_3$ [55].

Altered muscle contraction and relaxation have been reported in vitamin D-deficient animals [56]. Defective calcium uptake by the sarcoplasmic reticulum in skeletal muscle has been noted with vitamin D deficiency [57] and experimental uremia [58]; moreover, treatment of uremic animals with $1,25(OH)_2D_3$ reversed this abnormality [58]. Altered calcium transport by the sarcoplasmic reticulum of muscle could arise from abnormal vitamin D metabolism. The mechanism whereby $1,25(OH)_2D_3$ affects muscle function is unknown, because specific $1,25(OH)_2D_3$ receptors resembling those found in other target tissues, such as the kidney, intestine, and parathyroid glands, appear to be absent in muscle [59]. Why muscular weakness does not occur more often in uremia is uncertain, since low plasma levels of $1,25(OH)_2D_3$ are common in patients with advanced renal failure [23,24].

Some additional comments regarding the clinical and biochemical findings in this patient are worthwhile. He had no evidence of skeletal disease when his advanced, chronic renal insufficiency was first identified. Moreover, he developed significant osteitis fibrosa despite reasonable control of serum phosphorus levels. Careful maintenance of normal serum phosphorus levels clearly can reduce the incidence of secondary hyperparathyroidism [60], but significant symptoms still develop in some patients, perhaps because therapy is not initiated until long after parathyroid hyperplasia is well established. The elevation of plasma alkaline phosphatase, which occurs slowly over many weeks or months in patients with bone disease, has not been a useful differentiating factor for the type of bone disease.

Interpreting Serum PTH Assays

Before proceeding to the issues of diagnosis and management of renal osteodystrophy, a few comments about the determination of serum iPTH are necessary. Many clinically available assays for serum iPTH utilize antisera that primarily detect the carboxyl-terminal fragments of PTH. It now seems certain that the native PTH molecule, a single-chain peptide of 84 amino acids, is quickly cleaved by the liver into amino-terminal and carboxyl-terminal fragments [61,62]; the carboxyl-terminal fragments are inactive but remain in the circulation with a longer "half-life" than either the 1-84 intact PTH molecule or the biologically active, 1-34 amino-terminal fragment. Moreover, these carboxyl-terminal fragments are not degraded by the liver but rely entirely on the kidney for degradation and clearance from the blood [63]. The plasma half-life of carboxyl-terminal fragments is markedly prolonged when renal function is decreased, and serum iPTH levels, measured with antisera directed toward the carboxyl-terminal moiety of the PTH molecule, often are markedly elevated [64,65]. Serum iPTH in the patient under discussion today was measured in the research laboratory of Dr. Frederick Singer, with the Burroughs Wellcome antiserum 211/32. This antiserum is directed in large part toward the intact PTH molecule. Thus, the serum iPTH level that was fivefold higher than normal is quite significant; such a degree of elevation with an assay utilizing a carboxyl-terminal antiserum might be "normal" for uremia. A good correlation has been reported between serum iPTH levels, measured with a carboxyl-terminal antiserum, and morphometric changes in bone due to secondary hyperparathyroidism [65], unfortunately, such data are not available for many widely used assays of iPTH. For the appropriate use of serum iPTH measurements, the physician should know the degree of elevation of serum iPTH that occurs in uremic patients simply because of the retention in the circulation of biologically inactive fragments [63]. Ideally, one also should use a PTH immunoassay that correlates with the histomorphometric bone findings of secondary hyperparathyroidism; unfortunately, such data are not currently available.

Diagnosis of Renal Osteodystrophy

With the observation of high levels of serum iPTH and radiographic findings of subperiosteal resorption in our patient, the bone biopsy finding of osteitis fibrosa is not surprising. Although obtaining a properly undecalcified specimen from a bone biopsy is the most desirable way to diagnose skeletal lesions, appropriate radiographic techniques also can be very useful. The use of fine-grain x-ray film combined with magnification of the x-rays can greatly increase the sensitivity of x-rays in detecting abnormalities and can aid in the follow-up of patients, particularly when the films are viewed by a radiologist with expertise in metabolic bone disease [66,67]. The use of fine-grain, industrial-quality x-ray film is not popular with radiology departments because these films cannot be developed automatically; however, film ordinarily used for mammography can be a satisfactory substitute. Meema and his colleagues reported that the use of fine-grain x-ray film and magnification techniques remarkably improves the radiologist's ability to detect osteitis fibrosa [67–69]. In patients with secondary hyperparathyroidism, cortical striations frequently are seen in the shafts of the phalanges and metacarpals, and presumably represent enlarged haversian canals within the bone [67]. The x-ray techniques capable of detecting osteomalacia are far less sensitive; in our experience, pseudofractures or Looser's zones are unusual in uremic patients with osteomalacia [70]. Radiographic signs of rickets can develop in children, but such findings are not helpful after closure of epiphyses. The x-rays of patients with osteomalacia usually show only demineralization or osteopenia.

Recent data from laboratories in Germany [71], the United Kingdom [72], and this country [37,73] indicate the existence of distinct subcategories of metabolic bone disease in patients with kidney disease. Moreover, the type of skeletal disease is important in determining the patient's response to treatment with $1,25(OH)_2D_3$ or other active vitamin D sterols. Our work with these subgroups of bone disease was conducted in conjunction with Drs. Donald Sherrard, Arnold Brickman, Frederick Singer, Eugene Wong, and Anthony Norman. We evaluated bone bipsies by quantitative morphometric techniques in approximately 60 highly selected uremic patients who were treated with $1,25(OH)_2D_3$ or $1\alpha(OH)D_3$ [73–77]. Repeat bone biopsies were performed in many patients after 6 to 12 months. These patients, all of whom had advanced renal failure and most of whom were undergoing dialysis, were selected because of the presence of symptomatic bone disease, marked radiographic abnormalities, or both. The patients comprised four distinct categories (Table 3). One group, of which the patient presented today is representative, had osteitis fibrosa with substantial marrow-space fibrosis and increased bone turnover as measured by double tetracycline labeling. Biopsies from this group frequently exhibited an increase in unmineralized osteoid that lay beneath active osteoblasts; such unmineralized osteoid arises because of a lag in mineralization of newly formed matrix rather than because of defective mineralization.

A second group has been termed "mild." The bone biopsies in these patients revealed less than 0.1% of marrow space filled with fibrosis but showed increased resorption surface. These patients characteristically have increased serum iPTH levels. Few patients with symptom-

Table 3. Skeletal lesions in 50 patients with severe renal osteodystrophy.

	Fraction of Surface Area		
	Afflicted (%)	Mineralized (%)	Fibrosis (%)
Osteitis fibrosa	39	>80	>2.0
Mild	15	>85	<0.6
Osteomalacia	33	<80	<1.5
Mixed	13	<80	>2.0
Normal	–	>94	0

Source: Modified from Ref. 73.

atic bone disease have this type of skeletal pathology; most have responded favorably to treatment with $1,25(OH)_2D_3$.

Bone biopsy in a third subgroup showed osteomalacia with wide osteoid seams (greater than 20% of the bone surface not mineralized); tetracycline labeling revealed a delay in mineralization, with slow bone turnover. Biopsy in the fourth group showed "mixed lesions," with evidence of both osteitis fibrosa and osteomalacia; these patients had evidence of high bone turnover, but the areas of unmineralized osteoid were substantially greater than in patients with osteitis fibrosa alone. Serum iPTH levels measured with the antiserum described above correlated well with marrow fibrosis; strikingly elevated levels of serum iPTH were present only in the patients with osteitis fibrosa or "mixed lesions."

The patients with osteitis fibrosa or pure osteomalacia were separated into two subgroups on the basis of their response to treatment with $1,25(OH)_2D_3$ (Table 4). Patients with osteitis fibrosa, by far the largest subgroup, showed an improvement in symptoms and a decrease in serum iPTH and alkaline phosphatase. Sequential bone biopsies revealed substantial improvement, with reduction in marrow-space fibrosis and improved bone mineralization. The patient under discussion today is representative of this group. A smaller subgroup of patients with biopsy-proved osteitis fibrosa exhibited a rapid increase in serum calcium levels during treatment with $1,25(OH)_2D_3$; this hypercalcemia necessitated withdrawal of therapy. Neither serum levels of iPTH, alkaline phosphatase, nor the extent of bone abnormalities differed in these two subgroups. On the other hand, serum calcium levels exceeded 10.5 to 11.0 mg/dl before initiation of treatment with $1,25(OH)_2D_3$ in the patients who developed marked hypercalcemia. At subsequent surgery or at autopsy, the latter group of hypercalcemic patients was found to have massive parathyroid hyperplasia. These observations suggest that treatment with $1,25(OH)_2D_3$ might aid in the identification of patients needing parathyroid surgery [78].

The patients with pure osteomalacia also comprised two subgroups, which were determined by the response to treatment with $1,25(OH)_2D_3$. The patients in one subgroup showed no improvement of symptoms during treatment with $1,25(OH)_2D_3$; the serum iPTH levels were normal or undetectable and the bone biopsies disclosed no marrow-space fibrosis or increase in resorptive surface. These patients had a tendency to develop hypercalcemia during treatment with either $1,25(OH)_2D_3$, another form of vitamin D, or even oral supplements of calcium alone. Indeed, the marked propensity for developing hypercalcemia suggested that bone was not significantly contributing to the "buffering" of extracellular calcium [76]. Repeated bone biopsies showed no improvement after prolonged treatment with $1,25(OH)_2D_3$ even through the serum cal-

Table 4. Serum biochemical observation before and after treatment with 1,25-dihydroxy-vitamin D_3 in uremic patients.

Type of Bone Disease	No. of Patients	Response to Treatment	Serum iPTH[a] (ng/ml)		Calcium (mg/dl)		Phosphorus (mg/dl)		Alkaline Phosphatase (IU/ml)		25(OH)D (ng/ml)
			C[b]	T[c]	C	T	C	T	C	T	C
Ostetis fibrosa	21	R[d]	2.8 ± 0.3	1.0 ± 0.3	9.4 ± 0.2	10.1 ± 0.3	4.5 ± 0.2	5.0 ± 0.3	297 ± 61	139 ± 35	38 ± 4
	4	F[e]	3.1 ± 0.4	2.2 ± 0.5	11.1 ± 0.3	17.8 ± 0.9	5.8 ± 0.6	5.7 ± 0.9	173 ± 26	260 ± 109	-
Osteo-malacia	10	F	0.2 ± 0.1	-	10.5 ± 0.2	11.8 ± 0.2	4.7 ± 0.1	5.1 ± 0.2	174 ± 15	219 ± 23	58 ± 10
	6	R	1.5 ± 0.7	0.4 ± 0.1	8.7 ± 1.8	9.8 ± 0.9	5.9 ± 0.6	5.1 ± 0.7	259 ± 133	153 ± 76	31 ± 7
Mild	7	R	1.5 ± 0.3	0.4 ± 0.1	9.8 ± 0.1	10.3 ± 0.3	4.4 ± 0.5	5.0 ± 0.3	121 ± 34	80 ± 22	-
Mixed	8	R	2.1 ± 0.7	0.6 ± 0.2	7.2 ± 0.4	8.8 ± 0.3	4.6 ± 0.3	4.8 ± 0.3	501 ± 153	137 ± 41	25 ± 4

[a]Measured with Burroughs Wellcome antisera.
[b]C = control, pretreatment values.
[c]T = values at end of treatment.
[d]R = responders.
[e]F = treatment-failure group.
Note: All data are mean ± SE.
Source: Modified from Ref. 77.

calcium was sustained above normal. Plasma levels of 25(OH)D_3 were either normal or elevated, perhaps because of prior treatment with vitamin D_3. Thus, such patients appear to have defective bone mineralization that is related neither to levels of calcium or phosphorus in the extracellular fluid nor to treatment with vitamin D. These patients often had recurrent rib and hip fractures and back pain, and they experienced progressive debility. Patients from the Newcastle area of the United Kingdom have exhibited a similar clinical picture [79,80]; their skeletal disease has been attributed to excessive levels of aluminum in the tap water used for the preparation of dialysate [81]. Epidemiologic data from sporadic patients in the United States fail to implicate aluminum in tap water, and the cause of this disease remains obscure [76].

The other subgroup with predominant osteomalacia had pretreatment levels of serum calcium that were generally below 10.5 mg/dl, serum iPTH levels that were slightly above normal, and small areas of marrow fibrosis on bone biopsy. These patients exhibited clinical improvement during treatment with 1,25$(OH)_2D_3$, although the bone mineralization recovered only partially following treatment with 1,25$(OH)_2D_3$ for 6 to 12 months.

For the entire group of patients treated with 1,25$(OH)_2D_3$, the major pretreatment observations that were useful in predicting a favorable response to 1,25$(OH)_2D_3$ included a serum calcium level below 10.5 mg/dl and some elevation of serum iPTH levels (Table 4). A similar separation of patients with renal osteodystrophy during treatment with 1α (OH)D_3 has been reported by investigators in the United Kingdom [80,82,83].

Management of Renal Osteodystrophy

Before discussing the therapeutic use of 1,25$(OH)_2D_3$ (Rocaltrol) in the patient presented today, I should like to comment regarding general principles of managing altered calcium and phosphorus metabolism in uremia. The management objectives for altered divalent ion metabolism should be (1) maintaining the blood levels of calcium and phosphorus as near normal as possible; (2) preventing the development of parathyroid hyperplasia or, if secondary hyperparathyroidism is already established, suppressing PTH secretion; (3) restoring the skeleton to normal; and () preventing and/or reversing extraskeletal deposition of calcium. Of these factors, the control of serum phosphorus is probably the most important and can be accomplished by moderately restricting the dietary intake of phosphorus to 0.8 to 1.0 g/day and by administering aluminum hydroxide or aluminum carbonate to bind phosphate in the gut. Because of the variability of phosphorus absorption in patients with uremia, the dosage of aluminum-containing compounds must be adjusted on an individual basis. Serum phosphorus levels should be measured every 2 to 4 weeks to avoid either hyper- or hypophosphatemia, as the latter can predispose to osteomalacia. Dietary calcium intake should be adequate. We currently recommend oral calcium supplements that provide 1.0 g of calcium per day; calcium is prescribed only when the serum phosphorus level is controlled. The dialysate calcium concentration should be maintained at 6.0–6.5 mg/dl (3.0–3.25 mEq/liter) to prevent either the loss or gain of calcium during dialysis.

The indications for the use of vitamin D sterols are only currently being established. These compounds should not be given to patients who have uncontrolled hyperphosphatemia (i.e., serum phosphorus $>$ 6.0 mg/dl). After the serum phosphorus has been controlled, vitamin D sterols are indicated (1) in the presence of hypocalcemia unresponsive to calcium supplementation through diet or dialysis; (2) when there is evidence of overt secondary hyperparathyroidism, particularly when the serum calcium is below 11.0 mg/dl; (3) for osteomalacia, particularly when it coexists with secondary hyperparathyroidism; (4) in children with chronic renal failure [29]; (5) when the need exists for concomitant anticonvulsant therapy; and (6) in patients who exhibit symptoms of proximal myopathy. It is not yet known whether vitamin D should be used prophylactically in all patients with endstage renal disease.

Other management considerations include (1) the use of appropriate levels of dialysate magnesium (0.5–0.7 mEq/liter) to avoid hypermagnesemia [84]; (2) the use of water treatment in preparation of dialysate to remove fluoride and aluminum, and to regulate calcium and magnesium levels; (3) avoidance of unnecessary treatment with barbiturates, phenytoin, and comparable drugs; and (4) maintenance of normal acid-base status. The specific benefits of some of these measures have not been firmly established, however.

The man described today illustrates several characteristics of patients with severe osteitis fibrosa who respond favorably to treatment with $1,25(OH)_2D_3$. Symptoms usually improve within 1 to 2 months after initiation of treatment [74,77], although symptomatic improvement can be delayed on occasion [85]. Serum alkaline phosphatase can rise during the first few weeks of treatment and then slowly fall toward normal. The serum calcium level might not increase during the first several weeks or months of treatment, even with doses of $1,25(OH)_2D_3$ as large as 1.0 μg/day; this is particularly true in patients with radiographic evidence of extensive skeletal disease. The serum phosphorus levels, obtained immediately before each dialysis, often decrease significantly during the first month of treatment and slowly increase thereafter. After 8 months of treatment, our patient developed significant hyperphosphatemia despite an increase in the dosage of aluminum hydroxide. It is well recognized that $1,25(OH)_2D_3$ increases intestinal absorption of calcium and phosphorus [26,86]. Serum calcium and phosphorus might not increase during the initial period of treatment because of substantial remineralization of the skeleton. Later, when serum alkaline phosphatase has decreased, serum calcium and phosphorus levels commonly increase. This patient illustrates a significant relationship between the development of hypercalcemia and a decrease of serum alkaline phosphatase to normal during treatment with $1,25(OH)_2D_3$. A reduction in the dosage of $1,25(OH)_2D_3$ is indicated when the alkaline phosphatase decreases to normal. This patient exhibits another common finding seen during treatment with $1,25(OH)_2D_3$, a prompt fall in the serum levels of both phosphorus and calcium shortly after withdrawal of treatment. A major advantage of $1,25(OH)_2D_3$ over other forms of vitamin D is the short persistence of a biologic effect after the withdrawal of treatment [87,88]. Thus, this sterol can be used more safely than other forms of vitamin D that act for a longer time after the drug is discontinued [89].

Finally, parathyroidectomy should be reserved for patients with definite evidence of secondary hyperparathyroidism (subperiosteal erosions and significantly increased iPTH levels). Surgery might be indicated in these patients if they also have persistent hypercalcemia, progressive or symptomatic extraskeletal calcification, a persistently elevated serum calcium $\times$ phosphorus product that is recalcitrant to other therapy, or calciphylaxis [90].

Questions and Answers

Dr. Jerome P. Kassirer: Before $1,25(OH)_2D_3$ or $1\alpha(OH)D_3$ were available, a number of groups reported that patients who had substantial renal osteodystrophy, particularly osteitis fibrosa, responded effectively to vitamin D_2 or other vitamin D preparations. The problem was that these patients frequently developed sustained hypercalcemia. The questions are, what is the course of the hypercalcemia induced by $1,25(OH)_2D_3$? Does it typically respond promptly to reduction or elimination of therapy? Do you sometimes have to treat the hypercalcemia by other means?

Dr. Coburn: One of the major advantages of 1,25-dihydroxy-vitamin D over other forms of vitamin D is its relatively short half-life: the circulating half-life is probably 3–5 h, although its biologic effect might be somewhat longer. Nonetheless, when one discontinues the drug, the hypercalcemia usually abates within 2 to 3 days without special treatment. Only rarely are special procedures, such as dialysis with a calcium-free dialysate, needed.

Dr. Kassirer: The response in the patient discussed today is apparently typical of patients who receive $1,25(OH)_2D_3$; not only do their serum calcium levels rise, but their serum phosphorus levels rise as well. Why do you worry about the rise in serum phosphorus levels in these patients? Are you concerned about it only because of the possibility of metastatic calcification or do you have other reasons?

Dr. Coburn: The appearance of phosphate retention and hyperphosphatemia causes one to worry, not only because secondary hyperparathyroidism is aggravated but because an elevated calcium × phosphorus product increases the risk of extraskeletal calcification. We have seen no increase in serum iPTH when serum phosphorus is raised during therapy with $1,25(OH)_2D_3$, possibly because the serum calcium is usually slightly higher, and also because of the action of $1,25(OH)_2D_3$ on the parathyroid glands.

Dr. Jordan J. Cohen: You indicated that patients who have predominant osteomalacia histologically do not respond predictably to the administration of vitamin D preparations. Isn't it paradoxical that the one bony change thought to be the specific consequence of vitamin-D deficiency does not respond to hormone replacement as well as the bone disease due to parathyroid excess does?

Dr. Coburn: In patients with exlcusive osteomalacia and normal or increased plasma levels of 25-hydroxy-D, we have given $1,25(OH)_2D_3$ and raised their serum calcium levels to above normal for weeks or even months in an effort to improve their severe, symptomatic bone disease. We also have allowed serum phosphorus levels to increase in an effort to induce healing. If one increases serum calcium and phosphorus levels in the osteomalacia secondary to vitamin D deficiency, the unmineralized osteoid will calcify. We believe that the failure of healing in the uremic patient represents an abnormality of bone matrix that is unrelated to levels of serum calcium or phosphorus, or to an abnormality affecting vitamin D [91,92]. Morphologically, this disorder appears the same as one described in England in an area around Newcastle on Tyne. In England the condition has been blamed on the presence of excess aluminum in the tap water used to prepare dialysate [81,93]; however, the 18 or 20 dialysis patients we have seen with this disorder come from diverse areas of the country. Because many other patients who have undergone dialysis in the same units have not developed bone disease, I do not think one can justify blaming such sporadic cases on excess aluminum in the water supply. In a preliminary study, we have measured bone aluminum in several of these patients and in dialysis patients with other types of bone disease. The bone aluminum levels were above normal in all, but they were higher in patients with this mineralizing defect than in patients with other types of bone disease [94]. Serum iPTH levels also were lower than in other uremic patients. Thus, the accumulation of aluminum or other trace elements in bone, and the low levels of serum iPTH might contribute to defective mineralization. The source of aluminum is uncertain but might be related to ingestion of phosphate-binding antacids in the sporadically occurring cases. Such patients might have increased intestinal permeability to aluminum or an abnormality of bone matrix leading to aluminum accumulation; obviously, these comments are speculative.

Dr. Cohen: What you are calling osteomalacia, therefore, should not be interpreted as being related specifically to vitamin D deficiency.

Dr. Coburn: That is correct. Osteomalacia is a descriptive term used to indicate defective mineralization of bone, no matter what the cause.

Dr. Boris Senior *(Chief, Division of Pediatric Endocrinology, NEMC):* Two questions: Is a decreased response to 1,25$(OH)_2D_3$ ever caused by poor calcium absorption from the gut in patients with renal failure? Do uremic patients generate less calcium-binding protein in response to 1,25-dihydroxycholecalciferol?

Dr. Coburn: In an extensive study, we examined the relationship between the dose of 1,25$(OH)_2D_3$ and the change in intestinal calcium absorption during the oral administration of 1,25$(OH)_2D_3$ in patients with chronic renal failure and in normal individuals [86]. We could stimulate calcium absorption just as readily as in the uremic patients as in normals. Also, the patients with osteomalacia who do not improve readily become hypercalcemic when they are given small doses; thus, we conclude that their intestines are responding to 1,25$(OH)_2D_3$. It should be noted that we are giving a hormone by mouth that is normally produced in the kidney and then enters the bloodstream. It is possible that the intestinal cells might "see" the hormone first in larger amounts than might occur if the drug were administered intravenously. Perhaps the effect of 1,25$(OH)_2D_3$ should be evaluated using another route of administration.

Blood levels of 1,25$(OH)_2D_3$ have been measured only recently and only in occasional patients. One child, with typical osteitis fibrosa, responded sluggishly and had blood levels of 1,25$(OH)_2D_3$ that were lower than might be expected, suggesting poor absorption of the sterol. This problem obviously needs to be explored further.

Dr. Mark Molitch *(Division of Endocrinology, NEMC)*: Some patients with modest renal insufficiency have had an acceleration of renal failure when treated with 1,25$(OH)_2D_3$. I would like to hear your comments on this observation.

Dr. Coburn: One report from Denmark [95] indicates that patients with creatinine clearances of 15–40 ml/min who received 1,25$(OH)_2D_3$ experienced small but reversible increases in serum creatinine compared to a "placebo" group given only a very small dose of vitamin D. I wonder whether the augmented absoprtion of phosphorus or calcium that is stimulated by 1,25$(OH)_2D_3$ might worsen renal function. Animal experiments [96] and clinical studies by Walser and colleagues [97] suggest that glomerular filtration rate might improve in renal failure during phosphate depletion. These trials of 1,25$(OH)_2D_3$ should be repeated with careful attention to phosphate homeostasis; the researchers should ensure that phosphate retention does not occur.

Dr. Senior: Some have suggested that any adverse effect of 1,25-dihydroxycholecalciferol on renal function results from hypercalcemia. Do you agree?

Dr. Coburn: Certainly hypercalcemia could worsen renal function. However, the animal experiments that I cited indicate that renal failure progresses in a subtotally nephrectomized rat fed a regular diet. When the diet is depleted of phosphate, renal function improves. The serum calcium levels usually are higher in the phosphate-depleted rat than in the rat fed a normal diet. Thus, the change in renal function could arise from either calcium or phosphate retention.

Dr. Molitch: I am intrigued by the subgroup of uremic patients who have normal calcium levels and normal or low PTH levels. What is the explanation for these findings?

Dr. Coburn: That is a very interesting question. The regulatory mechanisms that control serum calcium and calcium balance in these patients are not understood. Several patients have exhibited a tendency to become hypercalcemic with oral calcium loads, very small doses of either vitamin D_2 or 1,25$(OH)_2D_3$, or exposure to high calcium-containing dialysates. Without the presence of functioning kidneys to excrete calcium, such patients have lost one mechanism for regulating serum calcium; the bone behaves as though it does not participate in the "buffering" of extracellular fluid calcium. Thus, these patients seem to have a very small miscible calcium pool and can develop protracted hypercalcemia when any calcium is administered because they have no means of excreting calcium. Why this should occur, I do not know. It would be well to test calcium kinetics to resolve the question of the pool size; this study has not been done because such patients are seen only sporadically and because regular dialysis would complicate such an evaluation.

Six or seven of our patients with these findings had undergone parathyroidectomy for preexisting well-documented osteitis fibrosa. In these patients, hyperparathyroid bone disease might have been converted to the less common disorder, osteomalacia. The tendency toward normal or even slightly increased serum calcium levels might be responsible for preventing hyperparathyroidism in the others; we are beginning to evaluate the parathyroid response to acute hypocalcemia in these patients. Thus, a primary failure of the parathyroid glands could exist, and the low levels of serum iPTH could contribute to the decreased bone turnover.

Dr. Serafino Garella *(Chief, Division of Renal Diseases, Rhode Island Hospital, Providence, Rhode Island)*: Do you use bone densitometry in diagnosing renal osteodystrophy?

Dr. Coburn: Bone densitometry only tells you the amount of bone mineral and provides no information about its cause. A low value can occur with osteoporosis, osteomalacia, or other bone disorders. I think bone densitometry is a useful adjunct in monitoring a patient's course of therapy, but it should be used with other studies such as careful bone x-rays to help explain the qualitative aspects of bone changes.

Dr. Garella: Except for its duration of action, the activity of dihydrotachysterol appears similar to that of 1,25-dihydroxy-vitamin D in treating some of these conditions. Do you know of another major difference?

Dr. Coburn: Dihydrotachysterol (DHT) is a nonnatural sterol, discovered somewhat by accident in the laboratory. Because physiologists and biochemists are less interested in thia quirk of the laboratory than in natural sterols, we know far less about the action of DHT on bone than we do about the more recently identified, naturally occurring sterols, Dihydrotachysterol must be 25-hydroxylated before it acts, and the dose required for action is larger than that needed for $25(OH)D_3$, and almost as high as that for vitamin D_2 itself. The action of DHT can be ineffective in patients with liver disease or those taking anticonvulsant medications. Also, there seems to be more variability in the doses needed to produce a given effect than is the case for $1,25(OH)_2D_3$. We have found beneficial effects of $1,25(OH)_2D_3$ in several patients who allegedly had received DHT in doses as large as 2 mg/day. However, a carefully controlled comparison of the effects of DHT and $1,25(OH)_2D_3$ has not been performed.

Dr. Garella: Do you have any suggestions regarding the treatment of patients who suffer primarily from osteomalacia?

Dr. Coburn: I wish I did. The results of various therapeutic maneuvers have been equivocal or negative in most patients. We have tried reducing the ingestion of aluminum hydroxide to ensure that there is no phosphate depletion. In some we have replaced the acetate in the dialysis bath with bicarbonate; in others we have tried lowering dialysate magnesium so that hypermagnesemia does not exist; and in some, we have initiated special treatment of tap water to reduce trace metals. There was no apparent benefit from any of these treatment modalities. The patients with osteomalacia often are bedridden, and some have actually died because of deformities of the chest or spine produced by their bone disease. We have given some of these patients 1,25$(OH)_2D_3$, and a few have exhibited decreased pain, improved muscle strength, and a decrease in serum alkaline phosphatase to normal. Improvement as shown by bone biopsy was negligible, however. The patients who had a clinical response to 1,25$(OH)_2D_3$ tolerated larger daily doses before developing hypercalcemia than did those who failed to respond [94].

We currently are evaluating another naturally occurring vitamin D sterol—24,25-dihydroxy-vitamin D_3[98]; this sterol is believed by some to stimulate bone formation, although others believe it is merely a degradation product of vitamin D. Preliminary results with 24,25$(OH)_2D_3$ in a few patients show a decrease in serum calcium and a greater tolerance for 1,25$(OH)_2D_3$ or DHT without causing hypercalcemia. Most such patients given 24,25$(OH)_2D_3$ with either 1,25$(OH)_2D_3$ or DHT have shown chemical, biochemical, and histologic improvement [99].

We have little idea about the pathogenesis of this type of osteomalacia. It might represent several different diseases; for example, cadmium excess might be a cause in one patient, aluminum excess in another, and deficiency of 24,25$(OH)_2D_3$ in yet another. Obviously, I am speculating.

Dr. Martin Gelman *(Renal Division, St. Elizabeth's Hospital, Boston, Massachusetts.)*: Slatopolsky has had some success treating osteomalacia using 25-hydroxy-vitamin D_3. Have you had a similar experience?

Dr. Coburn: In a multicenter trial with 25-hydroxy-vitamin D_3, the patients were separated into those who responded well—usually patients with secondary hyperparathyroidism—and those who didn't. Patients with osteomalacia who were treated with 25-hydroxy-vitamin D_3 failed to respond. The observation that serum levels of 25(OH)-vitamin D_3 were normal or high in our patients led us away from a therapeutic trial with this sterol.

Dr. Donald Hricik *(Renal Fellow, NEMC)*: Should we be using "phosphate binders" and dietary phosphate restriction in patients with progressive renal disease before overt hyperphosphatemia develops?

Dr. Coburn: You can marshall strong arguments for doing so; Slatopolsky, Bricker, and colleagues have presented convincing evidence that you should [2–5]. This program can reduce serum iPTH levels, but long-term studies have not evaluated its safety. In countries in which people eat diets lower in phosphate than those consumed in the U.S., a high incidence of osteomalacia has been reported. Thus, one might be trading secondary hyperparathyroidism for another type of bone disease. Studies are needed to evaluate this question.

Dr. Nicolaos E. Madias *(Renal Service, NEMC)*: Are there any data on the levels of 1,25$(OH)_2$-vitamin D in human acute renal failure?

Dr. Coburn: None of which I am aware.

Dr. Robert Rubin *(Chief of Nephrology, Lemuel Shattuck Hospital, Boston, Massachusetts)*: Your comments regarding treatment for uremic myopathy are interesting. Do you have any quantitative data in patients whom you have treated with $1,25(OH)_2D_3$?

Dr. Coburn: The data I presented are based on a clinical, retrospective analysis of patients who were identified because of symptoms thought to arise from bone disease. We are now carrying out a double-blind prospective study in dialysis patients, using clinical tests of muscle strength as an index of myopathy, but we do not yet have data available. I mentioned our experience because most physicians are not aware of the myopathy and its potential reversibility.

Dr. Cohen: Would you summarize what you regard as the indications for parathyroidectomy in patients with end-stage renal disease?

Dr. Coburn: Yes. Several syndromes can be improved with parathyroid surgery. Before parathyroidectomy is considered, secondary hyperparathyroidism must be verified by either (1) a bone biopsy showing osteitis fibrosa; (2) an x-ray showing subperiosteal absorption; or (3) markedly elevated serum iPTH levels, measured with an assay that correlates well with bone disease. When one of these criteria is met, surgery may be considered under several situations. When a uremic patient develops spontaneous hypercalcemia, I would consider parathyroidectomy. If a patient with documented secondary hyperparathyroidism rapidly develops symptomatic bone disease, e.g., serious fractures, I would proceed to parathyroid surgery. On occasion, patients have developed calciphylaxis with progressive ischemic necrosis of the fingertips, toes, and elsewhere [90]. This syndrome occurs in dialysis patients or in renal transplant recipients with normal renal function. The disease often pogresses rapidly, and patients can die as a consequence: given the observation that some of these patients improve dramatically following parathyroid surgery, surgery should be performed with haste. One also should consider parathyroidectomy in uremic patients with extensive soft tissue calcification when the hyperphosphatemia has been totally resistant to attempts to deplete phosphate stores. Serum phosphorus usually decreases transiently after surgery; then one must convince these patients to follow rigorous measures for phosphate restriction. Persistent hypercalcemia after successful renal transplantation might be another indication for surgery, particularly if renal function is deteriorating.

Dr. Cohen: When you do recommend parathyroidectomy, do you suggest that the surgeon perform autotransplantation of the gland?

Dr. Coburn: Total parathyroidectomy with autotransplantation of parathyroid tissue into the forearm has been recommended to avoid the need for subsequent neck exploration if hyperparathyroidism recurs, and to have the parathyroid tissue in a more accessible place should removal of more parathyroid tissue be necessary. Our parathyroid surgeon prefers not to perform the additional surgery; he rapidly freezes and stores the parathyroid tissue for subcutaneous implantation should evidence of persistent hypoparathyroidism appear. The internist or nephrologist involved should work closely with an experienced parathyroid surgeon to determine the best procedures to follow in patients who undergo parathyroid surgery.

Dr. Kassirer: With new hormonal insights into the pathogenesis of divalent cation and anion disturbances in uremia, do you have new insights into *tertiary* hyperparathyroidism?

Dr. Coburn: This is a term I prefer not to use because most data indicate that in most patients with uremia, serum iPTH levels will decrease when the blood calcium level is raised; thus, there is no evidence for autonomy of parathyroid function. One study has shown that one can produce persistent hypercalcemia in rats by transplanting the parathyroid gland from 40 normal rats into the subcutaneous tissue [99]. Hypercalcemia does not necessarily indicate that there is something different about parathyroid cell function. Research in cows has shown that basal PTH secretion persists even during marked hypercalcemia [100]. Thus, increased iPTH levels might exist in uremic patients with mild hypercalcemia on the basis of marked parathyroid hyperplasia. It would seem better to reserve the term "tertiary" hyperparathyroidism for patients who develop parathyroid adenomas, a rare occurrence.

Dr. John T. Harrington: Much has been written about parathyroid hormone as a uremic toxin. What are your thoughts about this notion?

Dr. Coburn: Data have been reported that suggest that PTH is a pathogenetic factor responsible for a number of clinical manifestations of uremia. Increased calcium content of several soft tissues, including skin, blood vessels, and brain, has been reported to be associated with marked secondary hyperparathyroidism. The accumulation of calcium in the brain might be a factor leading to an abnormal electroencephalogram, particularly in acute uremia; an increase in calcium content of peripheral nerves has been reported but there is disagreement. I already mentioned the occurrence of soft tissue necrosis or calciphylaxis; hyperlipidemia has been attributed in part to high levels of PTH; and anemia has been associated with secondary hyperparathyroidism. Whether the anemia is caused by a toxic effect of PTH, marrow fibrosis from osteitis fibrosa, or some other factor is uncertain. There are anecdotal experiences of an increase in libido and reversal of impotence following a decrease in PTH levels. However, controlled studies have not been done. It has been thought that the abnormal carbohydrate metabolism present in uremia might be related to high PTH levels. The evidence supporting the role of PTH in these conditions has only recently begun to accumulate, and this is an area that we will view with interest.

Dr. Cohen: Is there a role for measuring ionized calcium as opposed to total calcium levels in patients with renal failure?

Dr. Coburn: Unfortunately, few data are available. With the development of effective, specific ion electrodes for measuring calcium, some laboratories can now measure the ionized calcium readily. Uremia is a condition that can be associated with an increase in the complexed fraction of calcium, so there might be a decrease in ionized calcium level for any level of total blood calcium. Further investigation is needed to pursue this question.

References

1. Coburn JW, Llach F, Kurokawa K: Altered divalent ion metabolism in renal disease and renal osteodystrophy. In Maxwell MH, Kleeman CR. (eds.): Clinical Disorders of Fluid and Electrolyte Metabolism. New York, McGraw-Hill, 1980, p. 1153
2. Slatopolsky E, Caglar S, Pennell JP, Taggart DD, Canterbury JM, Reiss E, Bricker NS: On the pathogenesis of hyperparathyroidism in chronic experimental renal insufficiency in the dog. J Clin Invest 50:492–499, 1971
3. Slatopolsky E, Caglar S, Gradowska L, Canterbury JM, Reiss E, Bricker NS: On the prevention of secondary hyperparathyroidism in experimental chronic renal disease using "proportional reduction" of dietary phosphorus intake. Kidney Int 2:147:151, 1972
4. Slatopolsky E, Bricker NS: The role of phosphorus restriction in the prevention of secondary hyperparathyroidism in chronic renal disease. Kidney Int 4:141–145, 1973
5. Rutherford WE, Bordier P, Marie P, Hruska K, Harter H, Greenwalt A, Blondin J, Haddad J, Bricker NS, Slatopolsky E: Phosphate control and 25-hydroxycholecalciferol administration in preventing experimental renal osteodystrophy in the dog. J Clin Invest 60:332–341, 1977
6. Llach F, Massry SG, Singer FR, Kurokawa K, Kaye JH, Coburn JW: Skeletal resistance of endogenous parathyroid hormone in patients with early renal failure: A possible cause for secondary hyperparathyroidism. J Clin Endocrinol Metab 41:338–345, 1975
7. Coburn JW, Koppel MH, Brickman AS, Massry SG: Study of intestinal absorption of calcium in patients with renal failure. Kidney Int 3:264–272, 1973
8. Coburn JW, Popovtzer MM, Massry SG, Kleeman CR: The physiochemical state and renal handling of divalent ions in chronic renal failure. Arch Intern Med 124:302–311, 1969
9. Coburn JW, Hartenbower DL, Brickman AS: Advances in vitamin D metabolism as they pertain to chronic renal disease. Am J Clin Nutr 29:1283–1299, 1976

10. Ponchon G, DeLuca HF: The role of the liver in the metabolism of vitamin D. J Clin Invest 48:1273–1279, 1969
11. Smith JE, Goodman DS: The turnover and transport of vitamin D and of a polar metabolite with the properties of 25-hydroxycholecalciferol in human plasma. J Clin Invest 50:2159–2167, 1971
12. Fraser DR, Kodicek E: Unique biosynthesis by kidney of a biologically active vitamin D metabolite. Nature 228:764–766, 1970
13. Myrtle JF, Norman AW: Vitamin D: A cholecalciferol metabolite highly active in promoting intestinal calcium transport. Science 171:79–82, 1971
14. Boyle IT, Gray RW, DeLuca HF: Regulation by calcium of in vivo synthesis of 1,25-dihydroxycholecalciferol and 21,25-dihydroxycholecalciferol. Proc Natl Acad Sci USA 68:2131–2134, 1971
15. Henry HL, Midgett RJ, Norman AW: Regulation of 25-hydroxyvitamin D_3-1-hydroxylase in vivo. J Biol Chem 249:7584–7592, 1974
16. Booth BE, Tsai HC, Morris RC: Parathyroidectomy reduces 25-hydroxyvitamin D_3-1α-hydroxylase activity in the hypocalcemic vitamin D-deficient chick. J Clin Invest 60:1314–1320, 1977
17. Tanaka Y, DeLuca HF: The control of 25-hydroxy-vitamin D metabolism by inorganic phosphorus. Arch Biochem Biophys 154:566–574, 1973
18. Larkins RG, MacAuley SJ, Rapoport A, Martin TJ, Tulloch BR, Byfield PGH, Matthews EW, MacIntyre I: Effects of nucleotides, hormones, ions, and 1,25-dihydroxycholecalciferol on 1,25-dihydroxycholecalciferol production in isolated chick renal tubules. Clin Sci Mol Med 46:559–582, 1974
19. Malluche HH, Werner E, Ritz E: Intestinal absorption of calcium and whole body calcium retention in incipient and advanced renal failure. Min Electrol Metab 1:263–270, 1978
20. Slatopolsky E, Gray R, Adams ND, Lewis J, Hruska K, Martin K, Klahr E, DeLuca HF, Lemann J: Low serum levels of $1,25(OH)_2D_3$ are not responsible for the development of secondary hyperparathyroidism in early renal failure. Kidney Int 14:733, 1978
21. Portale AA, Boorth BE, Tsai HC, Morris RC: Reduced plasma concentration of $1,25(OH)_2D$ in children with moderate renal insufficiency. Kidney Int 16:922, 1979
22. Llach F, Massry SG, Koffler A, Malluche HH, Singer FR, Brickman AS, Kurokawa K: Secondary hyperparathyroidism in early renal failure: Role of phosphate retention. Kidney Int 12:459, 1977
23. Brumbaugh PF, Haussler DH, Bressler R, Haussler MR: Radip-receptor assay for 1α,25-dihydroxy-vitamin D_3. Science 183:1089–1091, 1974
24. Eisman JA, Hamstra AJ, Kream BE, DeLuca HF: 1,25-dihydroxy-vitamin D in biological fluids: A simplified and sensitive assay. Science 193:1021–1023, 1976
25. Brickman AS, Coburn JW, Norman AW: Action of 1,25-dihydroxycholecalciferol, a potent, kidney-produced metabolite of vitamin D_3, in uremic man. N Engl J Med 287:891–895, 1973
26. Brickman AS, Coburn JW, Massry SG, Norman AW: 1,25-dihydroxy-vitamin D_3 in normal man and patients with renal failure. Ann Intern Med 80:161–168, 1974
27. Henderson RG, Russell RGG, Ledingham JGG, Smith R, Oliver DO, Wal-

ton RJ, Small DG, Preston C, Warner GT, Norman AW: Effects of 1,25-dihydroxycholecalciferol on calcium absorption, muscle weakness, and bone disease in chronic renal failure. Lancet 1:379–384, 1974
28. Brickman AS, Sherrard DJ, Jowsey J, Singer FR, Baylink DJ, Maloney N, Massry SG, Norman AW, Coburn JW: 1,25-dihydroxycholecalciferol: Effect on skeletal lesions and plasma parathyroid hormone in uremic osteodystrophy. Arch Intern Med 134:883–888, 1974
29. Chesney RW, Moorthy AV, Eisman JA, Jax DK, Mazess RB, DeLuca HF: Increased growth after long-term oral 1α,25-vitamin D_3 in childhood renal osteodystrophy. N Engl J Med 298:238–242, 1978
30. Brumbaugh PF, Hughes MR, Haussler MR: Cytoplasmic and nuclear binding components for 1-alpha,25-dihydroxyvitamin D_3 in chick parathyroid glands. Proc Natl Acad Sci USA 72:4871–4875, 1975
31. Chertow BS, Baylink DJ, Wergedal JF, Su MHH, Norman AW: Decrease in serum immunoreactive parathyroid hormone in rats and in parathyroid hormone secretion in vitro by 1,25-dihydroxycholecalciferol. J Clin Invest 56:668–678, 1975
32. Tanaka Y, DeLuca HF, Ghazarian JG, Hargis GK, Williams GA: The effect of vitamin D and its metabolites on serum parathyroid hormone levels in the rat. Min Electrol Metab 2:20–25, 1979
33. Llach F, Coburn JW, Brickman AS, Kurokawa K, Norman AW, Canterbury JM, Reiss E: Acute actions of 1,25-dihydroxy-vitamin D_3 in normal man; Effect on calcium and parathyroid status. J Clin Endocrinol Metab 44:1054–1060, 1977
34. Oldham SB, Smith R, Hartenbowler DL, Henry HL, Norman AW, Coburn JW: The acute effects of 1,25-dihydroxycholecalciferol on serum immunoreactive parathyroid hormone (iPTH) in the dog. Endocrinology 104:248–254, 1979
35. Recker RR, Saville PD: Calcium absorption in renal failure: Its relationship to blood urea nitrogen, dietary calcium intake, time on dialysis, and other variables. J Lab Clin Med 78:380–388, 1971
36. Duursma SA, Visser WJ, Nijo L: A quantitative histological study of bone in 30 patients with renal insufficiency. Calcif Tissue Res 9:216–225, 1972
37. Sherrard DJ, Baylink DJ, Wergedal JE, Maloney N: Quantitative histological studies on the pathogenesis of uremic bone disease. J Clin Endocrinol Metab 39:119–135, 1974
38. Bordier PJ, Tun-Chot S, Eastwood JB, Fournier A, de Wardener HE: Lack of histological evidence of vitamin D abnormality in the bones of anephric patients. Clin Sci 44:33–41, 1973
39. Kanis JA, Adams ND, Earnshaw M, Heynen G, Ledingham JGG, Oliver DO, Russell RGG, Woods CG: Vitamin D, osteomalacia and chronic renal failure. In Norman AW, Schaeffer K, Coburn JW, DeLuca HF, Fraser D, Grigoleit HG, von Herrath D, (eds.): Vitamin D: Biochemical, Chemical and Clinical Aspects Related to Calcium Metabolism. Berlin, Walter de Gruyter 1977, p. 671
40. Massry SG, Coburn JW, Lee DBN, Jowsey J, Kleeman CR: Skeletal resistance to parathyroid hormone in renal failure: Study in 105 human subjects. Ann Intern Med 78:357–364, 1973
41. Massry SG, Stein R, Garty J, Arieff AI, Coburn JW, Norman AW, Friedler

RM: Skeletal resistance to the calcemic action of parathyroid hormone in uremia: Role of 1,25(OH)$_2$D$_3$. Kidney Int 9:467–474, 1976
42. Sommervile PJ, Kaye M: Resistance to parathyroid hormone in renal failure: Role of vitamin D metabolites. Kidney Int 14:245–254, 1978.
43. Hahn TJ, Avioli LV: Anticonvulsant osteomalacia. Arch Intern Med 135:997–1000, 1975
44. Hahn TJ: Bone complications of anticonvulsants. Drugs 12:201–211, 1976
45. Jubiz W, Haussler MR, McCain TA, Tolman KO: Plasma 1,25-dihydroxyvitamin D levels in patients receiving anticonvulsant drugs. J Clin Endocrinol Metab 44:617–621, 1977
46. Hahn TJ, Birge SJ, Scharp CR, Avioli LV: Phenobarbital-induced alterations in vitamin D metabolism. J Clin Invest 51:741–748, 1972
47. Pierides AM, Kerr DN, Ellis HA, O'Riordan JLH, DeLuca HF: 1α-hydroxycholecalciferol in hemodialysis renal osteodystrophy. Adverse effects of anticonvulsant therapy. Clin Nephrol 5:189–196, 1976
48. Pierides AM, Ellis HA, Ward M, Simpson W, Peart KM, Alvarex-Ude F, Uldall PR, Kerr DNS: Bartiturate and anticonvulsant treatment in relation to osteomalacia with haemodialysis and renal transplantation. Br Med J 1:190–193, 1976
49. Massry SG, Goldstein DA: Role of parathyroid hormone in uremic toxicity. Kidney Int 13:S39–S42, 1978
50. Rever BL, Brickman AS, Sherrard DJ, Coburn JW: Vitamin D responsive, proximal myopathy in chronic renal failure. West Dial Transpl Soc, 1979, p. 46
51. Schott GD, Wills MR: Muscle weakness in osteomalacia. Lancet 1:626–629, 1976
52. Mallette LE, Patten BM, Engel WK: Neuromuscular disease in secondary hyperparathyroidism. Ann Intern Med 82:474–483, 1975
53. Birge SJ: Vitamin D, muscle and phosphate homeostasis. Min Electrol Metab 1:57–64, 1978
54. Smith R, Stern G: Myopathy, osteomalacia and hyperparathyroidism. Brain 90:593–602, 1967
55. Schoenfeld PJ, Martin JA, Barnes B, Teitelbaum SL: Amelioration of myopathy with 25-hydroxyvitamin D$_3$ therapy [25(OH)D$_3$] in patients on chronic hemodialysis. Third Workshop on Vitamin D, Asilomar, California, 1977, p. 160
56. Rodman JS, Barker T: Changes in the kinetics of muscle contraction in vitamin D-depleted rats. Kidney Int 13:189–193, 1978
57. Curry OB, Basten JF, Francis MJO, Smith R: Calcium uptake by sarcoplasmic reticulum of muscle from vitamin D-deficient rabbits. Nature 249:83–84, 1974
58. Matthews C, Heimberg KW, Ritz E, Agostini B, Fritzsche J, Hasselbach W: Effect of 1,25-dihydroxycholecalciferol in impaired calcium transport by the sarcoplasmic reticulum in experimental uremia. Kidney Int 11:227–235, 1977
59. Haussler MR, McCain TA: Basic and clinical concepts related to vitamin D metabolism and action. N Engl J Med 297:974–983, 1041–1050, 1977
60. Johnson WJ, Goldsmith RS, Beabout JW, Jowsey J, Kelly PJ, Arnaud CD:

Prevention and reversal of progressive secondary hyperparathyroidism in patients maintained by hemodialysis. Am J Med 56:827–832, 1974
61. Canterbury JM, Levey GS, Reiss E: Activation of renal cortical adenylate cyclase by circulating immunoreactive parathyroid fragments. J Clin Invest 52:524–527, 1973
62. Martin K, Hruska K, Greenwalt A, Klahr S, Slatopolsky E: Selective uptake of intact parathyroid hormone by the liver. Differences between hepatic and renal uptake. J Clin Invest 58:781–788, 1976
63. Martin KJ, Hruska KA, Lewis J, Anderson C, Slatopolsky E: The renal handling of parathyroid hormone. Role of peritubular uptake and glomerular filtration. J Clin Invest 60:808–814, 1977
64. Freitag J, Martin KJ, Hruska KA, Anderson C, Conrades M, Ladenson J, Klahr S, Slatopolsky E: Impaired parathyroid hormone metabolism in patients with chronic renal failure. N Engl J Med 298:29–32, 1978
65. Hruska KA, Teitelbaum SL, Kopelman R, Richardson CA, Miller P, Depman J, Martin K, Slatopolsky E: The predictability of the histologic features of uremic bone disease by non-invasive techniques. Metab Bone Dis Rel Res (Paris) 1:39–44, 1978
66. Parfitt AM: Clinical and radiographic manifestations of renal osteodystrophy. In David DS (ed.): Calcium Metabolism in Renal Failure and Nephrolithiasis. New York, Wiley, 1977, p. 150
67. Meema HE, Oreopoulos DG, Meema S: A roentgenologic study of cortical bone resorption in chronic renal failure. Radiology 126:67–74, 1978
68. Meema HE, Rabinovich S, Meema S, Lloyd GJ, Oreopoulos DG: Improved radiological diagnosis of azotemic osteodystrophy. Radiology 102:1–10, 1972
69. Meema HE, Meema S: Microradioscopic quantitation of periosteal resorption in secondary hyperparathyroidism of chronic renal failure. Clin Orthop 130:297–302, 1978
70. Meema HE, Meema S: Improved roentgenologic diagnosis of osteomalacia by microradioscopy of hand bones. Am J Roentgenol Radium Ther Nucl Med 125:925–935, 1975
71. Delling G, Schulz A, Schulz W: Morphologische klassifikation der renalen osteopathie. Mels Med Mitt 49:133–140, 1975
72. Stanbury SW, Lumb GA: Parathyroid function in chronic renal failure: A statistical survey of the plasma biochemistry in azotaemic renal osteodystrophy. Q J Med 35:1–23, 1966
73. Sherrard DJ, Brickman AS, Coburn JW, Singer FR, Maloney N: Skeletal response to treatment with 1,25-dihydroxy-vitamin D in renal failure. Contrib Nephrol 18:92–97, 1979
74. Coburn JW, Brickman AS, Sherrard DJ, Singer FR, Baylink DJ, Wong EGC, Massry SG, Norman AW: Clinical efficacy of 1,25-dihydroxy-vitamin D_3 in renal osteodystrophy. In Norman, AW, Schaefer, K, Coburn JW, DeLuca HF, Fraser D, Grigoleit HG, von Herrath D (eds.): Vitamin D: Biochemical, Chemical and Clinical Aspects Related to Calcium Metabolism. Berlin, Walter de Gruyter, 1977, p. 657
75. Brickman AS, Sherrard DJ, Wong EGC, Singer FR, Norman AW, Schaefer K, Coburn JW. Renal osteodystrophy: Seperation of types by bone his-

tology and response to 1,25(OH)$_2$D$_3$. VIIth International Congress of Nephrology, 1978, p. D-29
76. Coburn JW, Sherrard DJ, Brickman AS, Wong EGC, Norman AW, Singer FR: A skeletal mineralizing defect in dialysis patients: A syndrome resembling osteomalacia but unrelated to vitamin D. Contrib Nephrol 18:172–183, 1979
77. Brickman AS, Coburn JW, Sherrard DJ, Wong EGC, Norman AW, Singer FR: Clinical effects of 1,25-dihydroxy-vitamin D$_3$ in uremic patients with overt osteodystrophy. Contrib Nephrol 18:29–41, 1979
78. Coburn JW, Brickman AS, Sherrard DJ, Singer FR, Wong EGC, Baylink DJ, Norman AW: Use of 1,25(OH)$_2$-vitamin D$_3$ to separate "types" of renal osteodystrophy. In Robinson BHB, Hawkins JB, Vereerstrachfen P (eds.): Dialysis, Transplantation, Nephrology. Kent, Pitman Medical, 1977, p. 442
79. Ellis HA, Peart KM: Azotemic renal osteodystrophy, a quantitative study on iliac bone. J Clin Pathol 26:83–101, 1973
80. Ellis HA, Pierides AM, Feest TG, Ward MK, Kerr DNS: Histopathology of renal osteodystrophy with particular reference to the effects of 1α-hydroxyvitamin D$_3$ in patients treated by long-term haemodialysis. Clin Endocrinol 7:31S–38S, 1977
81. Ward MK, Feest TG, Ellis HA, Parkinson IS, Kerr DNS, Herrington J, Goode GL: Osteomalacic dialysis osteodystrophy: Evidence for a water-borne aetiological agent, probably aluminum. Lancet 1:841–845, 1978
82. Kanis JA, Earnshaw M, Henderson RG, Heynen G, Ledingham JGG, Naik RB, Oliver DO, Russell RGG, Smith R, Wilkinson RH, Woods CG: Correlation of clinical, biochemical and skeletal responses to 1α-hydroxy-vitamin D$_3$ in renal bone disease. Clin Endocrinol 7:45S–50S, 1977
83. Kanis JA, Ruggell RGG, Naik RB, Earnshaw M, Smith R, Heynen G, Woods CG: Factors influencing the response to 1α-hydroxy-vitamin D$_3$ in patients with renal bone disease. Clin Endocrinol 7:51S–57S, 1977
84. Burnell JM, Teubner E: Effects of decreasing magnesium in patients with chronic renal failure. Proc Clin Dial Transplant Forum 5:191, 1976
85. Goldstein DA, Malluche HH, Massry SG: Long-term effects of 1,25-(OH)$_2$D$_3$ on clinical and biochemical derangements of divalent ions in dialysis patients. Contrib Nephrol 18:42–54, 1979
86. Brickman AS, Hartenbower DL, Norman AW, Coburn JW: Actions of 1α-hydroxy-vitamin D$_3$ and 1,25-dihydroxy-vitamin D$_3$ on mineral metabolism in man. I. Effects on net absorption of phosphorus. Am J Clin Nutr 30:1064–1068, 1977
87. Brickman AS, Coburn JW, Friedman GR, Okamura WH, Massry SG, Norman AW: Comparison of effects of 1α-hydroxy-vitamin D$_3$ and 1,25-dihydroxy-vitamin D$_3$ in man. J Clin Invest 57:1540–1547, 1976
88. Kanis JA, Russell RGG: Rate of reversal of hypercalcaemia and hypercalciuria induced by vitamin D and its 1α-hydroxylated derivatives. Br Med J 1:78–81, 1977
89. Frame B, Parfitt AM: Osteomalacia: Current concepts. Ann Intern Med 89:966–982, 1978
90. Gipstein RH, Coburn JW, Adams DA, Lee DBN, Parsa KP, Sellers A, Suki

WN, Massry SG: Calciphylaxis in man: A syndrome of tissue necrosis and vascular calcification in 11 patients with chronic renal disease. Arch Intern Med 136:1273–1280, 1976
91. Coburn JW, Llach F: Renal osteodystrophy and maintenance dialysis. In Drukker W, Parsons FM, Maher JF (eds.): Replacement of Renal Function by Dialysis. The Hague, Martinus Nijoff, 1979, p. 571
92. Nortman DF, Coburn JW: Altered calcium metabolism and osteodystrophy in end-stage renal failure. Postgrad Med 64:123–130, 1978
93. Ellis HA, McCarthy JH, Herrington J: Bone aluminum in hemodialysed patients and in rats injected with aluminum chloride; relationship to impaired bone mineralization. J Clin Pathol 32:832–844, 1979
94. Hodsman AB, Sherrard DJ, Wong EGC, Brickman AS, Lee DBN, Alfrey AC, Singer FR, Coburn JW: Vitamin D-resistant osteomalacia without secondary hyperparathyroidism in dialysis patients. Clin Res 28:560A, 1980
95. Christiansen C, Rodbro P, Christensen MS, Hartnack B, Transbol I: Deterioration of renal function during treatment of chronic failure with 1,25-dihydroxycholecalciferol. Lancet 2:700–703, 1978
96. Ibels LS, Alfrey AC, Haut L, Huffer WF: Preservation of function in experimental renal disease by dietary restriction of phosphate. N Engl J Med 298:122–126, 1978
97. Walser M, Mitch WE, Collier VU: The effect of nutritional therapy on the course of chronic renal failure. Clin Nephrol 11:66–70, 1979
98. Coburn JW, Wong EGC, Sherrard DJ, Brickman AS, Hodsman AB, Lee DBN, Singer FR, Norman AW: Use of 24,25-dihydroxy vitamin D_3 in dialysis osteomalacia: Preliminary results. Clin Res 28:532A, 1980
99. Gittes RF, Radde IC: Experimental model for hyperparathyroidism: effect of excessive numbers of transplanted isologous parathyroid glands. J Urol 95:595–603, 1966
100. Mayer GP, Habener JF, Potts JT Jr: Parathyroid hormone secretion in vivo. Demonstration of a calcium-independent non-suppressible component of secretion. J Clin Invest 57:678–683, 1976

Acute Hypophosphatemia

Principal Discussant
Eberhard Ritz

Case Presentation

Two weeks after admission to the hospital, a 53-year old woman with regional enteritis developed restlessness, paresthesias, weakness, abdominal distention, and hypoventilation.

The patient was well until years before admission, when she began vomiting daily. One year before admission she developed intermittent abdominal pain without relation to food intake or bowel movements. Her stools were loose but contained no blood or mucus. In association with these symptoms and a diet consisting almost exclusively of baked brains and raw liver, she began to lose weight and was admitted to another hospital. Anorexia nervosa was diagnosed at that time. In the 4 months prior to admission, weight loss accelerated and in that period the patient's weight fell from 55 to 40 kg.

On admission to the Klinikum der Universität Heidelberg, she appeared markedly malnourished. Blood pressure was 90/60 mmHg; pulse was 88/min. The liver was palpable but not tender. The spleen was not palpable. Bilateral pretibial edema was present. The right leg was markedly swollen but nontender on palpation, and Homan's sign was negative. Diffuse muscle wasting was prominent, but neurologic examination was normal. Laboratory findings disclosed the following: hemoglobin, 11.2 g/dl; white blood cell count, 11,500/mm^3, with 1% metamyelocytes and toxic granulations. Platelet count was 544,000/mm^3. The sedimentation rate was 12 to 19 mm/h. Serum electrolytes were sodium, 128 mEq/liter; potassium, 3.1 mEq/liter; chloride, 92 mEq/liter; and bicarbonate, 24 mEq/liter. Blood pH was 7.48; $PaCO_2$, 31 mmHg; serum calcium, 3.3 mEq/liter; serum phosphorus, 2.8–3.7 mg/dl; total serum protein, 3.0–3.8 g/dl; plasma urea nitrogen, 9 mg/dl; plasma creatinine, 0.6 mg/dl; plasma cholesterol, 76 mg/dl; and folate, 17 nM/liter. The plasma 25-OH-vitamin D concentration was 99 nM/liter (normal). Prothrombin time was 65%. Serum IgG was 817 mg/dl; IgA, 14 mg/dl; IgM, 88 mg/dl; plasma fibrinogen, 210 mg/dl (all reduced). Serum CH_{50} was 180 U. Serum iron was 22 μg, and iron-binding capacity was 101 μg/dl.

The patient was suspected of having deep-vein thrombosis in the right leg and was treated with urokinase, heparin, and indomethacin. An extensive gastrointestinal evaluation was performed to evaluate the cause of the weight loss and presumed malabsorption. Gastroscopy *revealed no ulcers or erosions, but gastric biopsy disclosed intestinal metaplasia of the gastric mucosa. An upper gastrointestinal series disclosed minor segmental narrowing of the distal jejunum and proximal ileum and spotty filling of the ileum. The findings were not thought to be consistent with regional enteritis, but were compatible with malabsorption. Studies of absorption showed xylose test, 3.34 g/5 h (low); fecal chymotryspin excretion, 62.4 U/g (normal, 120 U/g). Fecal fat excretion was 20.9 g/24 h (normal < 7 g/24 h). Excretion of ^{131}I-PVP was 1.47% of dose/4 days (normal). Stool examination for parasites, pathogenic bacteria, and fungi was negative.*

The patient failed to gain weight and on the 13th hospital day parenteral nutrition was initiated. The patient received 418 g of glucose/24 h, synthetic L-amino acids (8.03 g alpha-amino nitrogen/24 h), xylitol (100 g/24 h), lactate (11 mmol/24 h), acetate (59 mmol/24 h), regular insulin (24 U/24 h), sodium (75 mmol/24 h), potassium (65–145 mmol/24 h), phosphate (9 mM/24 h), and a polyvitamin preparation in a total volume of 2.5 liter/24 h.

On the 16th hospital day, the patient's temperature increased to 38.4 °C, but there were no shaking chills. At that time, the white blood cell count was 14,300/mm^3 without a left shift. Fever subsequently disappeared without antibiotic administration.

On the 19th hospital day, the patient became progressively restless and complained of circumoral and fingertip tingling followed by generalized numbness. She was lethargic and slightly disoriented, but otherwise mentation was normal. She had marked asthenia, was unable to sit up, and had difficulty swallowing. Respiration was labored and her speech had a nasal quality. On examination the temperature was 38.4 °C, blood pressure was 75/60 mmHg, pulse was 120/min, the abdomen was distended, and bowel sounds were scarce. Her speech had a nasal quality, she was unable to raise her head from the pillow, bilateral ptosis was present, and the gag reflex was diminished. Deep tendon reflexes were difficult to elicit, but there was a flexor plantar response and the sensory examination was normal.

An abdominal plain film showed excessive amounts of gas and several air-fluid levels in the small intestine. Hemoglobin was 6.6 g/dl; LDH, 160 IU; serum sodium, 114 mEq/liter; uric acid, 2.0 mg/dl; plasma creatinine, 0.4 mg/dl. Blood gases showed Pa_{O_2}, 88 mmHg; Pa_{CO_2}, 54 mmHg; pH, 7.40. Serum calcium was 3.1 mEq/liter, and serum phosphorus was 0.25 mg/dl. Creatinine phosphokinase was normal. Urinary myoglobin was not measured. Lumbar puncture was normal and the electroencephalogram showed only slowing of the rhythm and reduction of amplitude.

The patient was treated with hypertonic sodium chloride, albumin (400 ml), and macromolecular dextran (500 ml). On the 20th hospital day, treatment was instituted with intravenous potassium phosphate (20 mmol daily). By the 23rd day, hypotension, ileus, and the neurologic signs as well as hypercapnia had disappeared. Blood gases on that day showed Po_2*, 94 mmHg;* Pco_2, 28 mmHg; blood pH, 7.52; and bicarbonate, 25 mEq/liter.

Parenteral nutrition containing phosphorus was continued, but the patient failed to gain weight, and she left the hospital against medical advice. Two months later she died at home. Autopsy revealed regional enteritis of the upper jejunum with multiple ulcers, stenosis, and perforation.

Discussion

Prof. Med. Eberhard Ritz *(Head, Division of Nephrology, University of Heidelberg, Heidelberg, Federal Republic of Germany)*: The multisystem disorder of acute hypophosphatemia and acute ventilatory failure is rarely encountered today, but the underlying pathophysiology is highly instructive and merits detailed analysis.

The patient under discussion suffered from Crohn's disease. The diagnosis of anorexia nervosa was first entertained because of food idiosyncrasies and unusual personality traits, but nothing in her history suggested anorexia nervosa, and food faddism is not unusual in Crohn's disease. The findings that pointed to Crohn's disease were her history of abdominal complaints and weight loss with leukocytosis and thrombocytosis. The low sedimentation rate in this patient is unusual for Crohn's disease, but hypofibrinogenemia secondary to severe hypoproteinemia may account for this finding. Various tests pointed to malabsorption possibly caused by bacterial overgrowth. The diagnosis of Crohn's disease was not established during the patient's hospitalization because the small jejeunal segment involved escaped detection on the upper GI series. The diagnosis was unequivocally confirmed at autopsy, however.

It is interesting that many cases of acute iatrogenic hypophosphatemia with neuromuscular disturbances are described in patients with Crohn's disease [1,2] and in those with alcoholism [3]. Let us focus on the dramatic neuromuscular, cardiovascular, and hematologic alterations in this woman when parenteral hyperalimentation was instituted to treat the well-established malnutrition. Before doing so, I plan to discuss the diagnosis and mechanisms of phosphate depletion.

Diagnosis of Preexisting Phosphate Depletion

Let us explore first whether the patient was phosphorus depleted prior to receiving intravenous hyperalimentation. Unfortunately we are given conflicting clues. Evidence favoring such a contention can be adduced from the low plasma phosphorus value (2.9 mg/dl) before parenteral hyperalimentation was begun and from the low urinary phosphorus excretion on the first day of hyperalimentation (0.124 g/24 h or 0.277 g phosphorus/g creatinine). The response of the kidney to phosphate depletion provides an explanation for this assertion. Under ordinary circumstances, phosphate depletion is effectively prevented by the kidney's ability to conserve phosphorus in response to the body's need for it. It has been demonstrated in experimental studies that the net load of phosphorus absorbed from the gut [4], or more specifically the body's phosphorus requirements [5], are the most important determinants for the renal tubular phosphorus threshold. In the proximal tubule, the permeability of the luminal brush border membrane is modulated in response to changes of phosphorus balance [6]. As a result, urinary phosphate excretion is low in phosphate depletion, and this finding can be used to support the diagnosis. Indeed, in the classic study of Lotz et al., phosphorus vanished completely from the urine within a few days in human volunteers given a low-phosphorus diet and oral phosphate binders [7].

The low urinary phosphate level in this patient argues against a renal source of phosphate wasting but does not exclude it with certainty. Recent findings suggest that glucocorticoids can cause phosphaturia even in the presence of hypophosphatemia [8]; since glucocorticoid excess cannot be excluded entirely, it is possible that renal phosphate wasting contributed to depletion in this patient. Episodes of ketoacidosis also are known to cause phosphaturia [9] secondary to decomposition of organic phosphate within cells [10], and although it is possible that ketoacidotic episodes occurred in our patient, it seems quite unlikely.

One might argue that the low serum phosphorus levels provide only weak confirmatory evidence of phosphate depletion. It is known, for example, that hypocapnia tends to lower plasma phosphorus levels without affecting total-body phosphorus [11]. Because only 0.1% of total-body phosphate is contained in the extracellular compartment, loss of only a minute fraction of total-body phosphate from the extracellular compartment could cause significant hypophosphatemia. Thus, we could conclude that the patient was not phosphorus depleted before parenteral nutrition was instituted. This conclusion would be in line with previous clinical and experimental studies [12,13], which suggest that starvation is associated with "an orderly shrinkage of cellular mass so that the general relationships between nitrogen, phosphorus, potassium, and other intracellular components remain nearly normal" [13].

That more than 1 or 2 days elapsed between the introduction of parenteral alimentation in this patient and clinical manifestations of phosphate depletion also argues against preexisting phosphate depletion. Thus, in the presence of preexisting phosphorus deficiency (e.g.) in diabetic ketoacidosis and alcoholism), hypophosphatemia usually occurs within 1 or 2 days after hyperalimentation is begun, whereas in patients

Table 1. Conditions predisposing to phosphate depletion and hypophosphatemia.

1.	Parenteral hyperalimentation
2.	Alcoholism
3.	Recovery phase from diabetic ketoacidosis
4.	Recovery/diuretic phase after severe burns
5.	Recovery after starvation
6.	Overadministration of oral phosphate binders [$Al(OH)_3$]

not phosphate depleted, hypophosphatemia usually does not become manifest for 5–10 days. The patient under discussion today developed manifestations approximately 5 days after hyperalimentation was started.

Table 1 displays the many conditions in which hypophosphatemia can be observed [14]. In these various disorders, at what serum phosphorus level are clinical manifestations to be expected? Clinical manifestations usually are not observed until serum phosphorus falls below 1 mg/dl, and the phosphorus level in the patient discussed here was well below this concentration. Only a few clinical conditions lead to such severe hypophosphatemia [13,15,16].

Although we are concerned today about acute phosphorus depletion, it is worthy of note that chronic phosphorus depletion has been a problem to dairy farmers for decades [17]. Because they crave phosphorus when grazing on phosphorus-depleted pastures, cows devour animal cadavers. These animals often die of botulism after ingesting spores of *C. botulinum* because phosphorus depletion impairs their leukocyte function. Impairment of neuromuscular function secondary to phosphorus depletion also might be a contributing factor. In humans, despite isolated anecodotal observations [18], not until the report by Lotz et al. [7] did clinicians become interested in phosphorus depletion.

Serum vs. Total-body Phosphorus

So far, I have used little semantic caution is distinguishing hypophosphatemia from phosphorus depletion. The two are not synonymous, however, and hypophosphatemia may not necessarily be associated with phosphorus depletion. Cellular phosphorus content is the net result of different transmembrane fluxes [19]; a remarkable dissociation between ambient plasma phosphate concentration and cellular phosphorus content is, for instance, present in genetic disorders such as X-linked hypophosphatemia. Furthermore, cellular phosphorus shows remarkable compartmentation [20]. Erythrocytes lack mitochondria, which are a major intracellular repository of phosphorus in other cells; hence the intracellular phosphorus concentration in erythrocytes, but not in other cells, follows that of plasma [21]. In somatic cells that can draw on mitochondrial phosphorus stores, cytosolic phosphorus concentration can be maintained for a remarkably long period despite hypophosphatemia [22]. Consequently, if one uses plasma phosphorus concentration as an index of cellular phosphorus depletion, one must be aware that the relation between plasma phosphorus and intracellular phosphorus is variable. Even in advanced phosphorus depletion, intracellular phosphorus falls by no more than approximately 20% when measured in deproteinized tissue samples [22–24]. The possibility exists that these measurements of cellular phosphorus content are in error, however, since measurements by nondestructive techniques, such as nuclear magnetic resonance [25,26], give values lower by almost one order of magnitude. Consequently, it is conceivable that cytosolic phosphorus concentration is close to nil in phosphorus depletion.

Mechanisms of Phosphate Depletion

What was the mechanism by which phosphorus depletion occurred in the patient under consideration? First let us analyze the ways by which phosphorus depletion can occur, because several of them might have existed in this patient. Growing organisms develop phosphorus depletion on a low-phosphate diet; this fact prompted a protocol that has become a standard method of inducing phosphorus depletion in experimental animals [22]. In humans, premature babies develop rickets when raised on human milk containing relatively little phosphorus; the rickets heal readily when the infants are fed cow's milk containing a relatively large quantity of phosphorus [27].

In the adult, phosphorus depletion either can be due to negative external phosphorus balance, internal redistribution of phosphorus, or a combination of both. Negative external phosphorus balance with the attendant decrease of total-body phosphorus/nitrogen ratio may be caused by diminished intestinal net absorption (e.g., after ingestion of oral phosphate binders) [28] or by renal phosphorus loss [29]. Internal redistribution of phosphorus may lead to hypophosphatemia and phosphorus depletion in critical organs without necessary alteration of total-body phosphorus. Movement of inorganic phosphorus from the extracellular to the intracellular space can be due to utilization of phosphorus for synthesis of organic macromolecules (phosphoproteins, phospholipids, phosphorylated carbohydrates), as in refeeding after starvation or in parenteral hyperalimentation, or it can be due to intracellular trapping of phosphorus esters (hexose-phosphate, phosphorylated nucleotides, etc.), as in respiratory alkalosis or following the administration of carbohydrates such as fructose [15].

The hazards of refeeding starved individuals have been known for centuries [30]. When describing the horrors of the seige of Jerusalem, Joseph Flavius wrote that

> some of the deserters . . . fled to the Romans. Their fate was worse than if they had stayed in the City, and the hunger they had left behind was, as they discovered, less lethal than the plenty that the Romans provided. They arrived blown up by starvation as if by dropsy, then stuffed their empty bellies non-stop till they burst—except for those who were wise enough to restrain their appetite and take the unaccustomed food a little at a time.

Similarly, during World War II, many prisoners withstood years of starvation but died during hospitalization following release from captivity [1,31–34]. In such individuals, it was noted by some that refeeding with skim milk markedly reduced mortality [31]. Although detailed studies of blood and urine chemistry were not possible, it later was claimed that the phosphorus and potassium content of skim milk might have been important [13]; this view is supported by experimental studies [35].

Synthesis of protoplasm involves deposition of nitrogen in parallel with phosphorus in a ratio of 0.07 g phosphorus/g nitrogen. As shown during intravenous hyperalimentation of underweight adults [12], repletion of protoplasm is retarded or abolished if any one of the following elements is lacking: nitrogen, phosphorus, sodium, or potassium. Such weight gain as occurs when nitrogen, sodium, or phosphorus is not provided is due to enlargement of adipose tissue mass, for which the only requirement appears to be an abundant supply of glucose. After hyperalimentation was introduced, a virtual epidemic of hypophosphatemia was described in hyperalimented patients, at first in the United States [1], and after some delay in Europe, perhaps because of the continued use of phosphorus-containing solutions [36]. Acute hypophosphatemia is observed not only with intravenous hyperalimentation, but even when 5% glucose solutions are administered to malnourished alcoholics [3].

The first reason for hypophosphatemia that we can identify in the patient we are discussing today is the requirement for phosphorus during anabolism for synthesis of intracellular phosphoproteins, phospholipids, phosphorylated nucleotides, and carbohydrate phosphate esters. One additional factor can be identified, however. It has been known for decades that the plasma phosphorus level falls in response to glucose [37]; such a decrease is less pronounced in muscle disease and more marked in starvation or cirrhosis [38,39]. The amount by which phosphorus falls depends on the relative rates of glycogen synthesis (which requires little phosphorus), glycolysis, and utilization of glucose. In fact, changes in plasma phosphorus (and potassium) are primarily related to glycolysis, which is accompanied by esterification of organic phosphate within cells [40]. For maximum phosphorylation to occur in the glycolytic process, 1 mole of glucose must bind the equivalent of 4 moles of potassium phosphate. Whereas the fall of plasma phosphorus after glucose administration usually is modest and transient, a more pronounced and prolonged decrease of plasma phosphorus is observed after an infusion of fructose [41]. Phosphorus is trapped intracellularly in hepatocytes as fructose-1-phosphate (Fig. 1); this process produces profound hypophosphatemia. Inactivation of cellular phosphate in this bound form has profound effects. Phosphorus depletion in the cytosol of hepatocytes [16] is followed by depletion of hepatocellular ATP, activation of adenylate deaminase (with formation of inosine monophosphate and uric acid), inhibition of gluconeogenesis from lactate, and consequent lactacidemia [16]. This phenomenon is examplified by the particularly severe hypophosphatemia in patients with congenital fructose intolerance [42] and in fructose-galactose intolerance [43]. Although fructose was not given to our patient, these observations are pertinent because similar changes such as ATP consumption due to accumulation of alpha-glycerophosphate and depletion of hepatocellular phosphorus are observed with xylitol in the isolated perfused rat liver [44]. It is surprising that despite their known adverse effects on hepatocellular ATP, fructose and xylitol still are widely employed in some European countries as a source of energy, especially during the postoperative period [45]. In our patient, refeeding hypophosphatemia

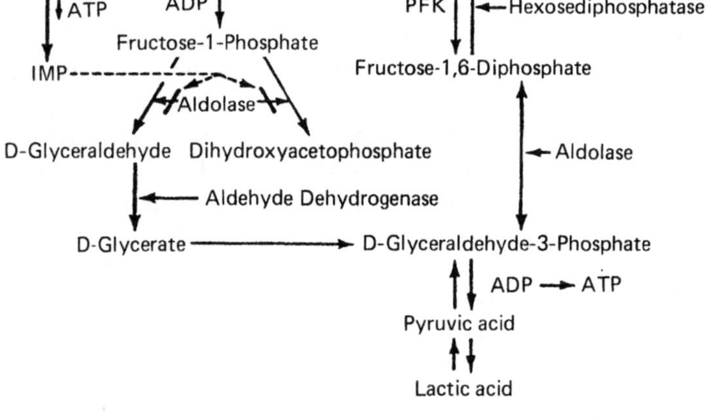

Fig. 1. Fructose metabolism in the liver (Ref. 69).

probably was compounded by the concomitant administration of xylitol. In this patient, serum uric acid did not increase, as commonly occurs after fructose or xylitol administration [16]; in fact, it actually decreased. Serum uric acid may be low [46] or high [47] during refeeding. In the absence of information about uric acid excretion, it is impossible for us to judge the extent to which uric acid production or renal excretion might have been abnormal in our patient. It is of note, however, that an increased clearance of uric acid can occur after administration of glucose and amino acids [46]. Disturbances of proximal tubular function also have been demonstrated in experimental phosphorus depletion [48–50], but there was no clinical evidence for such a disturbance in this patient, particularly no glycosuria.

Clinical Manifestations

Because phosphorus is a key element in cellular metabolism, one would expect that some disturbance of function will be found in every somatic cell. The clinical manifestations in acute or chronic hypophosphatemia, however, mainly concern the neuromuscular, cardiovascular, and hematologic systems. The factor or factors ultimately responsible for disturbed organ function in phosphorus depletion are currently unknown. Several possibilities have been discussed, such as depletion of cellular ATP; tissue hypoxia resulting from low erythrocyte 2,3 DPG; partial blockade of glycolysis because of lack of phosphorus as a crucial cofactor at the glyceraldehyde-phosphate-dehydrogenase step; and change of cytosolic calcium and hydrogen ion concentrations [13,15,16]. Let us now turn to an explanation of the clinical findings in this patient.

Neuromuscular

The presence of ptosis, dysarthria with nasal speech, difficulty in swallowing, and alveolar hypoventilation initially raised the suspicion of some form of partial bulbar palsy. Silvis [1], Newman [3], Oster [2], and Finck [51] have reported patients with remarkably similar findings. The most threatening feature of the syndrome, alveolar hypoventilation, may necessitate the use of mechanical ventilation [2,3]. Hypoventilation is not uniformly observed in acute hypophosphatemia, however. Indeed, some authors even have described hyperventilation [52]. Hyperventilation may have been the result of poor tissue oxygenation because of increased oxygen affinity of hemoglobin, i.e., a decrease of P_{50} secondary to low erythrocyte 2,3 DPG levels. This constellation contains the elements of a "vicious circle"; hypophosphatemia causes hyperventilation, which in turn leads to respiratory alkalosis, which provokes even more severe hypophosphatemia. When alveolar hypoventilation occurs, as in our patient, it points to a profound disturbance of efferent neuromuscular function. Also, despite hypercapnia, profound hypophosphatemia was maintained. One would expect that intracellular acidosis should cause egress of phosphorus from cells [10]. The normal arterial pH in our patient in the presence of hypercapnia points to a mixed type of acid-base abnormality or to laboratory error, but this possibility was not further pursued at the time.

What is the mechanism of neuromuscular dysfunction? An increase of intracellular water, sodium, chloride, and a decrease of transmembrane resting potential were found in the muscles of hypophosphatemic alcoholics [13]. Similar changes are present in hypophosphatemic dogs [26] but not in acutely [27] or chronically [53] hypophosphatemic rats. In chronically hypophosphatemic individuals, a myopathy occurs that involves predominantly proximal musculature [54,55]. This abnormality may be related to the changes of muscle composition described above [27,53–56]. Because of depletion of ATP and the fall in intracellular inorganic phosphorus activates AMP-deaminase, and because low ATP activates 5′-nucleotidase, the pool of adenylic acids shrinks and presumably makes muscle cells unable to withstand episodes of increased demand for ATP, e.g., during strenuous exercise or epileptic fits. Figure 2 describes the reversible elevation of serum creatine phosphokinase in an alcoholic with hypophosphatemia; indeed, rhabdomyolysis and acute myoglobinuric renal failure occur in such patients [13] and can

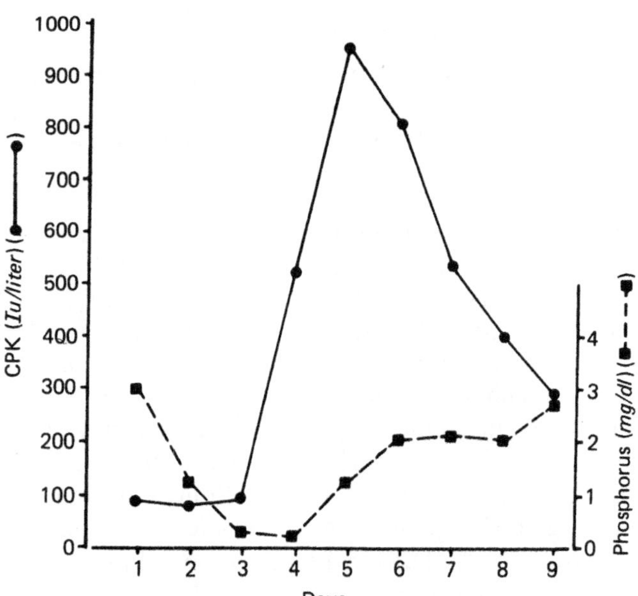

Fig. 2. Relationship between onset of hypophosphatemia and elevation of creatine phosphokinase activity (Ref. 13).

be reproduced in chronically phosphorus-depleted animals given intravenous hyperalimentation [56].

The muscular manifestations in our patient differ from the abovementioned syndromes in several respects. Although she had considerable weakness, the craniofacial involvement predominated over the proximal musculature affected. Furthermore, there was no muscle tenderness or elevation of serum creatine phosphokinase. I am therefore forced to look for alternative explanations for this type of neuromuscular dysfunction. Acute bulbar symptoms, remarkably similar to the ones in our patient, were observed in malnourished patients given hyperalimentation and in alcoholics given 5% glucose solutions [2,3,51,57,58]. A myopathic component is not definitely excluded, but I owe to Dr. Finck in Berlin the unpublished observation that one consistently finds in such patients evidence of neural disturbance at the radiculospinal level. Such disturbances are identified on the electromyogram as disturbed H reflexes and F waves without abnormalities of nerve conduction velocity or neuromuscular transmission. Evidence is overwhelming that central nervous system abnormalities, such as obtundation, seizures, tremors, disorientation, anisocoria, and ballismus result from phosphorus depletion [13,15,16]. The multilevel abnormalities of neuromuscular function in phosphorus depletion are poorly understood and present a fertile area for future investigation.

Ileus

Another noteworthy finding in our patient was ileus. Possibly Crohn's disease caused a latent abnormality of gastrointestinal motility that became apparent when the patient was critically ill. Disturbed smooth muscle function secondary to hypophosphatemia is a definite possibility, particularly in view of the recent demonstration in our laboratory of abnormalities of vascular smooth muscle function in hypophosphatemia [59].

Cardiovascular

I now would like to examine another aspect of the patient's clinical course. During the acute episode, she developed marked hypotension and tachycardia, which were attributed to ileus and hypovolemia. Recent findings suggest alternative possibilities, however. O'Connor et al. studied critically ill hypophosphatemic patients and found an increase of the cardiac index despite unchanged or even decreased preload when phosphorus was administered [60]. Furthermore, cardiac arrhythmias can occur in acutely hypophosphatemic patients [51]. Finally, congestive heart failure that responds to phosphate administration has been observed in individuals who ingested large amounts of oral phosphate binders [21]. A reversible depression in myocardial performance also can be demonstrated experimentally in phosphorus-deficient dogs; Fuller et al. observed a decrease of stroke volume, peak flow velocity, and maximum left ventricular dP/dt [61]. More recently, Dr. Kreusser in our laboratory observed decreased myocardial contractility (V_{max}) not only in the basal state, but also in response to cathecholaminergic stimulation (Fig. 3) [62]. This abnormality was completely reversible when phosphorus was administered. In addition, the hypophosphatemic dogs' failure to show an adequate pressor response to

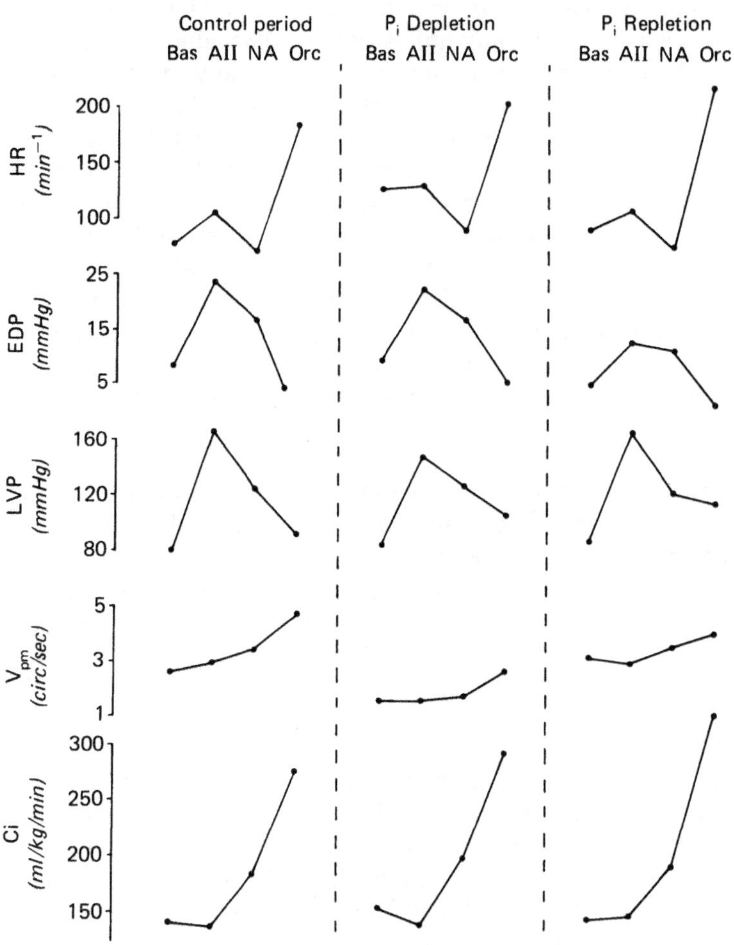

Fig. 3. Hemodynamics during control period, phosphate depletion, and phosphate repletion. The animals were studied under basal conditions (Bas) and after stimulation with angiotensin II (AII), norepinephrine (NA), and orciprenaline (Orc). *HR*, heart rate; *EDP*, left ventricular end diastolic pressure: *LVP*, left ventricular peak systolic pressure; V_{pm}, maximal contractile element shortening velocity (circ/s); *Ci*, cardiac index. (After Ref. 62.)

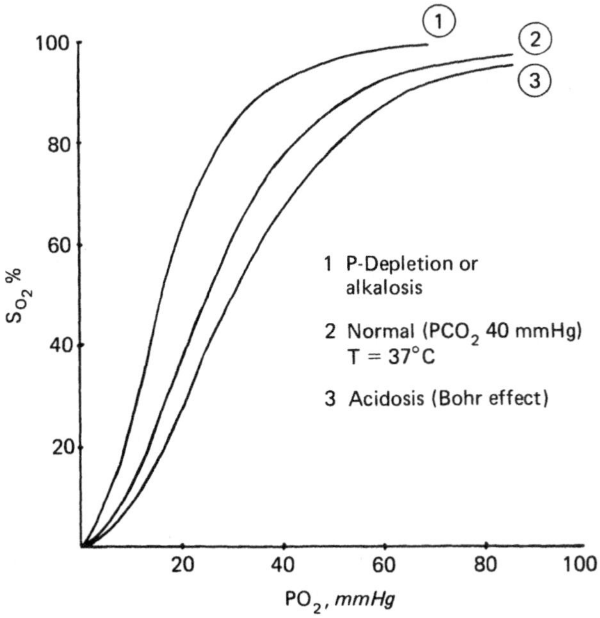

Fig. 4. Oxyhemoglobin dissociation and the effects of acidosis, alkalosis, and phosphate depletion. (After Ref. 15.)

angiotensin, and the reversal of this response with phosphate repletion, point to a vascular muscle abnormality induced by phosphorus depletion. In view of this experimental evidence, compromised cardiovascular function is likely an added risk in critically ill, acutely hypophosphatemic individuals, and although documentation is far from perfect, this situation may have been present in the patient under consideration.

Red Blood Cells

Let me comment on two findings in our patient that point to possible hematologic disturbances. Hemoglobin levels decreased from 9.2 to 6.6 g/dl. Although no further investigations were carried out in this patient, hemolytic anemia in severe hypophosphatemia has been documented [47,52,63]. Several abnormalities of erythrocyte function have been documented in hypophosphatemic patients and experimental animals [63]. Phosphate is a critical cofactor for the glyceraldehyde phosphate-dehydrogenase step of glycolysis [47,52]. In hypophosphatemia, a block of glycolysis occurs with a fall of 2,3 DPG and other intermediates distal to this step. Deficiency of ATP and particularly 2,3 DPG shift the position of the oxygen-hemoglobin equilbrium curve to the left (Fig. 4). This shift increases the affinity of hemoglobin for oxygen and deprives tissues of oxygen. Furthermore, fluidity and elastoviscous properties of the erythrocyte membrane crucially depend on the microfilamental system, which consists of actin and myosin analogs and which requires ATP for proper function. Loss of ATP causes rigidity and insufficient deformability of erythrocytes and leads to erthyrocyte fragmentation in the microvasculature. Hemolysis occurs when the serum phosphorus level falls below 0.5 mg/dl [13].

Leukocytes

The transient fever in our patient also deserves comment. Craddock et al, found a significant depression of chemotactic, phagocytic, and bactericidal activity of granulocytes of phosphate-depleted dogs [64]. The ATP concentration in granulocytes increases and the motility defect is corrected when phosphorus is repleted in vivo by supplementation of the diet or in vitro by incubation of the leukocytes with adenosine and phosphate. It appears likely that phosphorus depletion, by reducing ATP synthesis, interferes with the microtubular system that regulates the mechanical properties of leukocytes (pseudopod and vacuole formation) and also interferes with microfilaments that control surface movement. In addition, phosphorus depletion may impair the requirement for increased synthesis of phosphoinositides and other organic phosphate compounds of the cell membrane during phagocytosis. Synthesis of membrane material may be compromised; abnormalities of membrane phospholipids have been noted by Klock and Shohet in erythrocytes [65] and by our laboratory in subcellular muscle membranes [27]. The increased incidence of septicemia in patients on total parenteral hyperalimentation has been attributed to defective leukocyte function [13,64], but local hypertonicity at the site of the central catheter may be an added factor since phagocytic function is impaired by high osmolality. The potential importance of phosphorus for resistance to bacterial infection is well documented by experimental studies. Garner et al. demonstrated that phosphorus administration to hypophosphatemic animals with salmonella septicemia markedly reduced mortality [66].

Phosphorus is crucial for the function of every somatic cell. It is not surprising therefore that phosphate depletion alters the function of virtually every organ. A number of alterations in our patient, such as electrolyte changes and hepatic function, would merit further comment. But I would like to close on a short note concerning prevention of such unfortunate episodes.

Prevention

Dangerous hypophosphatemia during hyperalimentation can safely be prevented if potassium dihydrogen phosphate, 20–25 mEq/1000 kcal, is administered prophylactically [36]. Detailed guidelines for hyperalimentation of undernourished adults have been given by Rudman et al., who recommend 0.4 g/kg ideal body weight of sodium per day and 0.18

g/kg ideal body weight of phosphorus per day if no extrarenal losses of body fluid (diarrhea, vomiting, gastric suction, fistula) or hypermetabolic states (infection, trauma, fever) are present [12]. The practical details of phosphorus administration, particularly the prevention of dangerous hypocalcemia, recently have been dealt with in detail [67]. Suffice it to say that the kidney is usually wiser than the physician and signals adequate replacement by spilling phosphate into the urine when phosphate depletion has been reversed.

Questions and Answers

Dr. Jerome P. Kassirer: Thank you, Dr. Ritz. Given the complex clinical setting in which phosphate depletion develops, how can you identify whether the manifestations of such patients are caused by phosphate depletion?

Dr. Ritz: Clinical signs and symptoms of phosphate depletion usually are observed at serum phosphorus levels below 1 mg/dl, and such low levels usually indicate phosphorus depletion. When urinary phosphorus is low or absent in the presence of marked hypophosphatemia, phosphorus depletion is virtually certain. Although important symptoms usually are not observed at serum phosphorus levels above 1 mg/dl, lesser degrees of hypophosphatemia (2–3 mg/dl) still might indicate phosphate depletion severe enough to prevent maximum anabolism.

Dr. Kassirer: What is the best method of treating the patient acutely depleted of phosphate?

Dr. Ritz: One approach is oral administration of phosphorus. This route is preferable because it avoids some of the hazards associated with intravenous administration. If one gives phosphorus slowly, the body has time to adapt and self-correct the abnormalities that lead to such hazards. If the patient is unable to tolerate oral phosphate administration or if there is a medical emergency, one can administer phosphorus intravenously. One must be cognizant, however, of some potential complications. First, if a severely phosphorus-depleted patient is given phosphorus intravenously, profound hypocalcemia may ensue. For example, Drs. Rambusek and Kreusser administered phosphorus intravenously to chronically phosphorus-depleted rats and lost almost all of the animals; death was prevented by the simultaneous administration of calcium [68]. By administering radiocalcium they showed that phosphorus was translocated into cells of soft tissue, prdominantly muscle, and was accompanied by an equivalent amount of calcium. The most important consideration during intravenous administration of phosphorus is avoidance of severe hypocalcemia because it can be complicated by shock and cardiac arrhythmias. Of course, if calcium is administered intravenously, it is important that it not be given in the same venous line as phosphorus because precipitation will occur promptly. As I mentioned previously, detailed recommendations for dosage have been given in a recent report, and I refer you to that communication for details [67].

To ensure that the patient has been given an adequate amount of phosphorus, the clinician has available one simple procedure, determination of urinary phosphorus. In the absence of a renal tubular absorptive abnormality, urinary phosphorus is the best index of adequate phosphorus repletion.

Dr. Kassirer: Suppose you are dealing with an urgent situation: this patient, for example, became moderately hypercapnic and warranted rapid repletion of phosphorus. Would it be appropriate to give the patient intravenous sodium or potassium phosphate and follow the serum calcium level frequently?

Dr. Ritz: Yes, this is precisely what I would suggest in such a case.

Dr. Kassirer: Certain features in this patient raise the possibility that there might be a renal diluting defect. The combination of severe hypouricemia, hyponatremia, and a low serum creatninine level strongly suggests to me that the patient had the syndrome of inappropriate ADH secretion. If an excessively high water intake was not the cause (and there is no history to indicate that it was), then we must conclude that a diluting defect was present. Is there any evidence that phosphate depletion influences ADH production or release or the local effect of ADH on the kidney? Or does phosphate depletion affect the diluting mechanism independently of ADH?

Dr. Ritz: There is some experimental evidence of increased V/C_{in} and C_{H_2O}/C_{in} associated with increased fractional delivery out of the proximal tubule in phosphorus-depleted animals during acute water diuresis [48], and these abnormalities are promptly reversed by phosphorus repletion. There is no information, to the best of my knowledge, about ADH secretion and ADH response in chronic phosphorus depletion. I pointed out that phosphorus depletion has been investigated intensely only in the last few years; many aspects are still "terra incognita" for renal physiologists. In this particular patient documentation is poor, but the occurrence of ADH oversecretion as a result of nonosmotic stimuli is a good possibility.

Dr. Kassirer: Does phosphate depletion have important acid-base consequences? Because these depleted patients excrete little phosphate, their titratable acid excretion must be very low, and this disorder theoretically could lead to a defect in urinary acid excretion. Do these patients often have a mild metabolic acidosis, or does increased ammonia production make up for the reduction in titratable acid excretion?

Dr. Ritz: Titratable acid excretion, ammonia excretion, and bicarbonate reabsorption all are abnormal in phosphorus depletion. The bicarbonate threshold of the kidney is low, presumably because of increased cytosolic pH in proximal tubular cells, as suggested by measurements with the DMO technique [50]. Further, there is an abnormality of urinary ammonia excretion over and above diminished ammonia trapping as a result of alkaline urine pH [69]. Finally, titratable acid by necessity must be reduced because excretion of phosphate, the most important proton acceptor, is low.

To make a long story short, there is a tendency for proton retention in phosphorus depletion. Paradoxically, however, arterial pH usually is normal in the early phase of phosphorus depletion. Consequently, there must be some source of alkali that titrates the protons retained by the kidney. Bone hydroxyapatite presumably constitutes the source of such alkali [70]. I don't want to go through the stoichiometry, but dissolution of tertiary calcium phosphate consumes acid equivalents. On balance, this allows the body to maintain normal pH at the expense of consuming some skeletal alkali.

Dr. Kassirer: One other possibility, of course, is that the meager food intake greatly reduces acid production. Therefore, even though there is a defect in renal acid excretion, acidosis does not occur because the input of acid is so low.

Dr. Ritz: You are correct in pointing to this possibility. This consideration, however, does not apply to the experimental models of phosphorus depletion that demonstrate the abnormalities of tubular acid transport mentioned earlier.

Prof. Dr. Otto Mehls *(Associate Professor of Pediatrics, Heidelberg)*: Dr. Ritz, could you tell me how often and under what conditions hypercalcemia occurs in patients with hypophosphatemia? In the study on phosphorus depletion in healthy volunteers that you mentioned, hypercalcemia was not noted. I ask this question because I have observed marked hypercalcemia in two children with severe hypophosphatemia. Hypercalcemia in one child was so pronounced that we were unable to resolve it with peritoneal dialysis. This latter patient was on hemodialysis and had been treated with hyperalimentation without phosphorus supplementation.

Dr. Ritz: Am I correct in assuming that vitamin D intoxication, uncontrolled hyperparathyroidism, or hypercalcemia from immobilization cannot account for your observation?

Dr. Mehls: Yes.

Dr. Ritz: There are enormous species differences with respect to serum calcium levels in hypophosphatemia. In the phosphorus-depleted rat, hypercalcemia is constant, at least during the first 3 weeks of phosphorus depletion [71]. The serum calcium level later decreases for at least two reasons: first, indirect evidence exists for inappropriately low parathyroid hormone levels [72]; second, there is an abnormality of osteocyte ultrastructure in phosphorus depletion as shown in Kreusser's study.

Apparently, humans differ from rats with respect to serum calcium levels during phosphorus depletion. Humans usually are normocalcemic despite increased intestinal absorption of calcium and the development of hypercalciuria. I am aware of occasional phosphorus depleted adult patients who developed hypercalcemia during administration of thiazides (Massry S, personal communication), but this phenomenon seems to be the exception rather than the rule. But children may well differ from adults in this respect. I believe this issue has not been investigated. Finally, as the most likely explanation, I would propose that your children had marked (renal) secondary hyperparathyroidism; it is well known that if one lowers serum phosphorus in such individuals (for example, after transplantation), the serum calcium level will rise.

Dr. Mehls: The observation of hypercalcemia in hypophosphatemic children seems to be consistent, since I observed it in three children. A causal relationship is suggested by the observation that serum calcium levels promptly returned to normal upon administration of phosphorus, whereas hypercalcemia had been resistant even to peritoneal dialysis prior to phosphorus repletion.

Dr. Peter Gross *(Nephrologist, Division of Nephrology, Heidelberg)*: Could hypercalcemia be explained by an increased efflux of phosphorus and calcium from bone? According to Dr. Kreusser this disturbance is observed in phosphorus depletion.

Dr. Ritz: There is good experimental evidence in phosphorus depletion for bone mineral mobilization by osteoclasts independent of PTH [73], but increased bone mineral mobilization does not by necessity lead to hypercalcemia. This is well exemplified, for instance, by Paget's disease. We are certainly more at a loss to explain why humans do not develop hypercalcemia than to explain why rats do develop hypercalcemia.

Dr. Alexandra Kettner *(Nephrologist, Stiftung Rehabilitation, Heidelberg)*: I would like to pursue this point a bit further. The body has enormous phosphorus stores in bone. I wonder why such bone mineral phosphorus stores are not mobilized in individuals with phosphorus depletion so that normal phosphate levels are restored? Is it possible that the absence of hypercalcemia in humans, in contradistinction to its presence in rats, might point to inadequate bone mineral mobilization?

Dr. Ritz: With respect to mobilization of bone mineral, it is helpful to distinguish between acute and chronic hypophosphatemia. In acute hypophosphatemia usually due acute internal redistribution of phosphorus, bone is certainly too bradytrophic to mobilize the enormous amounts of calcium and phosphorus that would be required to correct hypophosphatemia. In chronic hypophosphatemia, bone mineral is mobilized by the action of osteoclasts and osteocytes even though PTH levels are low. The paradoxical activation of osteoclasts despite the absence of a PTH stimulus points to the lack of phosphorus as an important direct or indirect signal for bone cells [74]. Stimulation of bone cells through the signal of hypophosphatemia is homeostatically useful: phosphorus mobilized from bone is used to refill the phosphorus deficit of extracellular fluid and tissue stores, whereas calcium that is concomitantly mobilized is spilled into urine and accounts, at least in part, for hypercalciuria. As I mentioned before, bone mineral mobilization also is important for the provision of alkali and the correction of early metabolic acidosis resulting from abnormal tubular handling of acid.

Dr. Kettner: Are plasma $1{,}25(OH)_2$-vitamin D_3 levels normal in hypophosphatemic patients?

Dr. Ritz: Dr. Haussler found plasma $1{,}25(OH)_2D_3$ levels to be increased in hypophosphatemic rats [75,76]. This is not very surprising in view of the fact that phosphorus is one of the signals that controls the activity of 1-alpha-hydroxylase in the proximal tubule. Whether $1{,}25(OH)_2D_3$ plays a role as a PTH-independent signal to bone cells, as described above, has not been well established.

Dr. Kettner: You mentioned the danger of hypocalcemia during phosphorus depletion. Is there any evidence for a role of PTH in this condition? Does the incidence of hypocalcemia differ in parathyroidectomized animals?

Dr. Ritz: This issue has not been well investigated. Dr. Kreusser and Dr. Rambausek have evidence that PTH activity and fractional urinary cAMP excretion rise while plasma calcium levels fall during acute intravenous phosphorus repletion in phosphate-depleted rats [68]. The parathyroid glands are probably chronically suppressed in this condition as a consequence of hypercalcemia, so that the rise in plasma PTH concentration is inappropriate. In the above experiments, however, hypocalcemia could not be prevented by administration of exogenous PTH; this indicates that an element of PTH resistance also is involved. Radiocalcium studies showed that during phosphorus repletion, calcium is acutely translocated to muscle and internal organs and to a negligible extent to bone, in parallel with phosphorus.

Dr. Wilhelm Kreusser *(Nephrologist, Division of Nephrology, Heidelberg)*: Is there evidence that correction of hypophosphatemia is important for control of infection?

Dr. Ritz: Garner et al. studied guinea pigs with salmonella septicemia. Such animals hyperventilate and consequently have hypophosphatemia. If phosphorus is administered to such animals, mortality is dramatically reduced [66].

For obvious reasons, there exist no formal studies on this question in humans, but hyperventilation and hypophosphatemia are common consequences of gram-negative septicemia. Consequently, correction of hypophosphatemia should be part of the management of the septicemic patient. Whether such correction is beneficial only in severe hypophosphatemia or also in less severe hypophosphatemia is unknown.

Dr. Wolfgang Tschöpe *(Nephrologist, Division of Nephrology, Heidelberg)*: Can one readily calculate the phosphorus deficit in a hypophosphatemic patient prior to phosphorus repletion?

Dr. Ritz: There is no clear-cut linear relationship between serum phosphorus levels and the degree of phosphorus depletion for the reasons I outlined earlier. Erythrocyte phosphorus is of no help in assessing body phosphorus stores because erythrocyte phosphorus parallels plasma phosphorus levels [77–79]. What one really would like to know is the whole-body phosphorus:nitrogen ratio, but this information is not available in the clinical setting. So the only practical advice is, make an educated guess and treat the patient carefully with phosphorus until urinary phosphorus is restored to normal.

Dr. Kassirer: It seems to me that treating hypophosphatemia is analogous to treating hypokelmia or hypomagnesemia. When a patient's serum potassium or magnesium level is low, one doesn't know precisely the extent of the deficit. In both instances usually we cautiously administer potassium or magnesium until the plasma level rises. In the case of phosphate administration, one has to be careful not to give phosphate so rapidly that serum calcium falls to dangerously low levels.

Dr. Tschöpe: In patients on parenteral hyperalimentation, blood glucose levels can easily rise into the hyperglycemic range with consequent glycosuria and osmotic diuresis. In view of such an osmotic diuresis, is urinary phosphorus still a reliable indicator of body stores?

Dr. Ritz: You are correct that osmotic diuresis can cause phosphaturia. This mechanism is particularly important in causing latent phosphorus depletion in patients with diabetic ketoacidosis prior to therapy. In fact, neither osmotic diuresis nor PTH cause much phosphaturia in advanced phosphorus depletion. But your point is well taken that judging phosphorus repletion from the urinary phosphorus level is only valid if there is no osmotic diuresis and if no factors, such as volume expansion, diuretics, or glucocorticoids, are present that might interfere with proximal reabsorption.

Dr. Kreusser: Concerning osmotic diuresis, I wanted to add that according to the studies of Massry [80] and Frick [81], volume expansion does not cause phosphaturia in phosphorus depletion. Therefore, I question whether osmotic diuresis really can cause phosphaturia in an individual with phosphorus depletion. I suspect that a low urinary phosphorus level is still a good indicator of phosphorus depletion whether or not osmotic diuresis is present.

Dr. Ritz: From reverse balance studies, we know that prior to insulin therapy patients with diabetic ketoacidosis are phosphorus depleted and still have phosphaturia. The phosphaturia rapidly disappears, concomitant with the fall of serum phosphorus levels, when insulin therapy is begun, as demonstrated years ago by Seldin [82]. I agree that in advanced phosphorus depletion, the kidney has an enormous capacity to retain phosphorus, and that this ability is not overcome by volume expansion, osmotic diuresis, or PTH.

Dr. Michael Rambausek *(Nephrologist, Division of Nephrology, Heidelberg)*: I have a question with respect to low blood pressure in this patient. Could you comment on the possibility of diminished peripheral resistance in hypophosphatemia?

Dr. Ritz: There is no published information on total peripheral resistance in phosphorus depletion. Dr. Kreusser currently has a study underway in which he measured both the response of total peripheral resistance to pressor agents in intact phosphorus-depleted dogs and the response of resistance vessels to pressor agents in the isolated perfused hind limb of phosphorus-depleted rats. He found evidence for an attenuated rise of total peripheral resistance to pressor agents in intact phosphorus-depleted dogs in response to angiotensin II, and he observed similar findings in the perfused hind limbs. In addition, there is a possibility of impaired noradrenalin metabolism in the phosphorus-depleted rat with abnormal reuptake by the rat heart [59].

Dr. Gross: You have recommended assessing urinary or plasma phosphorus concentrations in judging repletion of phosphate stores. Since rhabdomyolysis occurs in phosphorus depletion, aren't you concerned that occasionally urinary phosphate would be high despite considerable phosphate depletion?

Dr. Ritz: Muscle phosphorus and nucleotide content is in the millimolar range, so necrosis of sizable amounts of muscle certainly could deliver phosphorus to the extracellular fluid space; this phenomenon is commonly observed in myoglobinuric acute renal failure. But this condition can be easily recognized on the basis of clinical findings and very high creatine phosphokinase levels. When muscle necrosis is present, the factors would have to be taken into consideration when assessing the need for phosphorus supplements.

Acknowledgment

Prof. Ritz wishes to thank Prof. Schlierf, Department of Internal Medicine, Heidelberg, for permission to study the patient's records.

References

1. Silvis SE, Paragas PD: Paresthesias, weakness, seizures and hypophosphatemia in patients receiving hyperalimentation. Gastroenterology 62:513-520, 1972
2. Oster P, Rieben FW, Schmidt-Gayk H, Schlierf G: Lähmungen bei Hypophosphatämie. Dtsch Med Wochenschr 102:1422–1423, 1977
3. Newman JH, Neff TA, Ziporin PH: Acute respiratory failure associated with hypophosphatemia. N Engl J Med 296:1101–1103, 1977
4. Troehler U, Bonjour JP, Fleisch H: Inorganic phosphate homeostasis. Renal adaptation to the dietary intake in intact and thyroparathyroidectomized rats. J Clin Invest 57:264, 1976
5. Bonjour JP, Troehler U. Mühlbauer R, Preston C, Fleisch H: Is there a bone-kidney link in the homeostasis of inorganic phosphate? Adv Exp Med Biol 81:319–323, 1977
6. Kempson SA, Shah SV, Werness PG, Berndt T, Lee PH, Smith LH, Know FG, Dousa TP: Renal brush border membrane adaptation to phosphorus deprivation: Effects of fasting versus low-phosphorus diet? Kidney Int 18:36–47, 1980
7. Lotz M, Zisman E, Bartter FC: Evidence for a phosphorus depletion syndrome in man. N Engl J Med 278:409, 1968
8. Knox FG, Dousa TP: Mechanism of regulation of phosphate transport in the renal tubule. In: Proc VIIIth Int Cong Nephrol, 1981, pp. 931–937
9. Haldane JBS, Wigglesworth DB, Woodrow CE: The effect of reaction changes on human inorganic metabolism. Proc R Soc Lond (Biol) 96:1, 1924
10. Relman AS: Metabolic consequences of acid-base disorders. Kidney Int 1:347–359, 1972
11. Parfitt AM, Kleerekoper M: Clinical disorders of calcium, phosphorus and magnesium metabolism. In Maxwell MH, Kleeman CR (eds.): Clinical Disorders of Fluid and Electrolyte Metabolism. New York, McGraw-Hill, 1980, pp. 947–1153
12. Rudman D, Millikan WJ, Richardson TJ, Bixler TH, Stackhouse WJ, McGarrity WC: Elemental balances during intravenous hyperalimentation of underweight adult subjects. J Clin Invest 55:94–104, 1975

13. Knochel JP: The pathophysiology and clinical characteristics of severe hypophosphatemia. Arch Intern Med 137:203, 1977
14. Lee DNB, Kleeman CR: Phosphorus Depletion in Man. Irvine, McGraw-Hill, 1976
15. Kreusser W, Ritz E: The phosphate depletion syndrome. Contrib Nephrol 14:162–174, 1978
16. Kreusser W, Ritz E, Boland R: Phosphate depletion. Klin Wochenschr 58:1–15, 1980
17. Riddell WH, Hughes JS, Fitch JB: The relation of phosphorus deficiency to the utilization of feed of dairy cattle. Kans Agr Expt Sta Techn Bull 36:54, 1934
18. Bloom WL, Flinchum D: Osteomalacia with pseudofractures caused by the ingestion of aluminum hydroxide. JAMA 174:1327, 1960
19. Scriver CR, Chesney RW, McInnes R: Genetic aspects of renal tubular transport: Diversity and topology of carriers. Kidney Int 9:149–172, 1976
20. Libanati CM, Tandler CJ: The distribution of the water-soluble inorganic orthophosphate ions within the cell: Accumulation in the nucleus. J Cell Biol 42:754–761, 1969
21. Travis SF, Sugerman HJ, Ruberg RL, Dudrick SJ, Delivoria-Papadipoulos M, Miller LD, Oski FA: Alterations of red-cell glycolytic intermediates and oxygen transport as a consequence of hypophosphatemia in patients receiving intravenous hyperalimentation. N Engl J Med 285:763–768, 1971
22. Kreusser W, Kurokawa K, Aznar E, Massry SG: Phosphate depletion. Effect of renal inorganic phosphorus and adenine nucleotides, urinary phosphate and calcium, and calcium balance. Miner Electrolyte Metab 5:30, 1978
23. Fuller TJ, Barter NW, Barcenas C, Knochel JP: Reversible changes of the muscle cell in experimental phosphorus deficiency. J Clin Invest 57:1019–1024, 1976
24. Kretz J, Sommer G, Boland R, Kreusser W, Hasselbach W, Ritz E: Lack of involvement of sarcoplasmic reticulum in myopathy of acute phosphorus depletion. Klin Wochenschr 58:833–837, 1980
25. Gadian DG, Radda GK: NMR studies of tissue metabolism. Annu Rev Biochem 50:69–83, 1981
26. Epstein FA: Nuclear magnetic resonance—A new tool in clinical medicine (editorial). N Engl J Med 304:1360–1361, 1981
27. Rowe JC, Wood DW, Rowe DW, Raisz LG: Nutritional hypophosphatemic rickets in a premature infant fed breast milk. N Engl J Med 300:293–296, 1979
28. Darsee JR, Nutter D: Reversible severe congestive cardiomyopathy in three cases of hypophosphatemia. Ann Intern Med 89:867, 1978
29. Ritz E, Kreusser W, Bommer J: Effects of hormones other than parathyroid hormone on renal handling of phosphate. In Massry SG, Fleisch H, (eds.): Renal Handling of Phosphate. New York, Plenum Press, 1980, pp. 137–179
30. Josephus: The Jewish War, translated by Williamson GA. Harmondsworth, Penguin Books, 1959, p. 300
31. Schnitker MA, Mattman PE, Bliss TL: A clinical study of malnutrition in Japanese prisoners of war. Ann Intern Med 35:69–96, 1951

32. Brozek J, Chapman CB, Keys A: Drastic food restriction. JAMA 137:1569–1574, 1948
33. Mollison PL: Observations on cases of starvation at Belsen. Br Med J 1:4–8, 1946
34. Rosencher H: Medicine in Dachau. Br Med J 2:953–955, 1946
35. Smith GS, Smith JL, Maneesh MS: Hypertension and cardiovascular abnormalities in starved-refed swine. J Nutr 82:173–182, 1964
36. Hypophosphatemia (editorial). Lancet 2:122–123, 1977
37. Harrop GA, Benedict EM: The participation of the inorganic substances in carbohydrate metabolism. J Biol Chem 59:683–697, 1924
38. Corredor DG, Sabeh G, Mendelsohn LV: Enhanced postglucose hypophosphatemia during starvation therapy of obesity. Metabolism 18:754–763, 1969
39. Danowski TS, Gillepsie HK, Fergus EG: Significance of blood sugar and serum electrolyte changes in cirrhosis following glucose, insulin, glucagon, or epinephrine. Yale J Biol Med 29:361–375, 1956
40. Bessman SP, Mandita P: Phosphate metabolic control of potassium movement—Its effect on osmotic pressure of the cell. Adv Exp Med Biol 128:175–186, 1980
41. Smith LJ Jr, Ettinger RH, Seligson D: A comparison of the metabolism of fructose and glucose in hepatic disease and diabetes mellitus. J Clin Invest 32:273–282, 1953
42. Froesch ER, Wolf HP, Bartsch H: Hereditary fructose intolerance. Am J Med 34:151–167, 1963
43. Dromandy TL, Porter RJ: Familial fructose and galactose intolerance. Lancet 1:1189–1194, 1961
44. Woods HF, Krebs HA: Xylitol metabolism in the isolated perfused rat liver. Biochem J 134:437–443, 1973
45. Baessler KH, Prellwitz W, Unbehaun V, Lang K: Xylitstoffwechsel beim Menschen. Zur Frage der Eignung von Xylit als Zuckerersatz beim Diabetiker. Klin Wochenschr 40:791–793, 1962
46. Metzger R, Burke P, Thompson A: Hypophosphatemia and hypouricemia during parenteral hyperalimentation with an amino acid-glucose preparation. J Clin Invest 50:65a–66a. 1971
47. Klock JC, Williams HE, Mentzer WC: Hemolytic anemia and somatic cell dysfunction in severe hypophosphatemia. Arch Intern Med 134:360–364, 1974
48. Goldfarb S, Westby GR, Goldberg M, Agus ZS: Renal tubular effects of chronic phosphate depletion. J Clin Invest 59:770–776, 1977
49. Gold LM, Massry SG, Friedler RM: Effect of phosphate depletion on renal tubular reabsorption of glucose. J Lab Clin Med 89:554–559, 1977
50. Gold LM, Massry SG, Arieff AI, Coburn JW: Renal bicarbonate wasting during phosphate depletion. A possible cause of altered acid-base homeostasis in hyperparathyroidism. J Clin Invest 52:2556–2562, 1973
51. Finck GA, Mai C, Gregor M: Passagere Polyneuropathie mit Hirnnervenbeteiligung durch Hypophosphatamie. Nervenarzi 50:778–782, 1979
52. Jacob HS, Amsden T: Acute hemolytic anemia with rigid red cells in hypophosphatemia. N Engl J Med 285:1446–1450, 1971
53. Kreusser W, Ritz E, Boland R, Brachmann J: Function of the sarcoplasmic

reticulum in hypophosphatemia myopathy. Adv Exp Biol Med 128:313-321, 1980
54. Baker LRI, Ackrill P, Cattell WR, Stamp TCB, Watson L: Neurogenic osteomalacia and myopathy due to phosphate depletion. Br Med J 3:150-152, 1974
55. Moser CR, Fessel WJ: Rheumatic manifestations of hypophosphatemia, Arch Intern Med 134:674-678, 1974
56. Knochel JP, Barcenas C, Cotton JR, Fuller TJ, Haller R, Carter NW: Hypophosphatemia and rhabdomyolysis. J Clin Invest 62:1240-1246, 1978
57. Boelens PA, Norwood W, Kjellstrand C: Hypophosphatemia with muscle weakness due to antacids and hemodialysis. Am J Dis Child 120:350-353, 1970
58. Furlan AJ, Hanson M, Cooperman A, Farmer RG: Acute areflexic paralysis. Association with hyperalimentation and hypophosphatemia. Arch Neurol 32:706-707, 1975
59. Kreusser W, Scholz H, Rascher W, Schömig A, Ritz E: Circulatory response to pressor agents in phosphorus depletion. Miner Electrol Metab 6:248a, 1981
60. O'Connor LW, Wheeler WS, Bethune JE: Effect of hypophosphatemia on myocardial performance in man. N Engl J Med 297:901-903, 1977
61. Fuller TJ, Nochols WW, Brenner BJ, Peterson JC: Reversible depression in myocardial performance in dogs with experimental phosphorus deficiency. J Clin Invest 62:1194-1200. 1978
62. Kreusser W, Vetter H, Mittmann U, Brückner U, Hörl H, Ritz E: Cardiac function and metabolism in phosphorus depleted dogs—Effects of hormonal stimulation. Miner Electrol Metab 6:248a, 1981
63. Yawata Y, Hebbel RP, Silvis S, Howe R, Jacob H: Blood cell abnormalities complicating the hypophosphatemia of hyperalimentation: Erythrocytes and platelet ATP deficiency associated with hemolytic anemia and bleeding in hyperalimented dogs. J Lab Clin Med 84:643-649, 1974
64. Craddock PR, Yawata Y, Senten L, Gilberstadt S, Silbis S, Jacob HS: Acquired phagocyte dysfunction. A complication of the hypophosphatemia of parenteral hyperalimentation. N Engl J Med 290:1403-1407, 1974
65. Klock JC, Shohet SB: Erythrocyte membrane lipid abnormalities in hypophosphatemia hemolysis. J Clin Invest 52:47a, 1973
66. Garner GB, Heubner PR, O'Dell BL: Dietary phosphorus and salmonellosis in guinea pigs. Proc Am Soc Exp Biol 26:799, 1967
67. Lentz RD, Brown DM, Kjellstrand C: Treatment of severe hypophosphatemia. Ann Intern Med 89:941-945, 1978
68. Kreusser W, Rambausek M, Ziegler T, Ritz E: Therapie der Phosphat-Depletion—Eine experimentelle Untersuchung Verh. Dtsch Ges Inn Med 85:630-632, 1979
69. Emmet M, Seldin DW: Disturbances in acid-base balance during hypophosphatemia and phosphate depletion. Adv Exp Biol Med 103:313-325, 1978
70. Emmet LM, Goldfarb S, Agus ZS, Narins RG: The pathophysiology of acid-base changes in chronically phosphate-depleted rats. J Clin Invest 59:291-298, 1977
71. Lee DNB, Brautbar N, Walling NW, Carlson HE, Golvin C, Coburn JW,

Kleeman CR: The biochemical indices of experimental phosphorus depletion: A re-examination of their physiological implications. Adv Exp Biol Med 103:381–394, 1978

72. Rambausek M, Kreusser W, Ritz E: PTH-resistant hypocalcemia and overshoot hyperphosphatemia in acute phosphorus repletion of chronically Pi-depleted rats. Miner Electrol Metab 6:260–261, 1981
73. Baylink D, Wergedal J, Stauffer M: Formation, mineralization and resorption of bone in hypophosphatemic rats. J Clin Invest 50:2519–2530, 1971
74. Cuisinier-Gleizes P, Thonosset M, Sainteny-Debove F, Mathieu T: Phosphorus deficiency, parathyroid hormone and bone resorption in the growing rat. Calc Tiss Res 20:235, 1976
75. Haussler M, Hughes M, Baylink D, Littledike ET, Cork D, Pitt M: Influence of phosphate depletion on the biosynthesis and circulating level of 1-alpha-25-dihydroxyvitamin D. Adv Exp Med Biol 81:233–250. 1977
76. Hughes MR, Brumbaugh PF, Haussler MR, Wergedal J, Baylink DJ: Regulation of serum 1-alpha-25-dihydroxyvitamin D_3 by calcium and phosphate in the rat. Science 190:578–579, 1975
77. Tsuboi KK, Fukunaga K: Inorganic phosphate and enhanced glucose degradation by the intact erythrocyte. J Biol Chem 240:2806–2810, 1965
78. Lichtman MA, Müller DR, Cohen J, Waterhouse C: Reduced red cell glycolysis, 2,3-diphosphoglycerate and adenosine triphosphate concentration, and increased hemoglobin oxygen affinity caused by hypophosphatemia. Ann Intern Med 74:562–570, 1972
79. Kurokawa K, Kreusser WJ, Massry SG: Phosphate depletion and adenine nucleotide metabolism in kidney and liver. Adv Exp Biol Med 103:327–341. 1978
80. Massry SG, Coburn JW, Kleeman CR: The influence of extracellular volume expansion on renal phosphate reabsorption in the dog. J Clin Invest 48:1237, 1969
81. Frick A: Reabsorption of inorganic phosphate in the rat kidney. I. Saturation of transport mechanism. II. Suppression of fractional phosphate reabsorption due to expansion of extracellular fluid volume. Pflüegers Arch Ges Physiol 34:351–364, 1968
82. Seldin DW, Tarail R: The metabolism of glucose and electrolytes in diabetic acidosis. J Clin Invest 29:552, 1950

Index

GPSR Compliance

The European Union's (EU) General Product Safety Regulation (GPSR) is a set of rules that requires consumer products to be safe and our obligations to ensure this.

If you have any concerns about our products, you can contact us on ProductSafety@springernature.com

In case Publisher is established outside the EU, the EU authorized representative is:

Springer Nature Customer Service Center GmbH
Europaplatz 3
69115 Heidelberg, Germany

Batch number: 10712228

Printed by Printforce, the Netherlands